Interpretation of Laboratory Results
for Small Animal Clinicians

Interpretation of Laboratory Results
for Small Animal Clinicians

B. M. Bush BVSc, PhD, FRCVS
Senior Lecturer in Small Animal Medicine, Royal Veterinary College, University of London

**Blackwell
Science**

© B. M. Bush 1991
Blackwell Science Ltd
Editorial Offices:
Osney Mead, Oxford OX2 0EL
25 John Street, London WC1N 2BL
23 Ainslie Place, Edinburgh EH3 6AJ
350 Main Street, Malden
   MA 02148 5018, USA
54 University Street, Carlton
   Victoria 3053, Australia
10, rue Casimir Delavigne
   75006 Paris, France

Other Editorial Offices:

Blackwell Wissenschafts-Verlag GmbH
Kurfürstendamm 57
10707 Berlin, Germany

Blackwell Science KK
MG Kodenmacho Building
7–10 Kodenmacho Nihombashi
Chuo-ku, Tokyo 104, Japan

The right of the Author to be
identified as the Author of this Work
has been asserted in accordance
with the Copyright, Designs and
Patents Act 1988.

First published 1991
Reprinted 1993, 1994, 1996, 1998, 1999

Set by Genesis Typesetting, Laser Quay
Rochester, Kent
Printed and bound in Great Britain by
MPG Books Ltd, Bodmin, Cornwall

The Blackwell Science logo is a
trade mark of Blackwell Science Ltd,
registered at the United Kingdom
Trade Marks Registry

DISTRIBUTORS

   Marston Book Services Ltd
   PO Box 269
   Abingdon
   Oxon OX14 4YN
   (Orders: Tel: 01235 465500
           Fax: 01235 465555)
USA
   Blackwell Science, Inc.
   Commerce Place
   350 Main Street
   Malden, MA 02148 5018
   (Orders: Tel: 800 759 6102
                781 388 8250
           Fax: 781 388 8255)
Canada
   Login Brothers Book Company
   324 Saulteaux Crescent
   Winnipeg, Manitoba R3J 3T2
   (Orders: Tel: 204 837-2987
           Fax: 204 837-3116)
Australia
   Blackwell Science Pty Ltd
   54 University Street
   Carlton, Victoria 3053
   (Orders: Tel: 03 9347 0300
           Fax: 03 9347 5001)

A catalogue record for this title
is available from the British Library

ISBN 0–632–03259–6

Library of Congress
Cataloguing-in-Publication Data

Bush, B. M.
Interpretation of laboratory results for small animal
clinicians/B. M. Bush
      p.   cm.
   Includes bibliographical references.
   Includes index.
   ISBN 0–632–03259–6
   1. Veterinary clinical pathology. 2. Dogs—
Diseases—Diagnosis. 3. Cats—Diseases—
Diagnosis—I. Title.
   [DNLM: 1. Animal diseases—diagnosis.
2. Diagnosis, laboratory—veterinary. SF771 B978i]
SF772.6.B87 1990
636.089'6075–dc20

For further information on Blackwell Science,
visit our website:
www.blackwell-science.com

Preface

Over the years veterinary surgeons in small animal practice have indicated the need for a book which would help them interpret the results of laboratory tests. The aim of this volume is to satisfy that need. Throughout the book, but especially in the first chapter, there is advice on the selection of tests and on avoiding the many traps for the unwary.

I trust that the reader will find the information of value. Regrettably it is almost inevitable that there will be errors and omissions. I should, therefore, be grateful if these could be drawn to my attention so that later they may be rectified.

Finally, I wish to thank my publishers, my family, and most especially my wife, for their patience and their cooperation. I hope it has been worth while.

B. M. Bush

Contents

Chapter 1

Aspects of interpretation

Introduction

This book is offered as a guide to interpreting the results of laboratory tests on blood and urine samples from dogs and cats. It should be emphasized that the information relates *only* to those species. The book is not intended to be a textbook of haematology or biochemistry, nor is it a manual of laboratory techniques (although in Appendix I, p. 466, certain test procedures are described because either they *must* be performed in the veterinary practice as opposed to the laboratory, or by custom and practice they almost certainly would be).

The information comprises:

- The known causes of abnormal test results (i.e. increases and decreases in the concentrations of cells and biochemical constituents etc.) listed in sections throughout the following chapters; to simplify checking the possibilities the majority of these sections are provided with summaries.

  Hopefully these lists will avoid having to rely on memory alone to select the most likely cause, with regard to the case history and clinical findings. To assist making the correct decision a short explanation is provided of how the change arises, wherever this is known.
- Comprehensive data on clinical topics, which usually require the performance of several laboratory tests, presented in the form of panels at the end of relevant chapters.
- Guidance in the choice of tests needed to establish a particular diagnosis; this is given specifically in the section 'Appropriate tests for various clinical signs' (p. 9) and subsequently at appropriate points in the text to assist in discriminating between possible diagnoses.

Although a number of tests are likely to be performed only by commercial laboratories, the interpretation of the results will be the same whether they are produced commercially or within the practice laboratory.

RELIABILITY OF TESTS

It is important to appreciate that *test results are not always reliable*. This may be because of:

- An inherent defect in the test method,
- An error in performing the test.
- Interference from other substances, e.g. drugs, or changes in the sample, e.g. haemolysis.

The clinician is advised to be especially cautious when a diagnosis appears to hinge solely on *one* test result. Consider what the effect would be if that result was inaccurate. Is there any supporting evidence for the diagnosis, i.e. from clinical signs, other tests etc.? If that single test result is the *only* thing that would support the diagnosis then some CHECK should be made, e.g.

* Have the crucial estimation repeated and, if the laboratory in question is suspected of some inaccuracy, have the test performed by another laboratory.
* Check the history of the case and if necessary re-examine the animal to obtain further clinical evidence.
* Perform any other test(s) that could confirm or refute the diagnosis.

Serial estimations are always valuable in double-checking results and in monitoring the progress of a disease or treatment, although of course if there is some fundamental flaw in the laboratory method, laboratory technique or sample collection then the error in the result is likely to be perpetuated.

Be suspicious – look for possible sources of error and consider the possible effects of any error.

The results of a number of laboratory tests can be altered by drugs, fear/excitement and by haemolysis and lipaemia. In humans much more is known about the effect of these factors on individual tests, especially in the case of drugs, but insofar as information is available or applicable to small animals, it is important to be aware of it. This is because:

* It may be possible to avoid the effect altogether, by collecting samples before (or after) drug treatment, avoiding excitement during collection, being especially careful in the taking of blood samples and ensuring that animals are fasted beforehand.
* It will avoid the abnormal result being incorrectly attributed to some other, potentially much more sinister, cause.

Other sections in this chapter deal with these effects.

The performance of tests on small animal samples by 'human' laboratories (i.e. laboratories which primarily test material from human patients) can present particular problems that it is well to be aware of, and so these are described under 'Problems that may arise using "human" laboratories' (p. 24). Furthermore features that will distinguish a *reliable* laboratory are worth bearing in mind and are considered in 'Features that distinguish a reliable clinical laboratory' (p. 15).

CLASSIFYING THE CAUSE OF ABNORMAL RESULTS

Difficulties are immediately encountered when classifying the causes of abnormal laboratory findings, e.g. whether such findings should be listed on the basis of:

* The underlying pathological changes, e.g. inflammation, fibrosis, necrosis, neoplasia etc. and physiological/pathological states, e.g. stress, parasitism, autoimmune disease etc.
* Clinical signs (e.g. diarrhoea, polyuria) and syndromes (e.g. malabsorption, chronic renal failure).
* Specific causes, e.g. lead poisoning or FeLV infection.

No single method of classification has been used in this text; all have been employed to some extent to assist with the need to provide both concise summaries and sufficient specific examples to be clinically useful. Inevitably this has resulted in some overlap of classifications but it is believed that this will be readily apparent and not prove confusing.

SI UNITS

The International System of Units, or SI unit system (Système International d'Unites) was adopted in the 1970s:

- To avoid the confusion inherent in using a variety of independent units.
- To provide a system which would be accepted and understood world wide.

All SI units are based on seven basic units of measurement, including the mole to indicate the amount of a substance in terms of molecules. The concentrations of all substances are now expressed in terms of a litre and, for biochemical substances, including electrolytes, this means their molar concentration per litre, usually expressed in the submultiples, millimoles per litre (mmol/l) and micromoles per litre (μmol/l). This has meant changes in the numerical values (i.e. in the normal reference ranges) of many substances.

However there are two important exceptions:

1. The concentrations of those substances whose molecular weight is variable and cannot be precisely determined, or is not universally agreed, continue to be expressed in gravimetric units, i.e. in terms of mass per litre rather than the amount per litre. This includes *globulin* (a collection of proteins having various molecular weights) and, in consequence, *total plasma protein*; hence, to keep all the plasma protein concentrations in the same units facilitating addition and subtraction, albumin (these are all in g/l). Also excepted are folate (in μg/l), and vitamin B_{12} (cyanocobalamin) (in ng/l).
2. Haemoglobin concentration is also measured in gravimetric units, but is generally expressed in terms of the decilitre (= 100 ml) rather than the litre, i.e. g/dl. At the time of writing the change to g/l is (slowly) under way.

Enzyme activity is currently still expressed in terms of international units per litre (iu/l) because the SI unit, the catal, has not been widely adopted. However, it is important to realize that because of variations in enzyme measurement between laboratories (depending upon the substrate, buffer and incubation temperature) most enzyme ranges will vary between laboratories despite *all* results being expressed in iu/l.

Very little modification of numerical values has been necessary in haematology, although some units have been altered.

Although of undoubted benefit in science generally, this system which was designed to eliminate confusion has instead created a good deal of it in human and veterinary medicine for reasons which it is well to be aware of:

- The changeover period from gravimetric units to SI units has been prolonged, and the USA (and Italy) are only just beginning to use SI units; American publications (including all the most recent quoted in the lists of References and Sources of information – pp. 487–90) continue to use the older units.
- All publications before 1975 employ the older units.
- Even in countries which are committed to SI units there are laboratory instruments still in use which produce results in the older units, e.g. the Unimeter system. Some commercial laboratories may at times also still employ them.

- To convert values expressed in older units to SI units (especially biochemical values) requires the use of conversion tables (see Appendix III, p. 482). In making the necessary calculation there is scope for error, principally by misplacing the decimal point and, if a clinician is unfamiliar with the order of the expected value when expressed in SI units, an erroneously calculated value may not be appreciated as such (although fortunately this is decreasingly the case).
- Even within the system of SI units there are a number of exceptions, i.e. measurements which are not expressed in SI units, either because it is not possible or has not yet become customary.
- In cases where the concentration of a substance is given *without* also stating the units (SI or gravimetric) in which it has been measured it may be impossible to know which units are intended, and consequently, whether the value is normal or abnormal.

Fortunately, increasing familiarization with the system, especially among new veterinary graduates, is resulting in less and less confusion as time passes. In this book all values possible are expressed in SI units but to facilitate comparison with other published work they are also provided in the older units.

NORMAL VALUES

Quoting normal reference ranges is frowned upon by some experts, but such ranges are stated throughout this book as a guide to the order of values which would normally be expected. However, such ranges should not be regarded as absolutely rigid and unalterable because variations in test methods will cause ranges to vary slightly between laboratories. Wherever possible the laboratory carrying out the testing should be consulted about its normal reference ranges (if they are not already provided on the laboratory's result sheet).

It is important to appreciate that:

- Not all the values from normal individuals will fall within the normal reference range.
- Some values from abnormal individuals (i.e. those suffering from disorders which would normally be expected to produce a change in the result) *will* fall within the normal range, especially around its upper and lower limits.

To develop these points further:

- When measuring the concentration of particular cells or of a substrate or metabolite, 1 in 40 of the values of normal animals will be above the normal range and likewise 1 in 40 values will fall below it (only 95% of values fall within the normal range – by definition). However four out of five of these 'across the border' values will be only slightly above or below the normal limits of the range (i.e. if the normal range is extended both upwards and downwards by 25% these values will now be included).

  The activity of plasma enzymes in normal individuals is not so evenly distributed and there are many more normal individuals that produce values *above* the normal range (sometimes considerably above) than produce values below it.

  These facts should be borne in mind when attempting to interpret values that inexplicably appear outside the normal range. In general, the further away from the normal range a value is, the more likely it is to be definitely abnormal, although enzyme activities have to show a much greater *degree* of increase before being regarded as significant.

- Values that are 'normal' for that species may not be normal for the individual concerned, i.e. before developing a disorder an animal may have a value which is in the lower part of the normal range and subsequently this may rise although still staying within the normal range. Alternatively the converse may occur, i.e. a value in the upper part of the normal range may fall with illness, although still remaining within the normal range. Consequently values around the upper and lower limits of a normal range may have significance and should be noted.

SAMPLE COLLECTION

Specific information on sample collection etc. is given in the introduction to the sections on haematology, plasma biochemistry and urinalysis, but in general:

- Collect blood samples from *'fasted'* animals (with the possible exception of those for bile acid determinations) wherever possible, but if *not* note the time and nature of the last meal.
- Ensure that *appropriate anticoagulants* are added to blood samples for the tests required (i.e. EDTA for haematological tests, heparin for plasma samples, fluoride–oxalate for glucose estimations, and *no* anticoagulant for serum samples). In particular failure to use an enzyme inhibitor (fluoride–oxalate) with blood samples undergoing glucose estimations can result in low (or no) values (but note that some glucose methods likely to be used in veterinary practices (e.g. the Glucometer, Seralyzer and Reflotron) will not give accurate results with samples preserved with fluoride–oxalate because, as well as inhibiting the glycolytic enzymes in the RBCs, it also inhibits enzymes in the test strips).
- Record the *use of any drug treatment or unusual diet*, which may be relevant in the subsequent interpretation of results.
- Record any *excitement/struggling* during sample collection, or the use of a general anaesthetic (i.e. excitement during induction) which again may affect test values.
- If a number of tests are to be performed it is desirable to *collect all the samples at essentially the same time*, rather than, for instance, to collect blood samples on one day and urine on another. This permits correlation of the findings and avoids the possibility that, between collections, the clinical situation could have changed producing apparent inconsistencies in the findings.
- When performing tests that require a number of samples to be collected in a particular sequence (e.g. an ACTH stimulation test or a glucose tolerance test) ensure that they are *correctly labelled*, at the time of collection, otherwise subsequently considerable confusion will ensue.

How to proceed in diagnosis

Establish clearly what the major concern of the owner is, discover the animal's past and present history and perform a clinical examination noting all abnormal signs. At this stage the nature of the problem may be obvious or the clinician may be left with a number of possible explanations – the differential diagnoses.

Laboratory examination of blood and urine samples (along with other diagnostic aids (especially radiography) will usually help to narrow the field, i.e. to eliminate some possibilities and to confirm or at least strongly indicate others, perhaps just a single one. At times clinicians may say things like 'I haven't a clue what's going on', which of course they do not really mean, although unfortunately if said to the owner it may be taken at face value. Generally what is meant is that there are a number of options from which to select a diagnosis and it is proving difficult to decide between them. However, almost always the clinician will be aware of the clinical area involved (be it large or small) and will want further information before coming to a conclusion. It is then a case of deciding which laboratory tests are capable of providing this information, and in this respect the section 'Appropriate tests for various clinical signs' (p. 9) offers suggestions about tests appropriate in various circumstances.

If the test values subsequently prove 'normal', this is not evidence of your failure as a diagnostician; it means that you have effectively ruled out one or more possible diagnoses, so that those which remain can be considered in more detail. (After all when a car is serviced you don't expect every check that is made to reveal some abnormality.)

Then the test results can be considered in relation to the whole clinical picture; do not discount laboratory findings if they do not fit with a particular theory; on the other hand, do not accept laboratory findings if they contradict something which you know absolutely to be true (such as the presence of external haemorrhage) – after all errors can occur. If possible look for ways of checking one result against another (this is one advantage of not confining the number of tests to the bare minimum) and, if there are anomalies that cannot be resolved, consider having the test performed again, or arranging other tests that will provide clarification.

There are some golden rules. Wherever possible:

- Collect samples after fasting (preferably 12 hours).
- Collect samples before starting treatment.
- Collect samples appropriate to the tests you want performed (i.e. use the correct anticoagulants).
- Collect and handle samples carefully to minimize haemolysis or unwanted clotting.
- Separate plasma and/or serum before despatch.
- Despatch all samples as soon as possible to reach the laboratory on a working day.
- Enclose all relevant details of the case, in particular the tests that you want performed.

How to check laboratory results

CHECK AGAINST NORMAL RANGE

Take the laboratory report and check the value obtained for each test against the normal reference range.

Make sure that:

- You use the correct range for the species in question, i.e. dog or cat.
- The units of measurement in the report and in the reference range are *identical* (preferably SI units). If they are not, then conversion will be required.

It is most desirable to use the 'normal' ranges given by the laboratory concerned, because there may be some idiosyncrasy in the methodology which produces slightly higher or slightly lower values than those stated elsewhere, including in this book. A good laboratory will provide its normal reference ranges (most conveniently on the report form itself alongside the test result).

If the laboratory's ranges are not available for some reason use those given in Appendix II (p. 478) of this book. But *enzyme activities* vary so much between laboratories, depending upon the test method, that no meaningful 'normal' range can be given. In the case of enzymes it is essential to obtain the normal reference range from the laboratory that has performed the estimation.

If a laboratory's reported reference range for a particular test is markedly different from ranges quoted elsewhere, it would be sensible to check the reason for this with the laboratory. It might be due to misprinting or mistyping, or be due to the use of an unorthodox method.

MARK ABNORMAL VALUES

Mark each abnormal value to indicate whether it is increased or decreased when compared to the normal reference range.

The use of upward- and downward-pointing arrows ($\uparrow \downarrow$) makes the change immediately apparent.

It is preferable *not* to mark all 'normal' values, e.g. with N, because this distracts attention from the abnormal values.

Helpful refinements are to mark:

1. *Slight* increases or decreases from the normal range as sl $\uparrow$ and sl $\downarrow$ respectively. These may or may not be significant, i.e. they may be values from normal animals that happen to fall just outside the 95% confidence limits of the normal range,
2. High 'normal' or low 'normal' values as $\uparrow$ N and $\downarrow$ N respectively. Again these may or may not be significant, although they could be abnormal values that overlap with the normal range.
3. Extremely high or extremely low values as $\uparrow \uparrow$ and $\downarrow \downarrow$ respectively (or even $\uparrow \uparrow \uparrow$ and $\downarrow \downarrow \downarrow$). This allows very marked changes from the normal to be recognized instantly.
   (a) Some commercial laboratories already mark results with symbols, letters or words in this way to indicate high and low results, but it is still valuable to check the findings personally using the 'normal' ranges for comparison because, (i) sometimes the person writing in the symbol for high or low gets it wrong, *and* (ii) there is often no indication as to *how* high or low the result is, i.e. whether the result is just outside the normal range or whether it is markedly outside the normal range; obviously the significance of the result will be very different. Computer-printed 'flags', i.e. symbols or words indicating high or low values, are particularly likely to lack discrimation since the printing is triggered by the entry of any abnormal value.

> **Note**
>
> If you have reason to alter the laboratory's 'interpretation' of the result do double check that you are correct in your assessment; in particular avoid comparing enzyme results from one laboratory with normal ranges obtained from another or that are applicable to an instrument being used within the practice.

   (b) Some laboratories have a confusing range of letter symbols for what appears to be the same type of change, e.g. I for increased, E for elevated, R for raised, H for high etc. Whilst these different adjectives may be used in papers and books (such as this) to provide some variety in description, their use in the same laboratory report suggests either that results are being graded in some way (it might be worth while checking what the system is) *or* simply that the laboratory has not bothered to standardize its reporting.

(c) Checking results is also a fairly painless way of becoming educated; you rapidly become familiar with the common normal ranges, even if you weren't already.

(d) When assessing differential WBC counts it is important to judge the value of each WBC type on the *absolute number* and *not* a percentage alone (only in assessing the presence or absence of a steroidal effect is the percentage count more helpful).

CHECK ABNORMAL VALUES

Where tests have produced abnormal values, refer to the tabulated causes of increased and decreased values in this book to help decide the most likely explanation with regard to the animal's history and clinical signs. Often other tests or features that may clarify the diagnosis will be indicated:

- Reference may be made to panels at the end of appropriate chapters, where information on some of the more complex diagnostic problems is brought together.
- Bear in mind that in any animal two (and sometimes more) conditions may be present simultaneously.
- Be aware that errors (e.g. poor sample collection, wrong choice of anticoagulant, time delays, drug interference, and errors in performing the test) can result in *falsely* increased or decreased values *or*, equally important and more likely to be overlooked, *falsely* normal values. Sources of error are described in the later chapters where appropriate.

Choice of tests

When it comes to choosing which laboratory tests should be performed, the obvious intention is to select those which will be most useful in arriving at a diagnosis. On the one hand, it is pointless (as well as expensive) to ask for every laboratory test that can be thought of, but, on the other hand, it is false economy not to ask for two or three additional tests that could yield pertinent information, particularly when the alternative for the client is to spend more on repeat visits, and on medication that is supplied 'on the off-chance' that it will work.

In this regard the use of 'profiles' offered by most clinical laboratories is valuable. A number of the most routinely useful tests can be carried out for a total cost that is considerably less than the sum of the individual charges. It may be that some of the tests in the profile are not immediately relevant to the condition being investigated, but usually the overall cost of the profile is much less than if the appropriate tests were requested individually. Some laboratories offer a number of different profiles and, when it comes to selecting one, care should be taken to ensure that the tests included in the profile match as closely as possible those which are required. Additional tests can always be added, and this should certainly be done if one or more tests that do not feature in the profile are judged to be essential or to offer considerable advantages over some that are included.

North American clinicians often refer to obtaining a 'minimum database', i.e. a basic amount of information from a number of routine haematological and biochemical tests.

The most useful *haematological information* will come from a combination of packed cell volume (particularly if other features of the haematocrit are also reported), the total WBC count and the differential WBC count (especially if the stained smear is used to provide information about the appearance of the blood cells and platelets). To these can be added, particularly in cases of anaemia, the RBC count and haemoglobin concentration in order to provide the haematological indices, mean corpuscular volume (MCV) and mean corpuscular haemoglobin concentration (MCHC), a reticulocyte count and (if possible) a platelet count. Where there are problems with blood coagulation, tests of haemostasis should be performed.

The most generally useful *biochemical tests* on plasma (or serum) are measurements of total plasma protein and albumin (and, by their difference, globulin), urea (and, if raised, creatinine) and the enzymes alanine aminotransferase (ALT) and alkaline phosphatase (ALP). If the plasma (or serum) is clearly jaundiced (i.e. yellow) it is helpful to estimate the level of total bilirubin and, if possible, the proportions that are conjugated and unconjugated. These few tests will provide a considerable amount of information relevant to a wide variety of clinical disorders. To them should be added other tests according to the nature of the clinical signs (see 'Appropriate tests for various clinical signs' below).

The value of the *examination of urine* should not be overlooked – not just the chemical tests performed using strips but also specific gravity, bacteriological culture and the examination of sediment.

Additional examination of other substances may at times be relevant (e.g. cerebrospinal fluid, intra-articular fluid, intraperitoneal or intrathoracic fluid, skin scrapings, hair, faeces, discharges etc.).

Appropriate tests for various clinical signs

The tests suggested are those judged to be of the greatest value and may be modified depending upon the features of individual cases. The lists should not be regarded as exhaustive; often more information on particular topics can be obtained by consulting the appropriate panels at the end of the appropriate chapters.

ABDOMINAL DISTENSION (INCLUDING OBESITY AND ASCITES)

- Routine haematology (splenomegaly, hepatomegaly, Cushing's syndrome, infection, pyometra, neoplasia, hypothyroidism etc.).
- Total plasma protein (nephrotic syndrome).
- Albumin (nephrotic syndrome) and globulin, especially fractions – electrophoresis (FIP).
- Glucose (diabetes mellitus, hyperinsulinism, acromegaly).
- Cholesterol (nephrotic syndrome, hypothyroidism, diabetes mellitus).
- ALP (Cushing's syndrome, acromegaly, liver disease).
- ALT (liver disease – neoplasia).
- Thyroxine – TSH stimulation (hypothyroidism).
- Cortisol – ACTH stimulation (Cushing's syndrome).
- Insulin (diabetes mellitus, hyperinsulinism, acromegaly).
- Urinary protein (nephrotic syndrome).
- FeLV test (splenomegaly, hepatomegaly with myeloproliferative disorders).
- Abdominal fluids, protein content, cell types and numbers.
- See *suspected renal disease* (later) if large kidneys are involved.

ABDOMINAL PAIN

- Routine haematology (inflammation – acute hepatitis, acute pyelonephritis).
- Urea/creatinine (ureteral obstruction, and to distinguish increases in lipase and amylase due to renal disease).
- ALT/ALP (hepatitis, acute pancreatitis).
- Lipase/amylase (acute pancreatitis).
- Calcium (acute pancreatitis).
- Bilirubin/bile acids (bile duct obstruction).
- Urine – WBCs, casts, bacteria (pyelonephritis).
- See later headings for *suspected liver disease* or *renal disease*.

ABNORMAL GROWTH AND DEVELOPMENT

- Routine haematology (anaemia, sepsis).
- Total plasma protein/albumin (hepatic encephalopathy, malabsorption).
- Urea (congenital renal disorders, hepatic encephalopathy).
- Creatinine (congenital renal disorders).
- Ammonia (hepatic encephalopathy).
- Calcium/inorganic phosphate (skeletal abnormalities, congenital renal abnormalities).
- Thyroxine – TSH stimulation (panhypopituitarism).

ALOPECIA

- Routine haematology (Cushing's syndrome, hypothyroidism).
- Cholesterol (Cushing's syndrome, hypothyroidism).
- ALP (Cushing's syndrome).
- CK (hypothyroidism).
- Glucose (diabetes mellitus – an unusual cause of alopecia).
- ANA test/LE cell test (immune-mediated disorders, e.g. systemic and discoid lupus erythematosus).

ANAEMIA (SUSPECTED)

In cases of pallor, spontaneous bleeding etc.

- Routine haematology.
- Haematological indices (MCV and MCHC).
- Examination of stained smear for cell morphology, platelet number estimate and inclusions (*Haemobartonella*, Heinz bodies, Howell–Jolly bodies).
- Reticulocyte count.
- Platelet count.
- Bilirubin (haemolytic anaemia).
- Coombs' test (autoimmune haemolytic anaemia).
- FeLV/FIV tests (in cat).
- Urine – for blood bilirubin and neoplastic epithelial cells.
- In cases of spontaneous bleeding, tests of haemostasis (see Panel 4.1, p. 205) and urea (uraemia).

COUGH

- Routine haematology (allergic pneumonia, infection, anaemia).
- Platelet count and tests of haemostasis – if there is persistent haemorrhage.
- Total plasma protein/albumin/electrophoresis (FIP).

- FeLV test/FIV test.
- ANA test/LE cell test (autoimmune origin).
- Serological tests for FIP, heartworm (not in UK).
- Faecal examination for lungworm larvae.
- Examine thoracic fluid (protein, cell types and numbers).

DIARRHOEA

- Routine haematology (malnutrition, lymphosarcoma, inflammation, eosinophilic enteritis, lymphangiectasia).
- Total plasma protein and albumin (malabsorption, protein-losing enteropathy, ulceration).
- Glucose (malabsorption).
- Cholesterol/triglycerides (malabsorption), also fat absorption test (EPI and bile salt deficiency).
- Urea/creatinine (uraemia, hypoadrenocorticism).
- ALT/ALP/bile acids (liver damage, bile salt deficiency).
- Lipase/amylase (acute pancreatitis).
- Sodium/potassium/cortisol – ACTH stimulation (hypoadrenocorticism).
- Calcium (low with low total plasma protein – malabsorption).
- Thyroxine (hyperthyroidism – cat).
- TLI (IRT) test (exocrine pancreatic insufficiency).
- Folate/vitamin B_{12} (malabsorption syndrome).
- Faecal fat determination (malabsorption – cat).

EPISODIC WEAKNESS (COLLAPSING/FAINTING)

See also Anaemia, Fever, Neurological signs, Neoplasia, Abdominal distension due to ascites and Weight loss.

- Routine haematology (anaemia, Cushing's syndrome, hypoadrenocorticism).
- Urea/creatinine (hypoadrenocorticism).
- Cholesterol (Cushing's syndrome).
- Glucose (hyperinsulinism, glycogen storage diseases).
- ALP (Cushing's syndrome).
- Sodium/potassium/chloride (diuretic therapy, hypoadrenocorticism).
- Calcium (hypoparathyroidism).
- Insulin (hyperinsulinism).
- Cortisol – ACTH stimulation (hypoadrenocorticism, Cushing's syndrome).

FEVER

See also Neurological signs (seizures).

- Routine haematology (*Haemobartonella*, autoimmune disorders, infection, neoplasia).
- Total protein/albumin/electrophoresis (infectious diseases, neoplasia).
- Amylase/lipase (acute pancreatitis).
- ALT/ALP (liver neoplasia).
- Calcium (eclampsia, lymphosarcoma).
- Urine – protein, WBCs, bacteria (pyelonephritis).
- FeLV test/FIV test.
- Titre against *Toxoplasma* (and *Brucella canis* and *Ehrlichia* – not in the UK).
- Blood culture (septicaemia).

HAEMATURIA

- Routine haematology (trauma causing anaemia, pyelonephritis).
- Platelet count/tests of haemostasis (anticoagulant poisoning, inherent defects).
- Total plasma protein/albumin (primary glomerular diseases).
- Urea/creatinine (acute renal failure).
- CK/AST/LD (myoglobinuria – muscle crush injuries and exertional rhabdomyolysis).
- Urine – casts, cells, crystals (acute renal failure, ?calculi).
- Bacterial culture of urine (urinary tract infection, pyelonephritis).

INAPPETANCE

See also Anaemia, Abdominal pain, Fever and Jaundice and suspected liver disease.

- Routine haematology (infectious diseases).
- Tests for the presence of FeLV/FIV/FIP/toxoplasmosis.
- Sodium/potassium/urea/cortisol – ACTH stimulation (hypoadrenocorticism).

JAUNDICE AND SUSPECTED LIVER DISEASE

- Routine haematology (anaemia – haemolytic or due to absence of clotting factors).
- Bilirubin – total, conjugated and unconjugated.
- Other haematological tests including platelet count, reticulocyte count, Coombs' test (and possibly haptoglobin concentration).
- Other tests associated with liver damage/dysfunction (see Panel 6.1, p. 333).
- Cholesterol, ammonia, bile acids, bromosulphthalein (BSP) (or indocyanine green) clearance, ALT and ALP (and, if desired, other liver enzymes).
- Urinary examination – bilirubin, bile salts, haemoglobin, specific gravity and, possibly, examination for leptospires and crystals of tyrosine and leucine.

NEOPLASIA (SUSPECTED)

Choice of tests is particularly related to the body organs or system suspected of being involved, but the following are valuable:

- Routine haematology (leukaemia, anaemia, i.e. in myeloproliferative and lymphoproliferative disorders), plus visual examination of blood smear and platelet count.
- Total plasma protein/albumin/electrophoresis (lymphosarcoma, paraproteinaemia).
- Urea (tissue necrosis).
- Creatinine (renal involvement).
- Cholesterol (obstruction of bile duct).
- Bilirubin (myeloproliferative disorders).
- ALT (liver damage).
- ALP (biliary obstruction, high levels of particular tissue isoenzymes released with degeneration).
- Calcium (lymphosarcoma).
- FeLV test.
- Test for faecal occult blood.

> **Note**
>
> Non-steroidal anti-inflammatory drugs (NSAIDs), e.g. flunixin meglumine (Finadyne), can increase the incidence of occult blood in the faeces.

- Blood in body cavities (abdomen, thorax).

NEUROLOGICAL SIGNS

These include seizures (convulsions), circling, head-pressing etc.

- Routine haematology (inflammation, anaemia, rarely polycythaemia, Cushing's syndrome).
- Urea (uraemic fits, hepatic encephalopathy).
- Ammonia (hepatic encephalopathy).
- Total plasma protein/albumin (hepatic encephalopathy).
- Glucose (insulinomas, glycogen storage diseases, diabetes mellitus).
- Cholesterol (hepatic encephalopathy).
- Calcium (eclampsia).
- ALT/ALP (hepatic encephalopathy/liver failure, Cushing's syndrome).
- Bile acids/BSP clearance (hepatic encephalopathy/liver failure).
- Insulin (insulinoma, diabetes mellitus).
- Urine – glucose, ketones (ketoacidosis), bilirubin (liver damage), haemoglobin (lead, chlorate poisoning), oxalate crystals (hepatic encephalopathy), specific gravity (very low with posterior pituitary tumour; isosthenuric with chronic renal failure – uraemic fits).
- Estimation of lead level in blood.

OEDEMA, PERIPHERAL AND GENERAL

- Routine haematology (lymphosarcoma causing obstruction).
- Total plasma protein and albumin (nephrotic syndrome, malabsorption, protein-losing enteropathy).
- Globulin fractions – electrophoresis (FIP).
- Cholesterol (nephrotic syndrome).
- Bile acids/BSP clearance/ALT/ALP (liver dysfunction).
- Thyroxine – TSH stimulation (hypothyroidism with myxoedema).
- ANA test/LE cell test (autoimmune disease).
- Tests for FeLV and FIP.
- Urine – protein (nephrotic syndrome).
- Abdominal fluids – protein content, cell types and numbers.

POLYURIA/POLYDIPSIA

- Routine haematology (toxaemia, e.g. pyometra, pyelonephritis, Cushing's syndrome, hypoadrenocorticism).
- Urea/creatinine (renal failure, hypoadrenocorticism).
- Total plasma protein/albumin (hyperviscosity syndrome, low protein diet).
- Glucose (diabetes mellitus, hyperinsulinism, acromegaly).
- ALT/ALP (liver damage, Cushing's syndrome).
- Sodium/potassium/bicarbonate (diuretics, hypoadrenocorticism, hypokalaemia due to excessive vomiting/diarrhoea).
- Calcium (pseudohyperparathyroidism, e.g. due to lymphosarcoma, chronic renal failure, hypoparathyroidism).

- Inorganic phosphate (chronic renal failure).
- Thyroxine (hyperthyroidism – cat).
- Cortisol – ACTH stimulation (Cushing's syndrome, hypoadrenocorticism).
- Insulin (hyperinsulinism, diabetes mellitus, acromegaly).
- Urine – glucose (diabetes mellitus, primary renal glycosuria, Fanconi's syndrome), protein (primary glomerular diseases), specific gravity (very low in diabetes insipidus, psychogenic polydipsia and Cushing's syndrome; isosthenuric in renal failure).
- Can check specific gravity after water deprivation and ADH tests.

UPPER RESPIRATORY TRACT SIGNS

For example sneezing, nose bleed, nasal discharge.

- Routine haematology (viral infections, anaemia, leukaemia).
- Platelet count and tests of haemostasis.
- Examination and culture of nasal discharge (bacteria, fungi).
- Isolation of viruses responsible for feline respiratory disease.
- See Neoplasia for other appropriate tests.

URINARY TRACT (APART FROM KIDNEY) AND GENITAL TRACT DISORDERS

- Routine haematology (pyometra, prostatitis, pyelonephritis).
- ACP (prostatic neoplasia?).
- Urine – blood, WBCs, bacteria (cystitis, prostatitis, pyometra, pyelonephritis), neoplastic epithelial cells, pH (urinary tract infection), crystals (possibly with calculi).

VOMITING, REGURGITATION

- Routine haematology (inflammation and toxaemia, e.g. pyometra and peritonitis, anaemia, neoplasia).
- Urea/creatinine (renal failure).
- Total plasma protein and albumin (to assess degree of debility).
- Glucose (ketoacidotic diabetes mellitus).
- ALT/ALP (liver disease, acute pancreatitis).
- Lipase/amylase (acute pancreatitis).
- Potassium (hypokalaemia – affecting gastric motility, acute renal failure).
- Sodium/chloride/total carbon dioxide content (assess severity of vomiting).
- Thyroxine – TSH stimulation (hypothyroidism).
- ANA test/LE cell test (autoimmune disease).
- FeLV test.
- Urine – glucose and ketones (ketoacidotic diabetes mellitus).

WEIGHT LOSS

See Neoplasia, Anaemia, Vomiting and Abnormal growth and development. Especially examine:

- Routine haematology (anaemia, evidence of neoplasia).
- Total plasma protein/albumin (malabsorption, protein-losing enteropathy).
- Glucose (diabetes mellitus).
- Folate and vitamin B_{12} estimation (malabsorption – may be present in the absence of diarrhoea).
- Urea/creatinine (renal failure).
- FeLV test/FIV test.
- Thyroxine (hyperthyroidism).
- Urine – glucose and ketones (ketoacidotic diabetes mellitus).

Features that distinguish a reliable clinical laboratory

Clinical laboratories, especially commercial ones, vary in their degree of professionalism. Apart from factors which improve a laboratory's service and make it more convenient to use (e.g. supplying sample containers plus packaging and address labels, arranging for sample collection, providing an emergency service and telephoning results etc.), there are a number of features which serve to distinguish reliable laboratories.

GENERAL

Normal ranges

A good laboratory will state its normal reference range for each test alongside the result. This is *essential* in the case of enzyme determinations where considerable variation is possible depending upon the method employed (i.e. incubation temperature, substrate and buffer).

Supplying the laboratory's normal range is more helpful to the clinician than simply marking results as high or low (although *both* stating the normal range *and* drawing attention to abnormal values is even better). With the normal range alongside, it is immediately apparent just *how* high, or low, the result is.

> **Note**
>
> Some laboratories use a bewildering array of designations, e.g. high, raised, elevated, increased, with no indication as to whether these represent degrees of change or are merely synonyms.

Terminology and units

An up-to-date laboratory will use modern terminology for its tests, e.g. ALT and AST instead of SGPT and SGOT, and will report its results in modern units, which nowadays means using SI units (see p. 3).

Beware of laboratories which submit results in a confusing mixture of SI units and the older gravimetric units or, worse, provide no units at all. A laboratory may intend one set of units, you may presume another; if you guess wrongly the result could be disastrous (e.g. a value of 35 for the plasma urea level would be regarded as quite normal if it was measured in mg/dl but very significantly elevated if in mmol/l). If no units are stated an entirely erroneous diagnosis is possible.

Also **CHECK** (if necessary by comparing the stated normal range, assuming it is provided, with that given in this book) that a laboratory is not confusing blood urea nitrogen (BUN) with urea (i.e. supplying values for urea whilst labelling them BUN – again a potentially disastrous practice since they differ by a factor of two).

Quality assessment

As well as making regular internal checks on its accuracy a responsible laboratory will often belong to an external quality assessment scheme (UKEQAS and NEQAS schemes for biochemistry and haematology which are run primarily for NHS hospital laboratories), and be achieving good scores. At the time of writing attempts are under way to establish a UK veterinary laboratory quality assessment scheme.

The accuracy of a laboratory's biochemical testing can be assessed by submitting a sample of a quality control serum (produced by many manufacturers) under the guise of being a patient sample.

Blood from an animal known to be receiving steroids, submitted for haematological examination, should result in a typical 'steroidal blood picture' being reported (i.e. an increased proportion of neutrophils, decreased proportions of eosinophils and lymphocytes and, in the dog, an increased proportion of monocytes).

Haemolysis, lipaemia, jaundice and clotting

The presence of haemolysis, lipaemia and/or jaundice in the sample when received should be reported, so that allowance can be made for the effects (see sections 'Effects of haemolysis' and 'Effects of lipaemia' on pp. 19 and 21). Ideally test results that are likely to have been affected should be identified.

Haematological samples that have clotted and on which it is pointless performing estimations should be identified and no attempt made to provide values that could be very misleading.

Note

Extremely low platelet values in otherwise normal animals are a sign which raises the suspicion that clotting has occurred.

Delays

If samples are delayed in reaching the laboratory (usually delays occur in the post but sometimes through forgetting to despatch samples promptly), a good laboratory would be expected to report this and to indicate which tests might give inaccurate results or even not be worth while performing (e.g. most haematological tests except the haemoglobin concentration).

Laboratory forms

A good laboratory will provide a form which is sensibly laid out, with the available tests grouped together logically (e.g. haematological, enzyme tests etc.) and not randomly arranged.

Ideally an indication would be given of the type of sample material required (i.e. whether an anticoagulant is required, and if so which one) and the amount.

Laboratory profiles (i.e. a collection of relevant tests provided at a reduced total charge) are a cost-effective way of obtaining basic information, but the components should be well chosen (see 'Appropriate tests for various clinical signs', p. 9) and small animal profiles should not contain tests that are seldom required or that are relevant mainly to large animals.

Typed vs written results

Written results on laboratory forms are sometimes recommended to avoid transcription errors, although usually the results have still to be copied from some master record book or work pad (and a technician's writing may prove difficult to decipher). Typed results certainly offer scope for error if the typing is done by secretarial staff unfamiliar with the tests and their meanings. Probably the best system is either a direct printout from an analyser, or a printout of values entered by the technician(s).

HAEMATOLOGICAL TESTS

Haematocrit

In addition to the packed cell volume a good laboratory will report any other useful features revealed by the haematocrit, e.g. 'streaming' of RBCs (indicating many immature forms), the appearance of the plasma and possibly an abnormal thickness of the buffy coat.

Reticulocyte count

When there is evidence of anaemia a good laboratory will either routinely perform a reticulocyte count or advise that one be performed (if it does not form part of the normal haematological profile).

Haematological indices

MCV and MCHC (and possibly the less useful MCH) should be ready calculated for the clinician (from the packed cell volume, RBC count and haemoglobin concentration), and the values checked to ensure that they are plausible, i.e. there is not an impossibly high MCHC value resulting from haemolysis or lipaemia.

Differential WBC count

- The diagnosis of disorders involving WBCs is most accurately based on the absolute number of each WBC type, rather than on its percentage of the total; almost the only exception is the recognition of a 'steroidal blood picture'. Absolute values should be ready calculated to assist the clinician (and should add up to the total WBC count).
- Percentage values that include half percentages (e.g. 7.5%) imply that 200 WBCs have been classified, which is recommended for accuracy, rather than only classifying 100, which is often done for speed.

Cell morphology

When performing the differential WBC count a good laboratory will also examine and comment upon the appearance of the RBCs, WBCs and platelets on the stained blood smear and draw attention to any significant features.

BIOCHEMICAL ESTIMATIONS

Protein values

A competent laboratory will use the total protein and albumin values to calculate the globulin level (by difference) and the albumin:globulin ratio. Also, where electrophoresis has been performed it will report the various globulin fractions not only in percentages but as the more meaningful absolute values.

URINALYSIS

Urinary bacteriology

Bacteriological testing of urine samples should include an assessment of the number of bacteria – the only effective way of distinguishing significant urinary tract infections from small numbers of bacteria being routinely washed from the urethra. Also an assessment of possible contamination should be made, e.g. if a few colonies of many different organisms are cultured. Antibacterial sensitivity testing should include drugs that might reasonably be used for routine treatment (e.g. nitrofurantoin, and nalidixic acid or cinoxacin), and in general exclude those that cannot be employed (i.e. exclude drugs which are very toxic when given systemically, give poor concentrations in the urine or are poorly absorbed when given by mouth, e.g. neomycin).

Haemolysis

The liberation of haemoglobin from the RBCs is termed 'haemolysis' and indicates damage to the cell membranes. This may occur within the body and, if extensive, results in haemolytic anaemia (see Panel 2.3, p. 95), but the majority of haemolysis arises during and after collection (see 'Causes of haemolysis' below).

It is a very undesirable effect that can seriously reduce the accuracy of many laboratory tests (see 'Effects of haemolysis' p. 19).

The RBCs of small animals appear to be more susceptible than those of other domesticated species.

It may not be apparent from inspection of a whole blood sample that haemolysis has occurred, although this becomes evident as soon as the plasma or serum is separated. Samples containing more than 0.02 g/dl haemoglobin appear grossly haemolysed.

Causes of haemolysis during and after blood collection

DIRECT TRAUMA

- Excessive suction to draw blood into a syringe (especially through a narrow needle).
- Excessive force to expel blood from a syringe (especially through a narrow needle).
- Drawing blood into a large volume evacuated tube (e.g. Vacutainer) due to the force with which it enters (especially through a narrow needle) and strikes the tube wall.
- Negative pressure applied to the blood already collected in a syringe while endeavouring to re-locate a vein which has been 'lost' (i.e. from which the needle has inadvertently been removed).
- Excessive stasis of venous blood when a vein is occluded during blood collection.
- Excessive pumping and squeezing of the limb to maintain blood flow when collection is directly into the sample container.
- Excessive shaking of the sample container to mix blood and anticoagulant.
- Freezing the blood sample.
- Centrifuging the blood at too high a speed and/or for too long.

LIPAEMIA

Increased mechanical fragility of the RBCs (related to changes in the lipid composition of the RBC membrane) causes lipaemic blood samples to haemolyse readily with handling.

CONTACT WITH A HYPOTONIC SOLUTION

This causes RBCs to rupture due to the osmotic effect, e.g. contact with water in a syringe, needle or sample container (including condensation or rain).

CONTACT WITH CHEMICALS

These may damage the RBC membrane, e.g. alcohol, ether, acids etc.

EXCESSIVE HEAT

For example, during storage.

LONG DELAY

Haemolysis can occur if there is a long delay before blood samples are despatched or examined, or before plasma or serum is separated.

If it is not possible to despatch or examine blood samples soon after collection, or to separate plasma or serum specimens, the entire blood sample should be refrigerated (although *not* frozen) to minimize haemolysis.

Wherever possible the serum or plasma should be separated before despatch rather than sending the complete blood sample to the laboratory.

Effects of haemolysis on laboratory tests

EFFECTS ON HAEMATOLOGICAL TESTS

The packed cell volume and RBC count are reduced by the loss of RBCs and the haemoglobin concentration then becomes the only accurate indicator of RBC mass.

Because haemoglobin concentration is unaltered, but packed cell volume is diminished, the MCHC is falsely elevated.

Assuming that haemolysis is not progressive and therefore of different degree when the PCV and RBC count are performed, the MCV might be accurate; unfortunately this cannot be relied upon.

CHANGES IN THE COMPOSITION OF PLASMA (OR SERUM)

These are due to the release of substances within the RBCs.

1. There are *significant increases* in the plasma activity of lactate dehydrogenase (due to the isoenzyme LDH_1) and aspartate aminotransferase (AST) which are present in the RBCs in high concentration.
2. There is a *lesser increase* in the level of inorganic phosphate and *marginal increases* in glucose and potassium. Unlike the situation in humans, potassium is not present in high concentration in the RBCs of cat or dog (except in the Akita breed).
3. There is a *reduction* in the plasma level of insulin due to the release of insulinases.

INTERFERENCE WITH PHOTOMETRIC BIOCHEMICAL ESTIMATIONS

This is caused by the strong red colour in the sample.

1. There are *false elevations* of the levels of a number of substances including
   (a) glucose,
   (b) cholesterol,
   (c) total plasma protein (if estimated by the Biuret method without using a sample blank),
   (d) the activity of lipase.
2. *False decreases* can occur (depending on the method) in the level of:
   (a) calcium (artefactual hypocalcaemia),
   (b) possibly in bilirubin,

(c) alkaline phosphatase (ALP) depending on the method,
(d) *possibly* the activity of lipase.

INCREASE IN TOTAL PLASMA PROTEIN ESTIMATED USING A REFRACTOMETER

This is due to decreased light transmission. If this value is combined with an albumin value obtained chemically, it can result in a falsely low albumin:globulin ratio.

HAEMOLYSIS OCCURRING BEFORE COLLECTION MAY BE OBSCURED

Subsequent haemolysis may obscure haemolysis occurring before collection. Haemolysis which is sufficient to cause an obvious red colouration of the plasma immediately after collection will almost invariably be intravascular in origin.

Lipaemia

Lipaemia (hyperlipaemia, hyperlipidaemia) when applied to samples refers to the clearly visible turbidity (milkiness) in freshly collected blood, and therefore plasma samples, caused by a high concentration of lipid. Blood samples are reported to look like 'cream of tomato soup'.

This *gross* lipaemia is due to the lipid *triglyceride*, present in the form of lipoproteins, notably chylomicrons or very-low-density lipoproteins (VLDLs) which consist mainly of triglyceride (see Triglycerides, p. 267).

Chylomicrons (the largest fat particles) are the form in which triglyceride is absorbed from the small intestine and transported in the blood. On chilling a plasma/serum sample, chylomicrons rise to the top to form a 'cream' with clear plasma/serum underneath. This type of lipaemia is termed 'exogenous lipaemia' because it is due to dietary fat.

Very-low-density lipoproteins (VLDLs) are synthesized in the liver and transported to other tissues in the blood and the lipaemia that they produce is termed 'endogenous lipaemia'. Following chilling of a sample the turbidity will still be uniformly present, i.e. lipid does *not* rise to the surface.

The two other lipoproteins (low-density lipoproteins (LDLs) and high-density lipoproteins (HDLs), containing lower proportions of triglyceride), are not responsible for gross lipaemia.

CAUSE

Usually *lipaemia* is due to collection of a blood sample too soon after a fatty meal. Large numbers of chylomicrons appear ½–6 hours (usually 1–3 hours) after feeding and can remain for 6–12 hours.

Lipaemia is best avoided by collecting samples after fasting (12 hours or longer, e.g. overnight).

Some dogs, e.g. Miniature Schnauzers, may require much longer fasting for lipaemia to disappear, even 3–4 days.

The triglyceride in the chylomicrons and VLDLs can be hydrolysed by the enzyme lipoprotein lipase which is activated in vivo by heparin. Therefore, to avoid lipaemic samples 90–100 units of heparin/kg body weight are given intravenously and a sample collected after 15 minutes.

Alternatively, lipid in a sample can be removed by chilling for 12 hours and decanting off the clear layer (where chylomicrons are involved), or with some tests diluting the plasma/serum with saline and correcting results by measuring a plasma/serum blank.

If a fasted sample continues to show lipaemia the cause can be determined by one of the following:

- Refrigerating the sample for 12 hours (as mentioned above); chylomicrons form a fatty layer on the surface whereas VLDLs remain dispersed.
- Measuring the levels of triglyceride and *cholesterol*. Both chylomicrons and VLDLs contain appreciable amounts of triglyceride, but the proportion of cholesterol is much higher in VLDLs (assuming cholesterol is not present in a high concentration from some other cause).

Less commonly available methods are:

- Lipoprotein electrophoresis which separates the types of lipoproteins in a manner similar to protein electrophoresis, enabling their relative proportions to be determined.
- Lipoprotein ultracentrifugation which separates and identifies the lipoprotein fractions on the basis of their molecular density.

Effects of lipaemia on laboratory tests

Lipaemia (hyperlipaemia, hyperlipidaemia) has a number of effects on laboratory tests, and the degree of abnormality is related to the severity of the lipaemia.

FALSELY ELEVATED BIOCHEMICAL VALUES

These are the result of the effect of the resultant turbidity on light transmission in photometric measurements. Substances which can be affected include:

- Total plasma protein (if estimated by the Biuret method without using a sample blank).
- Albumin.
- Glucose.
- Bilirubin.
- Calcium.
- Inorganic phosphate.

Values for total plasma protein obtained using a refractometer will also be falsely elevated due to the turbidity and, depending on the accuracy or otherwise of the albumin estimation, will produce an inaccurate albumin:globulin ratio.

FALSELY ELEVATED HAEMOGLOBIN CONCENTRATION

This is due to the effect of increased turbidity on photometric measurement. It would then result in a falsely elevated MCHC value.

FALSELY LOW AMYLASE ACTIVITY

This may be obtained depending on the analytical method employed (Zerbe, 1986). This would be an important consideration in the diagnosis of acute pancreatitis because lipaemia is very likely to be present.

FALSELY LOW SODIUM AND POTASSIUM LEVELS

The levels of sodium and potassium appear lower because these electrolytes are present only in the aqueous fraction of the plasma (or serum). Where there is a marked increase in the lipid (non-aqueous) fraction, this has the effect of 'diluting' the sodium and potassium contained in the volume of the particular sample used for the estimation.

Less obvious reductions may occur in the concentrations of other substances being measured.

HAEMOLYSIS

Lipaemia increases the tendency for haemolysis to occur following collection, i.e. during handling.

Other influences on test results

Effects of fear/excitement on laboratory tests

These effects are chiefly those of adrenaline, and they tend to be more pronounced in the cat than in the dog. The effects are transient, e.g. increases in the numbers of blood cells and platelets are due to their movement from the reserve pools into the circulation.

Particularly in the cat these effects may be associated with fear and struggling in the collection of blood samples, and they will also be obvious in blood samples collected under general anaesthesia if there has been a struggle during induction. These changes may also arise at other times (e.g. in dogs an increase in packed cell volume can occur with excitement at the time of feeding).

HAEMATOLOGICAL EFFECTS

Increases in packed cell volume, haemoglobin concentration and RBC count

These increases result from contraction of the spleen, squeezing out of more RBCs into the circulation, and last only a short time. (The value for glycosylated haemoglobin is unaffected.)

Increase in neutrophil count (pseudoneutrophilia)

Adult neutrophils from the marginal pool are temporarily redistributed to the circulating pool causing a modest increase in their number, an effect which lasts about 30 minutes.

This is not usual in dogs but occurs commonly in cats, especially those that are young and healthy (less often in sick animals). There is no accompanying shift-to-the-left.

Increase in lymphocyte count

A temporary increase in the number of lymphocytes in the circulation (which is often greater than the increase in neutrophils) occurs in cats but not in dogs.

It is seen especially in young healthy animals (less often in those that are ill) and again lasts for about 30 minutes.

Changes in eosinophil count

There is first a mild eosinophilia (peaking after about 1 hour), followed by a moderate eosinopenia, with the lowest values occurring after approximately 4 hours.

However, these effects of adrenaline occur too slowly to alter the eosinophil values in blood samples collected from excited animals, shortly after the period of excitement, i.e. this is essentially a late effect.

Increase in platelet count

Platelets are mobilized from the spleen following excitement (which in the cat may have lasted for as little as 3 minutes).

EFFECTS ON PLASMA BIOCHEMISTRY

Increase in glucose level (hyperglycaemia)

- In the *dog* the glucose level seldom exceeds 8 mmol/l (= 150 mg/dl) due to excitement, and therefore it is unusual for glycosuria to follow (renal threshold = 10 mmol/l).
- In the *cat* the glucose level in the blood can reach 16.5–22 mmol/l (= 300–400 mg/dl), or even more, with excitement and fear, and if high levels are obtained glycosuria will appear (renal threshold = 16 mmol/l).
- However, the fear/excitement has no effect on the proportion of glycosylated haemoglobin.

Possible decrease in total carbon dioxide content (bicarbonate)

This is a result of partially compensated respiratory alkalosis arising from hyper-ventilation due to fear/anxiety.

EFFECTS ON URINALYSIS

Glycosuria

This is likely to occur in the cat but not in the dog (see above).

Alkaline urinary pH

This *may* be the result of anxiety, causing panting (hyperventilation) and a loss of carbon dioxide.

Effects of drugs on laboratory tests

The effect of a drug on a laboratory test may be:

- Either a biological effect where the drug produces a change in the level of some constituent of the blood or urine, which consequently alters the value obtained.
- Or an analytical effect where the drug interferes with the analytical method producing an inaccurate result, i.e. one which does not represent the *true* level at that time of the substance being measured.

In most instances the effects of drugs are biological effects; very few analytical effects are recognized, although urine tests are subject to a higher proportion of this type of effect. Biological effects are usually constant within the same species, but may differ between species.

The effects of drugs vary in their severity but when these are extreme they can confuse the interpretation of laboratory results and may lead to erroneous diagnoses. Therefore, it would be desirable if the use of all drugs could be recorded and considered in relation to the test results. If information regarding drug usage was to be supplied to the laboratory concerned, then it could be possible to draw attention to values that could have changed as a result. Obviously, wherever possible it is preferable to collect samples for laboratory testing *before* starting drug therapy rather than the other way round.

Although not totally comprehensive, Table 1.1 includes the more commonly documented effects.

Problems that may arise using 'human' laboratories

Clinical laboratories established principally to test samples from humans may at times also examine samples from small animals. This can lead to problems in certain areas, as detailed below.

HAEMATOLOGY VALUES

Laboratories testing human blood routinely employ electronic instruments which both count the number of RBCs (RBC count) and measure their size (MCV).

RBC count

Canine RBCs are similar in size to human RBCs (just slightly smaller) and these electronic counts are generally accurate. Feline RBCs are substantially smaller than human RBCs and, unless the instrument is adjusted to take account of this, many feline RBCs are confused with platelets and are not counted, resulting in *falsely low counts*.

Mean corpuscular volume (MCV)

Measurements of canine MCVs by electronic instruments are usually reasonably accurate, although they may tend towards the upper limit of the normal range (which is close to the normal *human* range). But, as mentioned above, unless the instrument is re-set, many of the smaller feline RBCs are assumed to be platelets and the MCV is based only on the remainder, causing values to be *spuriously high*.

Packed cell volume (PCV)

In 'human' laboratories the measurements of RBC count and MCV are used to *calculate* the PCV, i.e. the PCV is *not* measured directly. It is often referred to as the 'haematocrit' (Hct). If the RBC count is falsely low (as is likely to be the case in cats, as explained above under 'RBC count'), this calculated PCV will also be *falsely low*.

Even if the RBCs are accurately counted the *calculated* PCV will be slightly lower than that obtained from a spun haematocrit, because in performing the haematocrit some slight trapping of plasma occurs between the RBCs which marginally raises the PCV.

PCVs which have been calculated can usually be recognized by the fact that they have more than two significant figures (e.g. 0.372 l/l or 37.2%), although occasionally

Table 1.1 Effects of drugs on laboratory tests

Drug	Effect
Acetazolamide	↓ Platelets, more alkaline urine
Acetylpromazine	↓ PCV etc.
ACTH	↑ Glucose, ↑ insulin
Adrenaline (epinephrine)	↑ Neutrophils, ↑ platelets, ↑ glucose, ↓ insulin
Alkylating agents	↓ PCV etc. (hypoproliferative anaemia)
Alloxan	↑ Glucose
Alphaxalone/alphadolone acetate (Saffan)	↓ PCV etc. (cat), ↑ glucose (cat)
Aluminium hydroxide	↑ Ca^{2+}, ↓ $InPO_4$
Aminoglycosides (e.g. streptomycin, neomycin, gentamicin) – toxic effects	↑ Urea, ↑ creatinine, ↓ Ca^{2+}, ↑ $InPO_4$, ↓ platelets, ↑ urinary protein, ↑ urinary glucose, ↑ urinary WBCs
Aluminium chloride	↑ Cl^-, more acid urine
Amphotericin B	↓ PCV etc. (hypoproliferative anaemia), ↑ urea, ↓ K^+, ↑ urinary protein
Ampicillin	See Penicillin
Anabolic steroids	↑ PCV etc., ↑ TPP, ↑ albumin
Androgens	↑ Glucose, ↓ T_4, ↑ insulin
Anti-cancer drugs	↓ PCV etc. (hypoproliferative anaemia), ↓ neutrophils, ↓ platelets (although vincristine causes ↑ platelets)
Anticoagulants	↑ Clotting time
Aspirin	↓ PCV etc. (hypoproliferative anaemia), ↓ platelets, ↑ clotting time, ↓ thrombin, ↑ urea (toxic effect), possible ↑ creatinine (A), possible ↓ albumin (BCG method) (A), ↓ glucose, ↑ ALT, ↑ TCO_2 content (metabolic acidosis), ↓ T_4, ↑ urinary glucose with Clinitest (A)
Barbiturates (e.g. phenobarbitone)	Slight ↓ PCV etc., ↓ platelets, ↑ clotting time, ↑ ALT, ↑ ALP, possible ↑ cortisol, ↓ T_4
Benzene	↓ PCV etc. (hypoproliferative anaemia)
Benzocaine	↑ Methaemoglobin (dog), ↑ clotting time, ↑ urinary Hb
Benzothiadiazine derivatives	See Chlorothiazide
Biguanides	↓ Glucose
Bromsulphthalein (BSP)	Red urine
Calciferol	↑ Ca^{2+}
Carbenicillin	See Penicillin
Carbimazole	See Methimazole
Carbonic anhydrase inhibitors	↑ Cl^-, ↓ TCO_2 content
Cephalosporins	↑ Creatinine (A), black urine with Clinitest (A), ↑ urinary protein with sulphosalicylic acid (A), ↓ urinary WBCs – with cephalexin (A)
Chloral hydrate	↑ Urinary glucose with Clinitest (A)
Chloramphenicol	↓ PCV etc. (hypoproliferative anaemia), ↓ reticulocytes, ↓ WBCs, ↓ neutrophils, ↓ lymphocytes, ↓ platelets, ↑ clotting time
Chlorpromazine (promazine tranquillizer)	↓ PCV etc., ↓ neutrophils, possible ↓ platelets (immune mediated), ↑ clotting time
Chlorpropamide	↓ Glucose, ↓ T_4
Chlorothiazide (and other benzothiadiazine derivatives)	↓ Platelets, possible ↓ Na^+, ↓ K^+, ↓ Cl^-, ↑ TCO_2 content, more alkaline urine
Cimetidine	Possible ↑ creatinine (A)
Clonidine	↑ Glucose, ↑ urinary glucose
Cyclophosphamide	↑ Urea, ↑ creatinine (toxic effects)
Dapsone	↓ PCV etc. (mild hypoproliferative anaemia), ↓ WBCs, ↓ neutrophils, ↓ platelets, ↑ ALT
Dextran (in large amounts)	↑ TPP (A), ↓ albumin:globulin ratio (A), ↑ clotting time
Dextrose	↑ Glucose, ↑ urinary glucose, ↓ Na^+ (with hypertonic dextrose solution)
Diazepam	↓ T_4

Table 1.1 (cont.)

Drug	Effect
Diazoxide	↑ Glucose, ↓ insulin
Digoxin (and digitalis compounds)	Possible ↓ platelets (immune mediated), ↑ K^+
Ethacrynic acid	↓ Neutrophils, possible ↓ Na^+, ↓ Cl^-, ↑ TCO_2 content
Ether (anaesthetic)	Slight ↑ PCV etc.
Flucytosine (= 5-fluorocytosine)	Possible ↓ PCV etc. (bone marrow suppression), ↑ urea, ↑ ALT (and other liver enzymes)
Fludrocortisone (and other mineralocorticoids)	Possible steroidal blood, i.e. haematological, picture (see Glucocorticoids), ↓ K^+
Fluids, intravenous	Possible ↓ PCV etc. by dilution
Frusemide (furosemide)	↓ Platelets, possible ↓ Na^+, ↓ K^+, ↓ Cl^-, ↑ TCO_2 content, more acid urine
Glucagon	↑ Glucose, ↑ insulin
Glucocorticoids (e.g. prednisolone)	Possible slight ↑ PCV etc., ↑ WBCs, ↑ adult neutrophils (less marked in cat, more likely with single injection), possible slight ↑ band neutrophils, ↓ eosinophils, ↓ lymphocytes, ↑ monocytes (unusual in cat), ↑ platelets, Howell–Jolly bodies (dogs), ↑ urea, ↑ glucose, ↑ ALT, ↑ AST, ↑ ALP (not in cat), ↑ bile acids, sometimes ↑ or ↓ amylase, possible ↑ lipase, ↓ K^+ (in high dose), ↓ Ca^{2+}, ↓ InPO$_4$, ↓ T_4, ↓ cortisol (endogenous), ↑ insulin, more acid urine
Gold compounds	↓ Neutrophils, ↓ platelets, possible ↑ urea, possible ↑ ALT
Griseofulvin	↓ PCV etc., ↓ WCBs, false positive to ANA test
Growth hormone	↑ Glucose, ↑ insulin
Halothane	Possible ↓ PCV etc., possible slight ↑ T_4
Hexamine	↑ Urinary glucose with Clinitest (A), ↓ urinary glucose with strip test (A), ↓ urinary urobilinogen (A)
Immunosuppressive drugs (e.g. azathioprine)	↓ Lymphocytes
Insulin	↓ Glucose, ↓ K^+, slight ↑ T_4
Iodide	↓ T_4
Ketamine	↓ PCV etc. (haemolytic anaemia), ↑ methaemoglobin (cat), ↑ glucose
Lactate	↓ K^+ (with increasing lactate therapy)
Levamisole	↓ Platelets
Local analgesics	See Benzocaine
Mannitol	↓ Na^+ (with hypertonic solution)
Mebendazole	Possible ↑ ALT, possible ↑ AST, possible ↑ ALP
Medroxyprogesterone acetate	↑ Glucose (in part due to (A) hexokinase method), ↑ insulin
Megestrol acetate	Steroidal blood picture – see Glucocorticoids (i.e. ↑ neutrophils and ↑ monocytes (unusual in cat) with ↓ eosinophils and ↓ lymphocytes), ↑ glucose, ↑ insulin (sudden withdrawal of megestrol acetate produces ↓ cortisol)
Methimazole/carbimazole (cat) (1 mg carbimazole is metabolized to 0.6 mg methimazole, i.e. weight for weight carbimazole is less toxic)	↑ Eosinophils, ↑ lymphocytes, possible ↓ WBCs, possible ↓ neutrophils, possible ↓ platelets, often ↑ ANA titre, ↑ ALT, ↑ AST, ↑ ALP, ↑ bilirubin, ↓ T_4
Methionine	More acid urine
Methotrexate	Possible ↓ PCV etc. (macrocytic/normochromic anaemia – folate antagonist)
Methotrimeprazine	See Chlorpromazine
Methoxyflurane	↑ Urea, ↑ creatinine
Methylene blue	↓ PCV etc. (hypoproliferative and haemolytic anaemia), blue/green urine
Metronidazole	Possible ↓ neutrophils, ↑ glucose (A)
Mitotane	↓ T_4, ↓ cortisol

Table 1.1 (cont.)

Drug	Effect
Morphine	↑ Glucose
Nalidixic acid	↑ Urinary glucose with Clinitest (A)
Nitrofurantoin	↑ Clotting time, slight ↓ neutrophils, bright yellow urine
Novobiocin	Slight ↓ neutrophils
Oestrogen	
Early effects	↑ Adult neutrophils, ↑ band neutrophils (shift-to-the-left, peaking after 3 weeks) ↑ lymphocytes, ↑ monocytes, ↑ platelets (peaking after 1 week)
Late effects	↓ PCV etc. (hypoproliferative anaemia), ↓ WBCs, ↓ adult neutrophils, ↓ platelets, ↑ bile acids, possible ↑ glucose, slight ↑ T_4, possible ↑ cortisol, possible ↑ insulin
Organic arsenicals	↓ PCV etc. (hypoproliferative anaemia)
Paracetamol (acetaminophen)	↓ PCV etc. (haemolytic anaemia), eccentrocytes or pyknocytes, ↑ methaemoglobin, ↓ platelets, ↑ bilirubin, ↑ ALT, ↑ AST, ↑ urinary Hb
Penicillin	↓ Platelets, false positive with ANA test, possible slight ↑ albumin (BCG method) (A), ↑ urinary protein with sulphosalicylic acid (A)
Phenacetin	↓ PCV etc. (haemolytic anaemia), ↑ urea, ↑ creatinine (toxic effects)
Phenazopyridine	↓ PCV etc. (haemolytic anaemia)
Phenolphthalein	Red urine
Phenolsulphonphthalein (PSP)	Orange-red urine (if alkaline) or bright yellow urine (if acid)
Phenylbutazone	↓ PCV etc. (hypoproliferative anaemia), ↓ neutrophils, ↓ platelets (in part immune mediated), ↑ clotting time, ↑ urea, ↑ creatinine
Phenytoin	Possible ↓ PCV etc. (macrocytic/normochromic anaemia – folate antagonist), ↑ MCV (dog), false positive with ANA test, ↓ albumin, ↑ cholesterol (A), ↑ ALT, ↑ AST, ↑ ALP, ↑ copper (cat), ↓ T_4, possible ↑ cortisol, ↓ insulin, red urine
Phosphate enemas	↓ Ca^{2+}
Polymyxin/bacitracin group of antibiotics	↑ Urea, ↑ creatinine (toxic effects)
Potassium citrate	More alkaline urine
Primidone	Possible ↓ PCV etc. (macrocytic/normochromic anaemia – folate antagonist), ↓ albumin, ↓ cholesterol, possible ↑ bilirubin, ↑ ALT, ↑ AST, ↑ ALP, ↓ T_4, possible ↑ cortisol, possible ↑ urinary bilirubin
Procainamide	↓ Neutrophils, false positive with ANA test
Progestogens (including megestrol acetate) and progesterone	↑ Glucose, possible ↑ cortisol, ↑ insulin, possible ↑ urinary glucose
Promazine tranquillizers	See Chlorpromazine
Propylthiouracil	↓ PCV etc. (haemolytic anaemia), ↓ neutrophils, ↓ platelets, ↓ T_4, ↑ urinary Hb
Pyrimethamine	↑ MCV
Reducing sugars (fructose, galactose, lactose, pentose)	Can be confused with ↑ glucose with Clinitest
Ribavirin	↓ Platelets
Riboflavin	Bright yellow urine
Ristocetin	↓ Neutrophils
Salicylates	See Aspirin
s/d diet	↑ ALP, more acid urine
Sodium acid phosphate	More acid urine
Sodium bicarbonate	↑ Na^+ (if deprived of water), ↓ K^+, ↑ TCO_2 content, ↓ Ca^{2+} (if excess given intravenously), more alkaline urine
Sodium chloride	↑ Na^+ (if deprived of water), more acid urine
Sodium lactate	More alkaline urine
Spironolactone	↑ Cortisol (fluorometric method) (A), possible ↓ Na^+, ↑ K^+

Table 1.1 (cont.)

Drug	Effect
Streptomycin	See Aminoglycosides
Streptozotocin	↑ Glucose
Succinylcholine	↑ K$^+$, ↑ TCO$_2$ content
Sulphonamides	↓ PCV etc. (long-term effects on folate synthesis giving macrocytic/ normochromic (i.e. hypoproliferative) anaemia and/or haemolytic anaemia), ↑ MCV, possible ↓ platelets (immune mediated), ↑ clotting time, ↑ thrombin, possible false positive to ANA test, possible ↑ urea (toxic effect), ↓ glucose, ↑ ALT, alkalosis (occasionally acidosis), ↑ urinary protein with sulphosalicylic acid (A), ↑ urinary urobilinogen (A)
Sulphonylureas	See Tolbutamide and Chlorpropamide
Tetracyclines	↓ Platelets, false positive to ANA test, ↓ urea, possible ↓ urinary WBCs (A)
Thiacetarsamide	↑ ALT, ↑ AST, ↑ ALP
Thyroid hormone	↑ Urea, ↑ glucose
Tolbutamide	↓ Glucose, ↓ T$_4$, ↑ urinary protein with sulphosalicylic acid
Trimethoprim	Possible ↓ PCV etc. (folate antagonist can give macrocytic/ normochromic anaemia), ↑ MCV, possible ↑ creatinine (A)
Vincristine	↑ Platelets (although most anti-cancer drugs cause ↓ platelets)
Vitamin C	↓ Cholesterol (A), ↓ glucose (inhibits GOD/POD method) (A), ↑ urinary glucose with Clinitest, ↓ urinary glucose with Clinistix (A), ↓ urinary Hb (A), ↓ urinary WBCs (A), ↓ urinary nitrite (A)
Vitamin D$_3$	↑ InPO$_4$ (if in excess)
Xylazine	↑ Glucose, ↑ urinary glucose

(A) – indicates analytical effects.
Note: ALP = alkaline phosphatase; ALT = alanine aminotransferase; ANA = antinuclear antibody; AST = aspartate aminotransferase; Ca^{2+} = calcium; Cl$^-$ = chloride; Hb = haemoglobin; InPO$_4$ = inorganic phosphate; K$^+$ = potassium; MCV = mean corpuscular volume; Na$^+$ = sodium; PCV = packed cell volume and, inevitably red blood cell count and haemoglobin concentration; T$_4$ = thyroxine; TCO$_2$ = total carbon dioxide; TPP = total plasma protein, WBCs = white blood cells.

the PCV read from a spun haematocrit may be read to half a per cent and therefore have 5 as a third figure (e.g. 0.425 l/l or 42.5%).

If the PCV has been calculated in this way, the most reliable guide to the red cell mass (e.g. in diagnosing anaemia) would be the value of the haemoglobin concentration.

Note

A falsely low calculated PCV (resulting from a falsely low RBC count) can produce a *falsely high* MCHC, although such a finding is most often attributable to haemolysis.

This method of obtaining the PCV is standard in 'human' laboratories and is currently being introduced into some of the large veterinary laboratories.

Total WBC count and platelet count

Human laboratories may not be aware that, particularly in feline blood:

- Total WBC counts may be *falsely elevated* because electronic counters include large platelets, clumps of platelets and clumps of Heinz bodies as if they were WBCs.

• Platelet counts may be falsely low because electronic counters may register a clump of platelets as a single platelet, *or* assume that large platelets or clumps of platelets are in fact WBCs and not count them at all.

Laboratories that are not aware of this problem are unlikely to check whether it is happening, i.e. by looking for large platelets and platelet clumps on a stained smear and, if necessary, checking the electronic count against a manual count.

Differential WBC count

Unfamiliarity with the appearance of non-human WBCs can lead to their erroneous classification and, in particular, to a reluctance to produce values which differ markedly from the reported normal reference ranges. For example, in a case of marked eosinophilia the finding of such a large number of eosinophils may be judged so improbable that it is assumed that a mistake has been made and the eosinophils subsequently re-classified as neutrophils.

Inclusion bodies in blood cells

A lack of familiarity with the inclusions found in small animal blood cells may result in them not even being mentioned or being wrongly attributed, e.g. *Haemobartonella felis* and distemper inclusion bodies.

BIOCHEMICAL ESTIMATIONS

Thyroid hormone

The levels of thyroxine (T_4) and tri-iodothyronine (T_3) in the normal dog are much lower than those found in humans (approximately a quarter and a half of the human values respectively), and these levels fall even lower in canine hypothyroidism. Methods designed to measure the level of hormones in human samples are not sufficiently sensitive, in the extremely low part of the range, to discriminate between the comparatively low canine normal values and the even lower canine hypothyroid values. In short, testing canine samples with a human test kit that has not been appropriately modified will not generate accurate results.

Occult blood in faeces

A 'human' laboratory *might* use a test which is *specific* for human haemoglobin and consequently produce a false negative result with a canine or feline faeces sample containing occult blood.

'Flagging'

Biochemical values, produced by autoanalysers, that fall outside the normal reference ranges are often highlighted on the printout by some indication to this effect (e.g. printing alongside HI or LO, or an upward-pointing or downward-pointing arrow etc.). However, the programmed 'normal' ranges will be those for humans, and values flagged as being abnormal may well be normal for the dog or cat, and conversely values that are abnormal in the dog or cat may not be distinguished because they fall within the normal human range. Such 'flagging' should therefore be disregarded and the values compared with normal ranges for the species in question if their interpretation is in any doubt.

Enzymes etc.

To interpret the result of a test it is important to know the normal range of values obtained using that particular laboratory's method; this is particularly true of enzymes where the normal range (even though always expressed in international units per litre) can vary enormously between laboratories. Unfortunately, human laboratories will usually not have developed normal ranges for dogs and cats because they examine so few samples from them. It can, therefore, prove difficult to interpret canine and feline enzyme activities.

It is assumed that enzyme activities in 'normal' dogs and cats will generally be within the normal human range, but this cannot be relied upon.

URINALYSIS

Clinical tests on urine will almost certainly be performed by 'dipstix' methods and it should be appreciated that, when testing canine or feline urine, the values obtained with the urobilinogen and nitrite tests, and particularly from the specific gravity test band, are *unreliable*. This may not be known by the laboratory concerned and therefore any interpretation based on such findings could be erroneous.

GENERAL

Choice of tests

Some tests of considerable value in small animal medicine (especially alkaline phosphatase and FeLV tests) may not be available from a human laboratory, whereas tests that are of little use, e.g. uric acid, may be routinely included in profiles.

Failure to detect errors

An erroneous result, e.g. due to a flaw in the test method, may not be recognized as such simply because the 'human' laboratory is not familiar with the range of values that might reasonably be expected in association with a particular history in (for them) an unusual species. In consequence the result is not checked and the error remains uncorrected.

Part 1 Haematology

Introduction

At the time of writing haematological examination is underemployed. The reason seems to be that haematological tests are considered less able than the organ-specific biochemical tests to pinpoint the source of a problem, and hence can be more difficult to interpret. Whilst there is some truth in this, a basic set of haematological tests (packed cell volume, total and differential WBC counts) will provide a wide variety of information to complement the biochemical findings. Even if most of the haematological results are normal, this has the considerable value of ruling out a number of differential diagnoses.

Interpretation of haematological results need not be difficult, although it is necessary to know which tests are most reliable.

Choice of test

The so-called routine haematology examination or haematological screen, haematological profile, full blood examination (FBE) or complete blood count (CBC) could include a number of tests but, in general, it will consist of the packed cell volume (and other information from performing the haematocrit), an RBC count and an estimation of haemoglobin concentration (to calculate the haematological indices), total and differential WBC count, and a report on a visual examination of a stained blood smear (usually that used for the differential WBC count).

The most useful and accurate test overall is the haematocrit and if only one test could be performed this would be the choice. (The reason for saying *would be* is that usually commercial laboratories use the haematocrit only to obtain the packed cell volume and do not report the salient features of the buffy coat or plasma.)

The combination of packed cell volume, total WBC count and differential WBC count will provide all the basic information about the RBCs and WBCs, and in all cases these three tests should be requested. By examining a Romanowsky-stained blood smear prepared for the differential WBC count, information can be obtained about the appearance of the RBCs as well as the WBCs, i.e. their size, shape and pigmentation, the presence and proportions of immature and abnormal cells and the presence of blood parasites etc. Also the appearance of the platelets can be observed and an *estimate* (though not an accurate count) of their numbers obtained. A good laboratory will make such an examination and report any significant findings.

Certain other features that might be revealed by a Romanowsky-stained blood smear show up more clearly (and can therefore be identified with greater certainty) when the smear is stained with a supravital stain – principally cell inclusion bodies that characterize particular disorders, and reticulocytes whose presence distinguishes regenerative and non-regenerative anaemias. A *reticulocyte count* is therefore important when establishing the cause and probable outcome of anaemia. Unfortunately, most commercial laboratories will not routinely pursue a line of enquiry by performing or recommending tests that have not been specifically requested, even when the value of such tests is clear (for example, advising a reticulocyte count and platelet count in cases of anaemia). Many will not routinely comment upon the appearance of cells and platelets when performing the differential WBC count.

The RBC count and haemoglobin concentration will generally only provide the same information about the RBC mass that can be obtained more accurately from the packed cell volume, and it should be appreciated that these are not three totally independent parameters but that inevitably they are related.

However, results of these tests used in conjunction with the packed cell volume permit the calculation of the haematological indices (primarily the MCV and MCHC). These indices give information about the size of the RBCs and their haemoglobin content and are of value in distinguishing types of anaemia. A good laboratory will calculate these indices for you. However, their accuracy depends entirely upon the accuracy of the test results that are used in the calculation and this should be borne in mind. The accuracy of these indices can easily be checked by looking at the stained blood smear and noting whether the observed size and staining of the RBCs are in agreement with the calculated values. Since these observations can always be made on a stained smear anyway, there is obviously no burning need to carry out the RBC count and the haemoglobin concentration.

The other test often described as part of a routine procedure is the erythrocyte sedimentation rate (ESR). Unfortunately, this has the dual disadvantages in small animals of requiring a comparatively large amount of blood and, in most cases, of adding very little information (in dogs the ESR is frequently 0 mm per 1 hour). Certainly the ESR is nowhere near so consistently valuable as it is in humans and, unless there is some special reason for performing it, the ESR is best omitted from the group of tests routinely performed.

Where necessary, specialized tests, e.g. for haemostasis or autoimmunity, should be requested.

SUMMARY

- The most useful tests overall are the packed cell volume (especially if other information is derived from the haematocrit), the total WBC count and the differential WBC count – particularly if other features of the smear are reported.
- Also useful in anaemia are the reticulocyte count (requiring a supravitally stained smear); the RBC count and haemoglobin concentration so that the haematological indices can be calculated.
- Of little use is the ESR.

Collection and preparation of blood samples

Fasting samples, i.e. ideally after 12 hours fasting, should be collected to decrease the risk of lipaemia which can lead to haemolysis.

In almost all species the jugular vein is an appropriate site for collection and recommended although in the dog and cat the cephalic vein is often employed because veterinary surgeons are familiar with using it when inducing general anaesthesia, and the saphenous vein is a very good alternative especially in nervous or aggressive animals, provided adequate assistance is available to restrain the animal on its side. Exceptionally in the cat, the marginal ear vein can be used to obtain sufficient drops of blood to perform a microhaematocrit.

As large a needle as is feasible should be used to speed collection and limit trauma to the cells. Smaller needles increase haemolysis; larger needles carry the risk of a haematoma. Appropriate sizes are 20–21 gauge in the cat or small dog and 19–20 gauge in other dogs.

A blood sample containing EDTA is appropriate for most haematological tests, including estimation of the fibrinogen level, but a citrated blood sample is required to obtain plasma for performance of the activated partial thromboplastin time (APTT), the prothrombin time (PT) and the thrombin time (TT). Other tests of haemostasis require specialized collection and/or immediate testing (see Panel 4.1, p. 205).

Large volumes of blood are not required for routine testing; aim to collect:

- 2.5 ml from medium-sized dogs or larger.
- 1 ml (or if necessary 0.5 ml) from cats and small dogs.

EDTA sample tubes are made in these standard sizes (i.e. 2.5 ml and the paediatric sizes 1 ml and 0.5 ml), as well as those for large volumes.

These quantities will be sufficient to perform all the *routine* tests mentioned previously with the exception of the ESR (for which alone at least 2 ml of blood should be collected).

Sample containers should be filled to the level indicated and the blood and anticoagulant mixed (by repeated gentle inversion of the container) immediately after replacing the cap. Failing to mix the sample with the anticoagulant immediately is likely to result in clotting.

Overfilling also carries the risk of clotting occurring; if a container is inadvertently overfilled the best immediate action is to take another container of the same type and to pour the blood back and forth gently from one container to another a few times to mix it with more anticoagulant.

This method of adding more anticoagulant may subsequently need to be resorted to when, despite everything connected with blood collection going smoothly, a sample collected into EDTA still clots. This can arise in cases of hypercalcaemia when there is insufficient anticoagulant to deal with the excess of calcium present.

Clotting may also arise during slow blood collection directly into the container.

Beware of containers that are knocked over after their caps have been removed (especially if they fall some distance, e.g. from table to floor) because the crystals of anticoagulant may be knocked out of them. These containers are best discarded and replaced.

Clotting renders all haematological values *meaningless*; once clotting has occurred it is pointless to proceed with testing – a fresh sample should be collected.

Method of collection

This can be:

- By direct collection through the needle into the container, although this can be slow and at times messy and, if prolonged, tends to distort cell numbers and encourage clotting.
- Into a syringe: if collection is slow clotting may begin in the syringe, and excessive suction can cause collapse of the vein, slow blood flow and haemolysis.
- Into an evacuated tube (e.g. Vacutainer): unfortunately, the larger sizes readily cause haemolysis in small animals, although the paediatric size tube (2 ml) usually proves satisfactory.
- Into a Monovette: used as a combination syringe and sample container; types are available containing all the usual anticoagulants.
- Into an S-Monovette, which can be used in the same way as the Monovette or as an evacuated tube.
- By incising the ear vein (e.g. in cats) for a few drops of blood to fill a microhaematocrit tube and/or produce a blood smear. Large amounts of blood will not be obtained.

Care should be taken not to withdraw blood from veins or cannulae recently used to administer intravenous fluids or drugs, because these can affect cell numbers (by dilution) as well as biochemical parameters.

Chapter 2

Red blood cells (RBCs)

Packed cell volume (PCV)

- Also known as the haematocrit index, or volume of packed red cells (VPRC).
- PCV is the fraction (or proportion) of the blood occupied by the RBCs. It does *not* include the WBCs or platelets.
- In general low values indicate anaemia and high values indicate dehydration.
- A number of other factors can cause changes (see 'Causes of increased PCV' and 'Causes of decreased PCV', pp. 38 and 40).
- The SI units for PCV measurement are litres per litre or l/l (sometimes written as ll^{-1}, e.g. $0.45\ ll^{-1}$).
- Previously PCV was reported as a percentage (e.g. 45%) and this is still very popular.
- Other units which have been used are ml/dl = ml/100 ml (e.g. 45 ml/100 ml) and some workers regard PCV simply as a ratio and do not apply units to it (e.g. 0.45).
- The two main ways of expressing results (as a fraction and a percentage) are so different that there is unlikely to be confusion, *but* care is needed in calculating haematological indices from the PCV, i.e. the MCV and MCHC.

NORMAL REFERENCE RANGE (ADULTS)

Dog

For dogs the normal reference range = 0.37–0.55 l/l (37–55%) for most breeds, although values are higher in the Greyhound/Whippet/Lurcher/Borzoi breeds (0.48–0.66 l/l = 48–66%). Values in Greyhounds are a further 8% higher immediately after racing.

PCV may also appear consistently high in some other breeds, i.e. in the upper part of the normal reference range or even above it, e.g. Poodles, German Shepherd Dogs, Boxers, Dachshunds, Chihuahuas, Dalmatians and Beagles, but it is due to nervousness causing splenic contraction.

Cat

For cats the normal reference range = 0.30–0.45 l/l (30–45%). Lower 'normal values' that are often reported occur chiefly in young cats (see 'Age' below).

Age

Dog
The lowest values are in puppies 4(–6) weeks old (0.24–0.34 l/l = 24–34%), gradually increasing to the adult range by 1 year of age.

Cat
The lowest values are in kittens 4(–6) weeks old (0.24–0.34 l/l = 24–34%), gradually increasing to the adult range by 6 months of age (4–7 months of age).

Sex

Values are *slightly* lower in females compared with males and this feature is more obvious in Greyhounds. There are significant falls associated with pregnancy.

Dog
During *pregnancy* PCV slowly falls and in the later stages can be below the normal range (e.g. as low as 0.32 l/l (32%) at parturition). This is probably mainly due to an *increase* in the plasma volume (i.e. a dilutional anaemia) rather than RBC loss or defective production. Values are restored to pre-pregnancy levels approximately 9 weeks after giving birth.

Cat
Likewise the PCV falls during pregnancy and in the last third can be below normal (e.g. as low as 0.24 l/l (24%) at parturition). Values are restored to normal within 1 week of giving birth.

In animals PCV is best obtained by performing the spun haematocrit (blood separation) and measuring the height of the RBC layer. When it is performed using a capillary tube the method is referred to as the microhaematocrit. A similar method, but yielding additional information, is the QBC-V Haematology System (see p. 470).

PCV obtained by the spun haematocrit method is the *most accurate* of the measurements of RBC mass and oxygen-carrying capacity, provided that there is no haemolysis. With the microhaematocrit method the error = ±1%.

The PCV is preferred to either a haemoglobin estimation (with an error of ±5%) or an RBC count (with an error of ±2–3% for an electronic counter or ±20% for 'manual' counts). The only indication for measuring haemoglobin concentration and the RBC count is when the PCV is abnormally low, i.e. when the animal is anaemic. From the PCV, haemoglobin concentration and RBC count, the MCV and MCHC, can be calculated, which may help in identifying the *type* and *cause* of anaemia (see 'Haematological indices', p. 54).

PCV values produced by 'human' laboratories on dog and cat blood will not be as accurate; they will be lower – probably falsely so in the case of cat blood. This is because the PCV values are *not measured* but are *calculated* from the RBC count and the mean corpuscular volume (see Note 3, p. 42). Such calculated PCVs can be detected because usually they will have more than two significant figures (e.g. 0.431 l/l or 43.1%). The use of similar methods in veterinary laboratories is beginning – hopefully they will be more aware of the problems arising with feline RBCs. As a result if a 'human' laboratory examines the blood sample the most accurate measurement of RBC mass is not the PCV but will be the *haemoglobin concentration*.

OTHER INFORMATION FROM THE HAEMATOCRIT

The spun haematocrit *also* yields information about the two other layers into which the blood is separated – buffy coat and the plasma. (Any abnormal features of these layers are less easily seen when using the microhaematocrit method, compared with methods using larger volumes of blood.)

Unfortunately veterinary laboratories seldom report this additional information.

Buffy coat

This consists mainly of WBCs with a (usually) thinner, whiter layer of platelets on top, and so a thicker buffy coat (>0.02 l/l = 2%) suggests leucocytosis, and an almost invisible one, leucopenia (although see mention of reticulocytes, below).

If the thickness of the buffy coat is measured, ignoring the platelet component, the total WBC count can be estimated. The first 0.01 l/l (1%) represents 1×10^9 WBCs/l (10 000 WBCs/µl), and each further 0.01 l/l (1%) represents a further 2×10^9 WBCs/l (20 000 WBCs/µl), but this is difficult to measure accurately.

Exceptionally thrombocytosis can result in platelets making up the bulk of the buffy coat.

Abnormal and immature RBCs (especially reticulocytes), being less dense, mix with the lower part of the buffy coat giving it a pink/reddish colour ('streaming'). If they are numerous the buffy coat, as an entity, is indistinct, and may even appear absent if these RBCs have coloured all of it red. This is seen in reticulocytosis, and can result in an over-estimation of the PCV (i.e. the buffy coat is included in the top of the RBC layer).

Colour of the plasma

The following colours can *also* be observed in plasma collected for biochemical tests, in which, because of the greater volume, they may be more obvious.

- Pale yellow/straw colour is normal indicating the presence of very small amounts of bilirubin.
- Colourless/clear plasma – seen in non-haemolytic anaemias where there are few RBCs old enough to be broken down, e.g. in acute blood loss and uraemia.
- Deep yellow plasma – indicative of hyperbilirubinaemia. The resultant jaundice may be haemolytic, hepatotoxic or obstructive (i.e. due to haemolysis, liver damage or obstruction to bile flow) – see 'Plasma bilirubin' (p. 254).
- Pink/red plasma due to the presence of free haemoglobin in the plasma arising from haemolysis (see 'Causes of haemolysis', p. 18).
- Milky white/turbid plasma due to lipaemia (see p. 20).
- Milky pink plasma ('strawberry milkshake') – the result of lipaemia leading on to haemolysis.

Total protein level in plasma

The plasma from a haematocrit tube can be (though usually isn't) used to estimate the level of total plasma protein using a refractometer. Values obtained are often slightly lower (e.g. 3–5%) than by the Biuret method using heparinized plasma because the anticoagulant (usually EDTA) removes some water from the RBCs which dilutes the plasma.

In cases of canine heartworm disease, if the plasma in the microhaematocrit tube, just above the buffy coat, is examined several hours after centrifugation, the microfilariae (of *Dirofilaria immitis*) may be seen.

Causes of increased PCV (haemoconcentration)

Summary

- Dehydration
- Fear/excitment
- Shock
- Strenuous activity
- Absolute polycythaemia: right-to-left cardiac shunts/chronic alveolar disease/renal tumours/endocrine disorders
- Hyperthyroidism (cats)
- Anabolic steroids
- Altitude

Errors: Evaporation/prolonged contact with EDTA

DEHYDRATION [USUAL]

Dehydration is the result of either or both of the following:

- Increased water loss (as with vomiting, diarrhoea and polyuric disorders, e.g. diabetes insipidus, chronic renal failure, diabetes mellitus, Cushing's syndrome, primary liver damage etc. where, despite polydipsia, water replacement cannot keep pace with its loss). It can also be present for 24 hours after very vigorous exercise, e.g. in racing Greyhounds.
- Reduced water intake; water may not be available in sufficient quantity *or* there may be difficulty in drinking it, *or* it may be vomited soon after being drunk.

Note

In the early stage of disorders in which there is very rapid water loss (e.g. haemorrhagic gastroenteritis in the dog), the PCV may be elevated *without* clinical signs of dehydration, e.g. skin turgor.

CHECK – confirm by CHECKING the total protein level, which (along with other metabolites) will be raised to the same degree as the PCV – see Note 1, p. 41.

FEAR/EXCITEMENT [COMMON]

Fear/excitement gives rise to splenic contraction which squeezes out blood cells into the circulation; this is a transient effect. (In the dog excitement associated with *feeding* can do this.)

SHOCK

Shock produces splenic contraction, so infusing more cells into the circulation, and shifting fluid to visceral organs, thereby causing an increase in PCV.

In hypovolaemic shock, caused by haemorrhage, there will be a subsequent dilution of the RBCs by fluid from the tissues which will mask this effect.

STRENUOUS ACTIVITY

Increased adrenaline output causes splenic contraction taking cells from the extravascular pool, e.g. an 8% increase in Greyhounds *immediately* after racing. However, this may not put the PCV above the normal range.

A rise in PCV due to dehydration or splenic contraction can be termed *relative* polycythaemia.

ABSOLUTE POLYCYTHAEMIA [RARE]

This is due to increased RBC production *without* an increase in total protein level – see Panel 2.6, p. 123.

It includes true (primary) polycythaemia (very rare) and secondary polycythaemia, in which cyanosis may be present (e.g. right-to-left cardiac shunts or chronic alveolar diseases) or absent (as with erythropoietin-producing renal tumours, acromegaly, feline hyperthyroidism (see below) and (usually) Cushing's syndrome).

HYPERTHYROIDISM IN CATS

About 50% of hyperthroid cats show an increased PCV although RBC count and haemoglobin concentration *may* be normal.

ANABOLIC STEROIDS

In Greyhounds these have been found to increase the PCV by up to 50%; some increase would be expected in all animals receiving anabolic steroids.

ALTITUDE

This is strictly included under 'Absolute polycythaemia'.

A significant increase in altitude will (eventually) raise all RBC parameters as a response to the fall in oxygen pressure.

ERRONEOUS CAUSES

Evaporation from blood sample

Leaving the cap off the sample container will allow evaporation, especially in a warm room, e.g. immediately after collection or while tests are being performed. It will have the same effect as clinical dehydration, i.e. there will be accompanying increases in total protein and other metabolite levels.

Prolonged contact with EDTA

This occurs, for example, in postal samples.

It can cause RBC swelling and raise the PCV by 2–5% (Tvedten, 1981). It can also cause MCV values 5–7 fl higher than in a recently collected specimen.

Causes of decreased PCV

Summary

- Anaemia [usual]
- Late pregnancy
- Tranquillization and anaesthesia
- Haemolysis at or after collection

Errors: excess EDTA/dilution/clots/electronic counters

ANAEMIA [USUAL]

PCV obtained by the spun haematocrit method is the most accurate measurement to detect anaemia – see Panel 2.1, p. 75.

In *compensated* extravascular haemolytic anaemia, where RBC production has increased to keep pace with a long-standing increased rate of RBC destruction, the PCV will be normal, although usually in the lower part of the normal range – see also Note 1: Anaemia and dehydration, p. 41.

LATE PREGNANCY

PCV (along with haemoglobin concentration and RBC count) gradually decreases in the last third of pregnancy to give a mild to moderate anaemia which is essentially normocytic/normochromic. In bitches it is most marked in those that are young or poorly nourished. The increase in plasma volume dilutes the RBCs.

However, at the end of pregnancy reticulocyte counts increase in response to the anaemia. PCV increases again after parturition, reaching normal values 6–9 weeks post partum in the bitch and 1 week post partum in the queen (Doxey, 1966; Berman, 1974).

TRANQUILLIZATION AND ANAESTHESIA

In blood withdrawn from cats during anaesthesia with ketamine (Vetalar) or alphaxalone/alphadolone acetate (Saffan), or from animals given phenothiazine tranquillizers, the PCV can be below the normal range because RBCs have been transferred from the circulation to the spleen – see Note 2: Anaesthetics and tranquillizers, p. 42.

HAEMOLYSIS [POSSIBLY ERROR]

This may be due to a clinical disorder, leading to *haemolytic anaemia*, (see 'Causes of haemolytic anaemia', p. 101), but is more likely to be due to *faults in collection or storage* which are *common* (see p. 18).

There needs to be a considerable amount of haemolysis to lower the PCV significantly.

CHECK – there will be a high MCHC because the haemoglobin concentration will be high relative to the PCV. A high MCHC is unlikely to occur from any *other* cause and strongly suggests the presence of haemolysis in the sample even if it has not been recorded by the laboratory.

If there is haemolysis the only RBC parameter which will be accurate is the haemoglobin estimation.

ERRONEOUS CAUSES

Excess EDTA

When an EDTA tube is less than half-filled (i.e. it contains >4 mg EDTA/ml blood), the osmotic withdrawal of water from the cells can reduce the PCV by 5–10%.

This discrepancy will lead to a slight reduction in MCV and a slight increase in MCHC.

CHECK – if the RBCs are examined on a stained blood smear, marked crenation is obvious.

Dilution of RBCs

Over-hydration due to the excessive administration of intravenous fluids could reduce the PCV by diluting the RBCs, but far more common is local dilution when blood samples are:

- Either withdrawn from an intravenous cannula after disconnecting the fluid-giving set.
- Or withdrawn from the *same* vein higher up.

The total protein level (and indeed the level of all metabolites) will be similarly reduced, mimicking an acute haemorrhagic anaemia.

Clots in the blood sample

This is due to insufficient EDTA, or incomplete or delayed mixing and will render all RBC parameters erroneous.

Electronic counter-sizers

Errors occur when using electronic counter-sizers that are calibrated for human RBCs to *calculate* the PCV for *cat* blood from the RBC count and MCV – see Note 3: Instrumentation, p. 42.

NOTE 1: ANAEMIA AND DEHYDRATION

Anaemia and dehydration have opposing effects on the PCV (and on the haemoglobin concentration and RBC count). If both are present the result could be a 'normal' PCV, or a PCV that does not show the full extent of a change from normal.

If the PCV is near the lower limit of the normal range and there are signs of dehydration, including an increased level of total plasma (or serum) protein, anaemia *may* exist.

However, if the animal is hypoproteinaemic, as well as being anaemic and dehydrated, it will be difficult to detect the disorders since the dehydration will tend to restore the PCV and total protein levels to normal.

NOTE 2: ANAESTHETICS AND TRANQUILLIZERS

Haematological samples may be collected from anaesthetized or tranquillized dogs and cats (perhaps because otherwise they are difficult to handle). Most of these drugs decrease the PCV, e.g.

● ACP (acepromazine=acetylpromazine), and other phenothiazine tranquillizers such as chlorpromazine, and also Immobilon, in the dog, because of its methotrimeprazine component.
    By blocking receptors these drugs relax the splenic capsule leading to enlargement of the spleen, an increased splenic uptake of RBCs, and thus fewer RBCs in the blood, i.e. a lower PCV.
● Alphaxalone/alphadolone acetate (Saffan) and ketamine hydrochloride (Vetalar) in the cat can depress PCV *below the normal range* by direct spasmolytic activity (Franckel and Hawkey, 1980).
● Barbiturates may have spasmolytic effects decreasing PCV slightly.
● Halothane has marginal effects on the PCV, if anything causing a slight decrease.

With all the above drugs any fall in PCV may also in part be due to the absence of stress.

● Anaesthetic ether by increasing sympathetic stimulation *slightly raises the PCV*.

NOTE 3: INSTRUMENTATION

● The PCV of cat blood determined by *electronic instruments* calibrated for use with human RBCs is unreliable. These instruments are used in human hospital laboratories and commercial laboratories that deal mainly with human samples. The instruments measure both the number of RBCs (RBC count) and their average size (i.e. mean corpuscular volume, MCV), and use these values to *calculate* the PCV (PCV = MCV × RBC count). The PCV is, therefore, *not* measured directly as with the spun haematocrit.
    Unless modified, i.e. unless their threshold is adjusted, such instruments will not accurately count different-sized cells from other species. Counts of canine RBCs, being of a similar size to human RBCs, will be much less affected than feline RBCs, which are considerably smaller.
    The result will be falsely low feline RBC counts and therefore low calculated PCVs on samples of cat blood.
● Even when the instruments have been modified to take account of the cell size in different species, this method of *calculating* the PCV tends to produce slightly *lower* PCV values. This is because no allowance is made for the trapping of plasma which occurs with the spun haematocrit method, and which marginally increases the PCV.
● The situation can be further complicated by the fact that, even when correctly set, these instruments may count large platelets and clumps of platelets in the blood as if they were RBCs, and this will tend to *raise* the calculated PCV. However, this effect is only significant with *anaemic blood* in which large platelets and platelet clumps are numerous – chiefly this will be cat blood.

Red blood cell count (RBC count, erythrocyte count)

● Currently the count of RBCs is expressed as the number in a litre of blood.
● In general low values indicate anaemia and high values indicate dehydration.

- The SI units for the RBC count are million millions per litre written as $10^{12}/l$ (e.g. $7.3 \times 10^{12}/l$). Numerically this is the same as expressing the RBC count in millions per microlitre ($10^6/\mu l$) or millions per cubic millimetre (million/mm^3) which were the units used previously. Consequently $7.3 \times 10^{12}/l = 7.3 \times 10^6/\mu l = 7.3$ million/mm^3.

NORMAL REFERENCE RANGE (ADULTS)

Dog

The range for dogs is $5.5–8.5 \times 10^{12}/l$ for most breeds. RBC counts in Greyhounds, Whippets, Lurchers and Borzois are higher, but in many cases not sufficient to put them outside the range for other dogs, e.g. in Greyhounds $6.5–9.5 \times 10^{12}/l$ with an 8% rise immediately after racing (Davis and Paris, 1983).

In some breeds the RBC count may appear consistently high, at or above the upper limit of normal, due to nervousness resulting in splenic contraction, e.g. Poodles, German Shepherd Dogs, Boxers, Dachshunds, Chihuahuas, Dalmatians and Beagles.

Cat

The range for cats is $5–10 \times 10^{12}/l$.

Age

Dog
The lowest values are in puppies 2(–3) weeks old ($3–4 \times 10^{12}/l$) gradually increasing to the adult range by 1 year of age.

Cat
The lowest values are in kittens 2(–3) weeks old (around $4.5 \times 10^{12}/l$) gradually increasing to the adult range by 3–4 months old.

Sex

Values tend to be only marginally higher in males, although in the Greyhound the difference is more marked.

During pregnancy, however, there is a slow fall in the RBC count (due to dilution in an increased plasma volume), and in the later stages RBC counts can be at or below the lower limit of normal.

Dog
At parturition most bitches have counts of well below $5 \times 10^{12}/l$, returning to pre-pregnancy values 8–9 weeks later.

Cat
The RBC count may be as low as $5 \times 10^{12}/l$ or less at parturition but is considerably increased only 1 week later.

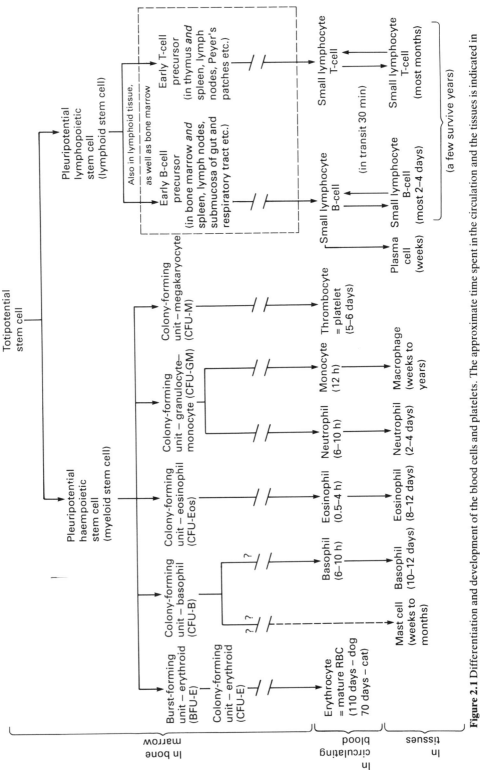

Figure 2.1 Differentiation and development of the blood cells and platelets. The approximate time spent in the circulation and the tissues is indicated in brackets. For details of developmental stages see p. 45 (RBCs), p. 144 (granulocytes and monocytes), p. 171 (lymphocytes) and p. 197 (platelets).

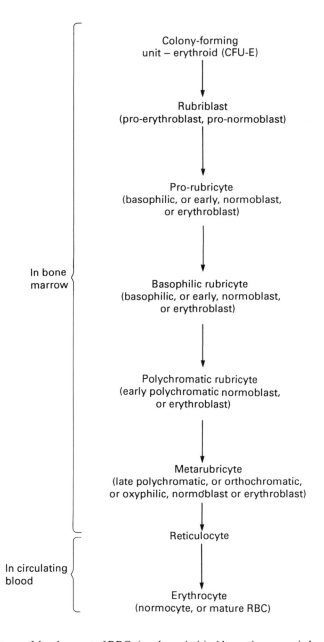

Figure 2.2 Stages of development of RBCs (erythropoiesis). Alternative names in brackets; see also p. 44 for relationship to other cells

ACCURACY

The accuracy of manual RBC counts (i.e. using a haemocytometer counting chamber) is low (±20%). Using electronic cell counters with the threshold properly set for the particular species accuracy is much greater (±2–3%).

However:

- Reliable counts of feline RBCs cannot be obtained using electronic counters which are set for the counting of human RBCs, although counts of canine RBCs are likely to be reliable (because they are of similar size).
- Even when instruments *are* properly calibrated, large platelets and clumps of platelets may be counted as if they were RBCs, giving falsely high counts, but the effect is only significant in extreme anaemia where there are numerous large platelets and/or platelet clumps – this is particularly likely in feline blood (see Note 3: Instrumentation, p. 42).

Note

Methods for estimating the RBC count by measuring light diffusion in a photometer are not recommended. The degree of diffusion produced by a diluted blood sample depends not only on the number of RBCs but on their MCV. The method assumes a standard MCV; if the actual MCV deviates from it this can result in errors of ±40%. Using a photometer much better estimates of oxygen-carrying capacity can be obtained by measuring haemoglobin concentration.

Causes of increased RBC count (haemoconcentration)

Summary

- Dehydration [usual]
- Fear/excitement [common]
- Shock
- Severe exertion
- Absolute polycythaemia
- Anabolic steroids

Error: evaporation.

These causes are dealt with more fully in the section 'Causes of increased PCV', p. 38.

DEHYDRATION [USUAL]

This is due to increased water loss and/or decreased water intake. The total protein levels will be raised to the same degree as the PCV – see Note 1: Anaemia and dehydration, p. 41.

FEAR/EXCITEMENT [COMMON]

Fear/excitement, which in the dog may be associated with feeding, produces splenic contraction, forcing RBCs out into the circulation and raising the RBC count. The effect is only transient.

SHOCK

This will cause splenic contraction and a shift of fluid to the visceral organs, which can raise the RBC count.

SEVERE EXERTION

By increasing the output of adrenaline this can result in splenic contraction and an increased RBC count (e.g. an 8% rise in Greyhounds immediately after racing).

ABSOLUTE POLYCYTHAEMIA

See Panel 2.6 (p. 123).
   This comprises:

* Primary polycythaemia (very rare).
* Secondary polycythaemia, e.g. right-to-left cardiac shunts, chronic alveolar diseases, erythropoietin-producing renal tumours, altitude, feline hyperthyroidism, acromegaly and Cushing's syndrome.

ANABOLIC STEROIDS

In Greyhounds as much as a 50% increase in RBC numbers has been reported.

ERROR

The *major error* is evaporation from the blood sample caused by leaving the cap of the container off for a significant period, particularly in warm surroundings.

Causes of decreased RBC count

Summary

* Anaemia
* Late pregancy
* Tranquillization and sedation
* Haemolysis (usually at/after collection)
Error: dilution with intravenous fluids/electronic counts/clotting

These causes are dealt with more fully in the section 'Causes of decreased PCV', p. 40.

ANAEMIA [USUAL]

Its diagnosis and differentiation are described in Panel 2.1 (p. 75).
   Dehydration may mask the presence of mild anaemia – see Note 1: Anaemia and dehydration, p. 41.

LATE PREGNANCY

The RBC count gradually falls throughout pregnancy to reach its lowest level at the time of birth.

The range of values returns to those of pre-pregnancy after 8–9 weeks in the bitch and 1 week in the queen. It is accompanied by *reticulocytosis* which is most prominent in late pregnancy and immediately post partum, particularly in the cat.

TRANQUILLIZATION AND SEDATION

These can lower the RBC count by transferring RBCs from the circulation to the spleen (see Note 2: Anaesthetics and tranquillizers, p. 42).

HAEMOLYSIS [POSSIBLE ERROR]

This may be caused by a disease (and could lead to haemolytic anaemia) but it is *more likely* to be the result of faulty collection and/or storage. There would need to be considerable haemolysis before it reduced the RBC count significantly.

CHECK – the MCHC in haemolysis will be falsely high, even impossibly so. In this situation the only accurate RBC parameter would be a haemoglobin estimation.

ERRONEOUS CAUSES

These include the following.

Dilution of RBCs

The overzealous administration of intravenous fluids will over-dilute the RBCs, but it is more important where blood samples are:

- Either withdrawn from an intravenous cannula after disconnecting the fluid-giving set.
- Or withdrawn from the same vein higher up.

Electronic counting equipment

Errors occur when using electronic counting equipment whose threshold has not been set for RBCs of the correct species (especially the cat) – see Note 3: Instrumentation, p. 42.

Clots in the blood sample

Errors occur when there are clots due to insufficient EDTA, incomplete or delayed mixing, or a very high calcium level. This will render all RBC parameters inaccurate.

Haemoglobin concentration

Haemoglobin concentration is the amount of haemoglobin in a stated volume of blood, either 1 litre or 1 decilitre (= 100 ml).

In general low values indicate anaemia and high values indicate dehydration.

Approximately 2 years before publication of this book the SI units for haemoglobin concentration were changed from grams per decilitre (g/dl, alternatively written as g/100 ml) to grams per litre (g/l). This change confers uniformity since all measurements of concentration in haematology are now expressed in terms of the litre.

Numerically, values expressed as g/l are 10 times greater than those expressed as g/dl, e.g. 14.5 g/dl (= 14.5 g/100 ml) = 145 g/l.

However, it seems likely that the use of the previous units, i.e. g/dl (= g/100 ml), will persist for some time yet.

Note

Sometimes haemoglobin concentration can be found expressed as millimoles per litre (mmol/l), e.g. dog: 7.5–11.5 mmol/l, and cat: 5–9.5 mmol/l.

This is *unnecessary* and *incompatible* with the measurement of other blood proteins in grams per litre (g/l) and, because there are different types of haemoglobin, there can be uncertainty about its precise molecular weight. In general:

- To convert mmol/l to g/dl multiply by 1.61.
- To convert mmol/l to g/l multiply by 16.1.
- To convert g/dl to mmol/l multiply by 0.62.
- To convert g/l to mmol/l multiply by 0.062.

NORMAL REFERENCE RANGE (ADULTS)

Dog

For most breeds the range is 12–18 g/dl (= 120–180 g/l) although the values are higher in the Greyhound, Whippet, Lurcher and Borzoi breeds (70–23 g/dl = 170–230 g/l), and it is significantly higher (8% in Greyhounds) immediately after racing.

Haemoglobin concentration can also appear consistently high in some other breeds, i.e. in the upper part of the normal reference range or even above it (e.g. Poodles, German Shepherd Dogs, Boxers, Dachshunds, Chihuahuas, Dalmatians and Beagles) due to nervousness causing splenic contraction.

Cat

The range for the cat is 8–15 g/dl (= 80–150 g/l).

Age

Dog
The lowest values are in puppies 4–6 weeks old (8–11 g/dl = 80–110 g/l), gradually increasing to the adult range by 1 year of age.

Cat
The lowest values are in kittens 4–6 weeks old (7–8 g/dl = 70–80 g/l), gradually increasing to the adult range by 5–6 months of age.

Sex

Values are only marginally higher in males although in Greyhounds this difference is accentuated. There is a *gradual fall during pregnancy* and in the later stages the haemoglobin concentrations can be below the normal range.

Dog
At parturition the values can be 11 g/dl (= 110 g/l) or less but return to pre-pregnancy values 8–9 weeks later.

Cat
At parturition the haemoglobin concentration may be as low as 7 g/dl (= 70 g/l) but rapidly increases within the following week.

ACCURACY

This is ±5% by the usual cyanomethaemoglobin method. Other methods are not recommended because a major problem is devising a *stable* standard with which to compare the sample.

Haemoglobin estimation is likely to be less accurate than measuring PCV by the spun haematocrit method, but is more accurate than the calculated PCV derived (from the RBC count and MCV) by laboratories dealing with human samples. If the blood has been examined by a 'human laboratory', base the assessment of anaemia on the haemoglobin concentration.

Haemoglobin concentration is the only RBC parameter which can be accurately measured using a haemolysed blood sample, or one containing a gross excess of EDTA.

Haemoglobin values will be falsely high if the blood is lipaemic or contains RBCs bearing large numbers of Heinz bodies, both of which decrease light transmission in a photometer. Look for comments about these features in the laboratory report. Lipaemia (evident 'milkiness' or turbidity) of the plasma may be noted between collection and despatch of the sample, e.g. after overnight storage. (Heinz bodies can be removed by centrifuging the blood–reagent mixture prior to haemoglobin measurement.)

If it is possible to obtain a spun haematocrit PCV value, the haemoglobin concentration is best reserved solely for calculation of the MCHC.

Causes of increased haemoglobin concentration

Summary

- Dehydration [usual]
- Fear/excitement [common]
- Shock
- Severe exertion
- Absolute polycythaemia – many disorders
- Anabolic steroids

Error: evaporation/lipaemia/Heinz bodies

These causes are dealt with more fully in the section 'Causes of increased PCV', p. 38.

DEHYDRATION [USUAL]

This is due to increased water loss and/or decreased water intake. The total protein level will be raised to the same degree as the haemoglobin alone (see Note 1: Anaemia and dehydration, p. 41).

FEAR/EXCITEMENT [COMMON]

Fear and excitement, which in the dog may be associated with feeding, produces splenic contraction forcing RBCs out into the circulation and raising the haemoglobin concentration. The effect is only transient.

SHOCK

This will cause splenic contraction and a shift of fluid to the visceral organs which can raise the RBC count and the haemoglobin concentration.

SEVERE EXERTION

By increasing the output of adrenaline, this can result in splenic contraction and again an elevated haemoglobin concentration (e.g. in Greyhounds, 8% immediately following racing).

ABSOLUTE POLYCYTHAEMIA

See Panel 2.6, p. 123.
   This comprises:

- Primary polycythaemia [very rare].
- Secondary polycythaemia – e.g. right-to-left cardiac shunts, chronic alveolar diseases, erythropoietin-producing renal tumours, altitude, feline hyperthyroidism, acromegaly and Cushing's syndrome.

ANABOLIC STEROIDS

In Greyhounds, as much as a 50% increase in haemoglobin concentration has been reported following their use.

ERRONEOUS CAUSES

These include the following.

Evaporation from the blood sample

This occurs as a result of leaving off the cap of the sample container for a significant period, especially in warm surroundings.

Lipaemia

By reducing light transmission, lipaemia gives rise to elevated readings with a photometer.

Large numbers of Heinz bodies

This is particularly likely in the cat and will increase the optical density of the blood sample, so falsely elevating the reading of haemoglobin concentration.

Causes of decreased haemoglobin concentration

Summary

- Anaemia
- Late pregnancy
- Tranquillization and sedation
- Haemolysis (usually at/after collection)

Error: dilution with intravenous fluids/clotting

These causes are dealt with more fully in the section 'Causes of decreased PCV', p. 40.

ANAEMIA [USUAL]

Its diagnosis and differentiation are described in Panel 2.1, p. 75.

Dehydration may mask the presence of mild anaemia – see Note 1: Anaemia and dehydration, p. 41.

LATE PREGNANCY

The haemoglobin concentration gradually falls throughout pregnancy to reach its lowest value at the time of birth. The range of values returns to normal after 8–9 weeks in the bitch and around 1 week in the queen. It is accompanied by *reticulocytosis* which is most prominent in late pregnancy and immediately post partum, particularly in the cat.

TRANQUILLIZATION AND SEDATION

These can lower the haemoglobin concentration by transferring RBCs from the circulation to the spleen (see Note 2: Anaesthetics and tranquillizers, p. 42).

ERRONEOUS CAUSES

These include the following.

Dilution of RBCs

The over-zealous administration of intravenous fluids will over-dilute the RBCs; however, dilution is more important where blood samples are:

- Either taken from an intravenous cannula after disconnecting the fluid-giving set.
- Or withdrawn from the same vein higher up.

Clots

Errors are caused by clots in the blood sample, due to insufficient EDTA, incomplete or delayed mixing, *or* a very high plasma calcium level. Clotting will render all RBC parameters inaccurate.

Glycosylated haemoglobin (glycohaemoglobin)

This is a variant of normal haemoglobin which is progressively synthesized from normal haemoglobin during the lifespan of each RBC (about 110 days in the dog). The amount which is formed (by an irreversible reaction between glucose and haemoglobin) depends upon the plasma glucose level over this period. Consequently, the *proportion* of the total haemoglobin which has been 'glycosylated' is a reflection of the glucose level over the previous 4 months. In diabetic dogs (as in diabetic humans), its measurement can be used to check whether the diabetes mellitus has been successfully controlled throughout that period.

Measurement is made using a heparinized blood sample.

NORMAL REFERENCE RANGE

Dog

The normal range of glycosylated haemoglobin is 4–8% of total haemoglobin.

It rises to 10–18% in poorly managed diabetics.

Cat

The test is not reliable.

The percentage of glycosylated haemoglobin is a measure of what the plasma glucose level *has been* over the last 4 months in the dog, *not* what the glucose level is at the time of collecting the blood sample. It is unaffected by surges of adrenaline due to fear or excitement which can temporarily and misleadingly elevate plasma glucose levels (see p. 280).

It *cannot* replace plasma glucose estimations in the initial stabilization of a diabetic or in determining the need for daily adjustments to the insulin dosage. It *can* be used to monitor long-term control of stable diabetics with or without daily glucose measurements on blood or urine (Chastain and Nichols, 1984).

ACCURACY

- Direct chemical measurements are more reliable.
- Chromatographic measurements can be altered by the presence of salicylates, protein-breakdown products and certain antibodies.
- Since older RBCs (containing the highest proportion of glycosylated haemoglobin) are preferentially destroyed in haemolytic anaemia, the percentage of glycosylated haemoglobin inevitably falls in that condition.

Methaemoglobin

This is a brownish compound of haemoglobin formed by the oxidation of iron from the ferrous to the ferric state, which when present in an appreciable amount in the blood gives a muddy, cyanotic colour to the mucous membranes.

Normally it accounts for less than 1.1% of all the haemoglobin (certainly <2%). The level can be measured (heparin is the preferred anticoagulant), but its presence is demonstrated by the dark-brownish (chocolate) colour of a blood sample and the chocolate brown colour of a spot of blood on filter paper (which is especially obvious when compared with normal blood).

INCREASED LEVELS

These are due to the following.

Oxidant poisons and drugs

Mild to moderate oxidants (e.g. ketamine in some cats) cause only methaemo-globinaemia. Stronger oxidants (paracetamol, the weedkiller sodium chlorate and raw onions) also denature and precipitate haemoglobin as Heinz bodies in the RBCs, especially in the cat, and their subsequent phagocytosis can result in extravascular haemolytic anaemia. Benzocaine applied as a local analgesic to skin ulcers can be a cause of methaemoglobinaemia in dogs (see Panel 2.3, p. 101).

Congenital methaemoglobinaemia

This occurs as a result of a deficiency of the RBC enzyme NADH-methaemoglobin reductase.

Haematological indices (MVC, MCHC and MCH)

MEAN CORPUSCULAR VOLUME (MCV)

This is a measure of RBC size and represents the volume of a single RBC.
It is calculated as:

$$\frac{\text{PCV (in l/l)} \times 1000}{\text{RBC count (in } 10^{12}/\text{l)}}$$

It is expressed in femtolitres (fl), which were termed 'cubic micrometres' (μm^3). One femtolitre = 10^{-15} litre. Using older units the calculation becomes:

$$\text{MCV (in fl)} = \frac{\text{PCV (in \%)} \times 10}{\text{RBC count (in } 10^6/\mu l)}$$

MEAN CORPUSCULAR HAEMOGLOBIN CONCENTRATION (MCHC)

This is a measure of the concentration of haemoglobin in the red blood cells. It indicates the weight of haemoglobin (in grams) in one decilitre (i.e. 100 ml) of RBCs (not in one decilitre of whole blood).

Therefore, MCHC is expressed in grams/decilitre (g/dl). Previously it was expressed as a percentage, and numerically the two are the same since one per cent is defined as 1 g/dl.

$$\text{MCHC} = \frac{\text{Hb (in g/dl)}}{\text{PCV (in l/l)}} = \frac{\text{Hb (in g/l)}}{\text{PCV (in l/l)} \times 10}$$

Or, using older units,

$$\text{MCHC} = \frac{\text{Hb (in g/dl)} \times 100}{\text{PCV (in \%)}}$$

MEAN CORPUSCULAR HAEMOGLOBIN (MCH)

The other remaining haematological index, the MCH, is seldom used. It also indicates the haemoglobin content of the RBCs (being the weight of haemoglobin in an average RBC), but it is less accurate than the MCHC since it is calculated from the two least accurate measurements, RBC count and haemoglobin concentration. It is expressed in picograms (pg). There is little advantage in knowing or reporting it, except that it usually changes in proportion with the MCV, and any disproportionate alteration in the MCH suggests an error in the RBC count or Hb estimation. But in late iron deficiency, the fall in MCH is greater than the fall in MCV.

$$\text{MCH} = \frac{\text{Hb (in g/dl)} \times 10}{\text{RBC (in } 10^{12}/\text{l)}} = \frac{\text{Hb (in g/l)}}{\text{RBC (in } 10^{12}/\text{l)}}$$

NORMAL REFERENCE RANGES (ADULT)

	MCV (fl)	*MCHC (g/dl)*	*MCH (pg)*
Dog	60–77	32–36	19.5–24.5
Cat	39–55	30–36	12.5–17.5

Note

If haemoglobin concentration is expressed in mmol/l then MCHC will also be expressed in mmol/l (dog: 20–22.5 mmol/l; cat: 18.5–22.5 mmol/l) but these are not standard SI units.

The smaller cat RBCs are often confused with platelets by electronic counting and sizing instruments. Consequently, the MCV for cat RBCs provided by these machines is best disregarded and the MCV calculated from the number of RBCs and the PCV (derived from a spun haematocrit).

Age

MCV
- Dog – at birth the RBCs are large (MCV = 95–100 fl). The MCV falls to adult values by 2 months of age.
- Cat – at birth the RBCs are also large (MCV averages 90 fl) but reduce to adult size at 1 month of age.

MCHC
- Dog – this index stays within the adult range all the time.
- Cat – the low MCHC at birth increases for 2 weeks, but then falls again and does not attain adult values until 4 months of age.

Breed
MCV

- Japanese Akita has smaller RBCs than other dogs (MCV = 55–65 fl). Occasionally Miniature and Toy Poodles have macrocytic RBCs (MCV = >80 fl, i.e. 85–95 fl), which are normochromic (i.e. MCHC is in the normal range) plus occasional RBCs with features of immaturity (e.g. polychromasia or many Howell–Jolly bodies). This change resembles those of vitamin B_{12} and folate deficiencies, although there is *no anaemia*.
- In the Greyhound/Whippet/Lurcher breeds, the indices are generally similar to other breeds, although exceptionally the RBCs are larger, i.e. MCV is >77 fl.

MCHC
MCHC is usually below the normal range in Alaskan Malamute dwarfs.

CONSTANCY OF HAEMATOLOGICAL INDICES

Changes in RBC size and pigmentation, and consequently changes in MCV and MCHC, are unusual, so that normally:

- For the dog – Hb concn = PCV × (100/3), RBC count = PCV × (100/6) and Hb concn = 2 × RBC count.

Note

In dwarf Alaskan Malamutes, a diagnostic feature is a change in the PCV:Hb ratio from 3:1 to 4:1 or 5:1 (Fletch et al., 1973).

- For the cat – Hb concn = PCV × (100/3), RBC count = PCV × (100/5) and Hb concn = 1.6 × RBC count.

In the above formulae, PCV is in l/l, Hb concn is in g/dl and RBC count is in × 10^{12}/l.

Changes from normal

An *increase in MCV* implies abnormally large cells, i.e. macrocytes. These are principally immature cells – reticulocytes and possibly nucleated red blood cells, in regenerative anaemias; less often they are nucleated red blood cells which result from neoplastic change in myeloproliferative disorders, or large RBCs produced in folate and vitamin B_{12} deficiences – the so-called macrocytic (megaloblastic) anaemias.

A *decrease in MCV* implies abnormally small cells, i.e. microcytic. These are seldom seen and are principally due to well-developed iron deficiency. Cells with a *normal MCV* are termed 'normocytic'.

A *decrease in MCHC* implies cells with a reduced haemoglobin content, termed 'hypochromic'. The most commonly encountered are reticulocytes, but also the RBCs in the later stages of iron deficiency are hypochromic. Cells with normal haemoglobin content, i.e. with *normal MCHC*, are termed 'normochromic'.

An *increase in MCHC* probably indicates an error in one or both of the measurements (haemoglobin concentration and PCV, most probably the former), since it is not possible for cells to hold more than the maximum amount of haemoglobin, although a slight increase in MCHC above normal may occur where there are large numbers of spherocytes (small, spherical cells occurring in immune-mediated haemolytic anaemias).

An *apparent increase in MCHC* (as calculated) arises with haemolysis (either intravascular or during collection or handling). Lysis of the RBCs results in a fall in the PCV, although the total haemoglobin concentration remains unaltered; the net effect is an increase in calculated MCHC.

Almost all true changes from normal haematological indices arise in particular types of anaemia (see 'Distinctive features of each type of anaemia', p. 84). But abnormal values can often result from errors in measuring the parameters from which they are calculated, especially the RBC count and haemoglobin concentration.

If there is not an abnormal PCV, abnormal MCV and MCHC values that cannot be checked microscopically are best disregarded. Significantly elevated MCHC values should always be dismissed as erroneous.

Abnormal MCV and MCHC values *can* be checked by examining a stained blood smear (e.g. that made for the differential WBC count). It is possible to assess the *size* of the RBCs (compared with the size of the various WBCs which vary very little) and the *degree of pigmentation* and hence staining, of the RBCs especially in the centre area which is their thinnest part. Where there appears to be discrepancy between the calculated value and the cell appearance, what is actually seen is always more reliable.

GENERAL NOTE

Abnormal values for the MCV and MCHC reflect changes that involve a significant proportion of the RBCs *but* not every RBC needs to change in that way. If only a few RBCs show a change in size or pigmentation, the overall effect may be insufficient to shift the MCV or MCHC from its normal range, i.e. these indices simply represent *mean* values.

Although changes in size and pigmentation affecting only a minority of RBCs will probably not alter the MCV and MCHC, the changes *will* be evident when a stained blood smear is examined. (Variation in size, i.e. RBCs of different sizes in the same smear, is termed 'anisocytosis'.)

Causes of an increased MCV

Dog >77 fl.
Cat >55 fl.

This implies the presence in the blood of a significant number of larger RBCs (macrocytes).

First see the General note above.

Summary

- Reticulocytosis
- Large mature RBCs
- Hyperthyroidism
- Nucleated RBCs
- Inherited macrocytosis
- Age related

Error: EDTA/low RBC count/high PCV

RETICULOCYTES [USUAL]

In regenerative anaemias (haemorrhagic or haemolytic), a large number of reticulocytes appear constituting reticulocytosis (see Panel 2.5, p. 115).

They take about 3 days to appear in significant numbers. They appear polychromasic/hypochromic with Romanowksy staining – their reticulum becomes obvious with supravital staining. Their appearance is a short-lived response to a sudden lack of RBCs; consequently, the increase in MCV is also transient (regenerative anaemias may therefore be termed 'pseudo-macrocytic anaemias'). This finding is associated with a low MCHC.

The MCV will return to normal within 2–3 weeks, unless the reticulocytosis continues due to persistence of the underlying cause.

LARGE MATURE (i.e. NON-NUCLEATED) NORMOCHROMIC RBCs [VERY RARE]

These RBCs of varying sizes (derived from large rubricytes = megaloblasts) occur in *megaloblastic anaemia*.

Their presence is caused by a dietary deficiency of folate due to chronic malabsorption or more usually to long-term treatment with folate antagonists such as methotrexate, pyrimethamine, trimethoprim, and phenytoin (in dogs) or drugs which inhibit folate synthesis, e.g. sulphonamides. Onset is slow (i.e. takes several days).

Experimentally a dietary deficiency of niacin, causing black tongue, also gives this effect, but anaemia due to vitamin B_{12} (cyanocobalamin) deficiency, which is well recognized in humans, is not recorded in dogs or cats, although cyanocobalamin deficiency may be a feature of small intestinal malabsorption in the dog (see Panel 6.3, p. 344).

Lack of these vitamins interferes with nucleic acid synthesis inhibiting cell division, thus producing larger RBCs.

When the deficiency is corrected the MCV returns to normal. Macrocytic anaemia from this cause can be distinguished from the pseudomacrocytic anaemia due to reticulocytosis (see above) by finding a normal MCHC; with reticulocytosis the MCHC is low.

HYPERTHYROIDISM [OCCASIONAL]

Approximately half of cats with hyperthyroidism show macrocytosis and an increased MCV. (This could be due to the direct effect of thyroid hormones on the bone marrow and also to an increase in erythropoietin production which reduces the RBC maturation time.)

NUCLEATED RBCs [GENERALLY UNCOMMON]

Myeloproliferative disorders

Nucleated RBCs occur where there is neoplastic proliferation of bone marrow cells, which is usually associated with a non-regenerative anaemia.

Reticulocytes are few or absent (see Panel 3.2, p. 189).

- Nucleated RBCs are *prominent* when proliferation involves the erythroid cells, as in erythroleukaemia and erythraemic myelosis in the cat.
- Nucleated RBCs arise in most other myeloproliferative disorders and *might* possibly increase the MCV, e.g. in monocytic leukaemia and in myelofibrosis (sometimes a terminal event in myeloproliferative disorders).
- Primitive cells which are formed in reticuloendotheliosis and *resemble* early erythroid precursors (i.e. immature developmental RBCs) could *contribute* to an increased MCV.

Severe regenerative anaemias

There would be insufficient nucleated RBCs to increase MCV alone but their presence enhances the increase in MCV due to the prominent reticulocytosis, i.e. in severe acute haemorrhagic or haemolytic anaemias.

Nucleated RBCs that arise in other situations

These (see Panel 2.5, p. 115) will seldom be sufficient to increase the MCV – e.g. in chronic lead poisoning, with reduced splenic function, with infection or septicaemia, with extramedullary haemopoiesis and in myelophthistic diseases.

INHERITED MACROCYTOSIS [BREED RELATED]

Poodles

In some Poodles, Toy and Miniature, macrocytosis occurs sometimes with numerous nuclear fragments (in nucleated RBCs) and Howell–Jolly bodies (in mature RBCs). MCV = >80 fl. These dogs are *not anaemic.*

Alaskan Malamutes

In Alaskan Malamutes, macrocytosis can be due to *hereditary stomatocytosis.* RBCs are also hypochromic throughout life but only puppies less than 6 months old are anaemic.

Siamese cats

Erythropoietic porphyria occurs with macrocytic/normochromic anaemia.

Greyhound/Whippet/Lurcher

In these breeds, the MCV is exceptionally over 77 fl.

AGE RELATED

Dog

MCV is large at birth (95–100 fl), then reduces to adult size at 2–3 months old.

Cat

MCV is large at birth (90 fl) reducing to adult size at approximately 2 months old (punctate reticulocytes *can* at times comprise up to 50% of the RBCs at 2–3 months old).

ERRONEOUSLY HIGH MCVs

These can be due to the following.

Prolonged contact of RBCs with EDTA

This can increase MCV by 5–7 fl due to RBCs swelling.

Falsely low RBC count

Autoimmune haemolytic anaemia

The RBCs and spherocytes are more fragile and, if counted electronically, the diluent can result in some of them haemolysing, i.e. the RBC count is reduced. But there is no haemolysis when measuring the PCV by spun haematocrit (so that the PCV is *relatively* higher) giving a *higher MCV*.

To distinguish an increased MCV due to this haemolysis in the RBC count, from an increased MCV due to reticulocytosis alone, examine the MCHC; *with this haemolysis* neither the PCV nor the haemoglobin concentration is affected and therefore the MCHC is normal, or very slightly low – *with reticulocytosis* the haemoglobin concentration is low, because the cells are hypochromic, and therefore the MCHC is also low.

Agglutination

Agglutination (clumping) of RBCs or *small clots* in the sample. Electronic counts of RBCs will be erroneously low *but* PCV will be unaffected so MCV will be increased.

CHECK – it can be distinguished from the increased MCV due to reticulocytosis in the same way as described above.

Incorrect setting of electronic counter

In the cat, if the threshold is incorrectly set for the RBC size, smaller RBCs (microcytes and leptocytes) may not register, giving a low RBC count and an apparently high MCV.

Falsely high PCV value

If haematocrit fails to pack RBCs adequately, i.e. trapping more plasma between them, the PCV will be high giving a high MCV (and of course a low MCHC also).

This can happen if centrifugation is for too short a time or at too low a speed.

Causes of a decreased MCV

Dog: <50 fl.
Cat: <39 fl.

This implies the presence in the blood of a significant number of smaller RBCs (microcytes).

First see the General note on p. 57.

Summary

- Iron deficiency
- Pyridoxine deficiency
- Feline haemobartonellosis
- Age related
- Breed related

Error: electronic count of cat RBCs

IRON DEFICIENCY – LATER STAGES [USUAL CAUSE (THOUGH NOT COMMON)]

In the *early* stages of iron deficiency the MCV is in the normal range, i.e. there is initially a normocytic/normochromic anaemia which, if the deficiency continues, then progresses through normocytic/hypochromic *or* microcytic/normochromic to microcytic/hypochromic anaemia.

The lack of iron limits haemoglobin formation but cell division only ceases in the bone marrow when the haemoglobin concentration reaches a certain level. This means that in *prolonged* iron deficiency an *extra cell division* occurs producing smaller RBCs.

Prolonged, i.e. chronic, blood loss

This is the most usual cause of iron deficiency – as in blood donor animals bled too frequently, or a continuously bleeding tumour, e.g. in the gastrointestinal or urinary tracts. (This means the increased MCV of regenerative anaemia can change to the decreased MCV of iron deficiency if there is persistent blood loss.)

Chronic inflammatory disease, chronic infection or necrotizing neoplasia

These can impair the transfer of iron.

Dietary deficiency of iron

This is usually in young growing animals on a solely milk diet.

CHECK – to confirm, measure the serum iron level and the total iron-binding capacity in serum (see p. 381).

Impaired iron uptake and utilization

For example, this occurs in some anaemic dogs with portosystemic shunts.

PYRIDOXINE DEFICIENCY (VITAMIN B_6 DEFICIENCY) [RARE]

Lack of pyridoxine in the diet reduces haemoglobin formation producing the same effects as iron deficiency. (Also riboflavin (vitamin B_2) deficiency experimentally results in a decreased MCV.)

FELINE HAEMOBARTONELLOSIS (FELINE INFECTIOUS ANAEMIA = FIA) [OCCASIONAL]

A few cats with FIA show an abnormally low MCV indicating a lack of remission of the anaemia.

AGE RELATED

Temporary microcytosis

This can arise in kittens especially at 1 month old due to iron deficiency in their mother's milk.

BREED RELATED

Japanese Akita

This breed of dog generally has a smaller RBC with an MCV of 55–65 fl.

ERRONEOUSLY LOW MCVs

These can be due to counting feline RBCs with electronic counters – clumps of platelets or abnormally large platelets may register as RBCs giving a falsely increased RBC count, and a falsely low MCV. This may be important in severe anaemia.

Causes of an increased MCHC

An increased MCHC (in dog and cat >36 g/dl) is almost always due to error since it is not really possible to increase the RBC's normal haemoglobin capacity much further.
  However, it can (rarely) arise with *large numbers of spherocytes* (spherical RBCs associated with immune-mediated haemolytic anaemias). Their shape causes a lower PCV than usual and with a high haemoglobin concentration the MCHC is increased, usually only slightly but *possibly* above the normal range.

Erroneously high MCHCs

Erroneously high MCHCs (which are far more common) may be due to:

1. Haemolysis, occurring either
    (a) intravascularly (uncommon), or
    (b) during or after collection (common), will cause a fall in the PCV, although all the haemoglobin remains in the blood so that the MCHC is elevated.

CHECK – examine the plasma in the microhaematocrit tube for haemolysis. Even if there is haemolysis, the remaining RBCs may genuinely be *hypochromic* and this may be checked by examining a stained blood smear.

2. Increased optical density of blood plasma will falsely increase the readings for haemoglobin concentration, thereby elevating the MCHC. Factors, other than haemolysis, that may cause this are:
    (a) lipaemia (most commonly),
    (b) increased numbers of Heinz bodies in cat RBCs. (Heinz bodies may be present in over 50% of the RBCs, although usually no more than 10%.)

Causes of a decreased MCHC

Summary

- Reticulocytes [most usual]
- Nucleated RBCs [rare]
- Iron deficiency [unusual]
- Pyridoxine deficiency [very rare]
- Protein deficiency [rare]
- Inherited hypochromia [rare]
- Age related

Error: erroneously low MCHCs due to falsely high PCV

A decreased MCHC is: in the dog, < 32 g/dl; in the cat, < 30 g/dl. This implies RBCs with a reduced haemoglobin content (hypochromic). First see General note, p. 57.

RETICULOCYTES [MOST USUAL]

These occur in regenerative anaemias (haemorrhagic/haemolytic) that are in remission. Their haemoglobin content is less in relation to their increased volume than in mature RBCs and in sufficient numbers they can result in a slightly lower MCHC. The fall in MCHC takes several days to develop and, as the reticulocytes mature and the anaemia is corrected, the abnormal haematological indices (lower MCHC, higher MCV) return to normal.

NUCLEATED RBCs [RARE]

These would lower the MCHC for the same reasons as reticulocytes, but they would seldom occur in sufficient numbers to reduce appreciably the MCHC.

IRON DEFICIENCY (LATER STAGES) [UNUSUAL]

This results in diminished haemoglobin production. Initially, in iron deficiency the MCHC is in the normal range, i.e. there is first a normocytic/normochromic anaemia which progresses through normocytic/hypochromic and microcytic/normochromic to microcytic/hypochromic anaemia.

Iron deficiency may be caused by:

- Chronic persistent blood loss causing a regenerative anaemia (chronic haemorrhagic) to become a non-regenerative (iron deficiency) anaemia. This is the most common cause of iron deficiency.
- Chronic inflammatory disease, chronic infection or necrotizing neoplasia which impair the transfer of iron from iron stores to plasma
- Dietary deficiency: this is seldom recognized; if it occurs it is usually in young animals on a milk diet. There is a transient deficiency in cats around 1–2 months of age.
- Impaired iron uptake and utilization, e.g. in some anaemic dogs with portosystemic shunts.

PYRIDOXINE DEFICIENCY [VERY RARE]

Pyridoxine or vitamin B_6 deficiency in the diet limits haemoglobin production resulting in the same effects as iron deficiency. (Also experimentally riboflavin, i.e. vitamin B_2, deficiency gives a decrease in MCHC.)

PROTEIN DEFICIENCY [RARE]

Maldigestion, malabsorption and protein-losing conditions, e.g. enteropathies, can produce anaemia of moderate severity (with a poor reticulocyte response and possibly a slightly decreased MCHC), accompanied by a moderate hypoproteinaemia.

INHERITED HYPOCHROMIA [RARE]

This occurs in Alaskan Malamutes with hereditary stomatocytosis, and in Siamese cats with erythropoietic porphyria (Parry, 1987).

AGE RELATED

At birth the MCHC is generally just below the normal adult range (i.e. <27 g/dl). It fluctuates over the next few weeks entering the normal range at 5–6 months of age.

Table 2.1 Anaemia classified by MCV and MCHC

	Microcytic (↓ MCV)	Normocytic (normal MCV)	Macrocytic (↑ MCV)
Hypochromic (↓ MCHC)	Iron deficiency – later stage Usually chronic haemorrhage Possibly lack in diet of young Rarely chronic inflammation or malignant neoplasia Rarely impaired uptake, e.g. portacaval shunt Pyridoxine (B_6) deficiency	Early iron deficiency Protein deficiency or loss	Haemorrhage ⎫ Haemolysis ⎬ Severe regenerative anaemia with reticulocytosis i.e. after first 2–3 days = anaemia in remission* Pyruvate kinase deficiency in Basenji and Beagle Stomatocytosis in chondrodysplastic Alaskan Malamute puppies (less than 6 months old, adults are not anaemic) ERROR – inadequate RBC packing in haematocrit (= PCV estimation)
Normochromic (normal MCHC)	Iron deficiency – intermediate stage Feline infectious anaemia not responding to therapy Japanese Akita dogs ERROR (cat) – electronic counters counting platelets or clumps of platelets as RBCs (could make normocytic anaemia appear microcytic)	Initially after haemorrhage or extravascular haemolysis (first 2–3 days) Initial iron deficiency Pure red cell aplasia – FeLV or immune-mediated Secondary anaemias Chronic inflammation Chronic infections Malignant neoplasia Chronic renal failure Chronic liver disease Endocrine disorders	Less severe regenerative anaemia – haemorrhage or haemolysis Hyperthyroidism in cats Folic acid deficiency – usually drug antagonists Niacin deficiency (black tongue) Some myeloproliferative disorders Erythraemic myelosis and erythroleukaemia primarily; also at times with monocytic leukaemia and myelofibrosis Erythropoietic porphyria in Siamese cat

Aplastic anaemia
  Chemical and drug toxicity
  Infections (bacterial toxins, viruses, *Ehrlichia*)
  Radiation
Myelophthistic anaemia – bone marrow tissue replaced by:
  Primary neoplasm (most myeloproliferative disorders)
  Metastatic neoplasm
  Granulomatous tissue

ERROR (cat) incorrect threshold setting for electronic counter
ERROR – RBCs destroyed in performing RBC count (with autoimmune haemolytic anaemia)*
ERROR – RBC agglutination*
ERROR – prolonged contact with EDTA (could make normocytic anaemia appear macrocytic)

Hyperchromic
(↑ MCHC)

ERRORS (which will make RBCs appear hyperchromic):
Increased optical density of plasma
Haemolysis – intravascular or faults in collection and/or handling*
Lipaemia (in anaemic animal)
Cat – large numbers of Heinz bodies (oxidant poisons)*
? Possible in immune-mediated haemolytic anaemia with large numbers of spherocytes*

Spherocytes, being spherical RBCs (associated with immune-mediated haemolytic anaemia), appear microcytic on blood smears, but have a normal MCV.

*More than one of the factors marked * might, although very rarely, be present concurrently in a case of haemolytic anaemia (most probably one that is immune-mediated).

Some changes in MCV or MCHC are not associated with anaemia – notably the decreased MCHC and/or increased MCV in the first few months of life and the inherited condition of macrocytosis in some Poodles.

ERRONEOUS CAUSES

Erroneously low MCHCs may be due to a falsely high PCV. Incomplete packing of RBCs in the microhaematocrit tube (due to insufficient centrifugation) elevates the PCV and gives a falsely low MCHC.

Abnormal RBCs and RBC inclusions

Haematology reports may mention the presence of one or more abnormal types of RBCs and/or inclusions in the RBCs. The implications of such findings are described below.

Abnormal RBCs

CRENATED RBCs (ECHINOCYTES)

These shrunken 'RBCs' show an irregular outline with several evenly spaced blunted points. Some occur in all blood smears and are usually considered an artefact due to withdrawal of water from the cell by anticoagulants, pH changes and defects in drying (e.g. slow drying of a thick smear). They are particularly prominent in:

- *Old* blood samples (as RBCs lose ATP).
- Uraemia.
- Cats' blood samples, due to incomplete filling of the collecting tube with resultant high EDTA concentration.

Markedly crenated cells are termed 'burr cells' (see below).

BURR CELLS

These are markedly crenated cells (see above) and, apart from being an artefact, are often a feature of:

- Severe uraemia in dog or cat (arising from impaired glycolysis in the RBC).
- Disseminated intravascular coagulation (DIC).

ACANTHOCYTES (SPUR CELLS)

These non-biconcave RBCs show a small number (3–12) of prominent, irregular and unevenly spaced spicules, due to increased cholesterol in the RBC membrane.

They are seen in dogs, especially those with splenic haemangiosarcomas or haemangiomas, and also some with severe diffuse liver disease, e.g. those with increased levels of plasma bilirubin (hyperbilirubinaemia) and with portosystemic shunts.

SPHEROCYTES

These are small darkly staining spherical RBCs. They have lost their biconcavity and central pale area and appear smaller (microcytic). They are easily distinguished in the dog, but not in the cat where the RBCs are *normally* smaller and stain more densely.

They generally result from RBCs being encoated with antibody or complement and then being partially phagocytosed by macrophages (especially in the spleen). They are associated with immune-mediated haemolytic diseases (see 'Causes of haemolytic anaemia', p. 101):

- Primarily autoimmune haemolytic anaemia (AIHA) where there may be large numbers present.
- Drug-induced immune haemolytic anaemia.
- Alloantibody-induced haemolytic anaemia (incompatible blood transfusion and haemolytic disease of the newborn).

Because they cannot readily deform, spherocytes are removed from the circulation prematurely by macrophages in the spleen.

Note

Old RBCs in stored blood (e.g. stored for blood transfusion) may become spherocytes.

POIKILOCYTES

These are *any* abnormally shaped RBCs. Most of them can be more precisely described (e.g. as crenated RBCs, acanthocytes, spherocytes, schistocytes etc.) and therefore this non-specific term is best reserved for RBCs which do not fit into other categories.

In general they are the result of:

- Either a defect in production, as with chronic blood loss (iron deficiency anaemia).
- Or premature destruction, i.e. fragmented RBCs resulting from haemolysis, e.g. due to immune-mediated diseases or disseminated intravascular coagulation (see 'Causes of haemolytic anaemia', p. 101).

LEPTOCYTES

These are thin flat RBCs, i.e. with increased diameter and decreased thickness.

Stained with Romanowsky stains they may appear:

- Hypochromic (overall poorly staining), where there is reduced haemoglobin production as in iron deficiency anaemia.
- Polychromic (variable staining, otherwise termed 'polychromasic', 'polychromatic' or 'polychromatophilic') – these are essentially reticulocytes due to a regenerative response, i.e. primarily in haemorrhagic and haemolytic anaemias, but also in association with basophilic stippling in the rare condition of lead poisoning.
- Or orthochromic – these are found in conditions which lead to non-regenerative anaemia such as chronic debilitating diseases, end-stage renal disease, liver disease, obstructive jaundice, hypothyroidism, bone marrow suppression and following splenectomy.

Being thin cells leptocytes readily fold and distort, and may be reported as:

- Folded cells (knizocytes), i.e. looking like the head of a screw, with a central dark bar and pale areas on either side.
- Bowl-shaped cells.

- But particularly as target cells (codocytes), i.e. looking like a shooting target, with a central dark area surrounded by a circular pale zone and outside that a circular dark zone at the periphery. This seems to be the most common shape for leptocytes associated with disease.

Leptocytes can be an artefact if the plasma is hypertonic.

SCHISTOCYTES (SHIZOCYTES)

These are irregular fragments of RBCs that arise from mechanical damage occurring within the blood vessels. They are a particular feature of haemolysis attributable to disseminated intravascular coagulation and malignant tumours (especially haemangiosarcomas).

Schistocytes may also arise in congestive heart failure, myelofibrosis, glomerulonephritis, chronic iron deficiency and where there is turbulent blood flow (as with valvular heart lesions, patent ductus arteriosus and cardiomyopathy).

Normally less than half of one per cent of the RBCs are schistocytes.

OVAL RBCs (OVALOCYTES/ELLIPTOCYTES) AND TEARDROP-SHAPED RBCs (DACROCYTES)

These distorted shapes are seen in myeloproliferative disorders, myelofibrosis and myelophthisis.

Dacrocytes can also be an artefact at the 'feather edge' of a blood smear.

STOMATOCYTES (MOUTH-SHAPED CELLS)

Those with a slit-like opening near the centre are principally associated with the rare disease of hereditary stomatocytosis in Alaskan Malamutes.

Exceptionally they may develop in dogs with chronic anaemia and certain liver disorders.

Distorted leptocytes (bowl-shaped cells) can appear similar.

TOROCYTES

These are ring-shaped or 'punched out' RBCs having a clear centre and dark rim, seen in hypochromic anaemia (e.g. iron deficiency anaemia).

SIDEROCYTES

These are RBCs containing blue-black iron-containing granules (Pappenheimer bodies). Usually they are associated with regenerative anaemia (especially haemolytic) but they are also seen in lead poisioning.

ECCENTROCYTES OR PYKNOCYTES

These are RBCs where the haemoglobin has coalesced together in one area. They develop in dogs poisoned with paracetamol (acetaminophen) or onions.

ROULEAU FORMATION

This needs to be distinguished from agglutination.

A rouleau consists of a number of RBCs that have stuck together, looking like a stack of coins that has toppled over. Some rouleaux are normally present in dog and cat blood, and are more common in the latter. Increased numbers are a feature of hyperproteinaemia and can be prominent in inflammatory and neoplastic diseases.

AGGLUTINATION

This is the spontaneous clumping of RBCs that indicates the presence of antibodies against them, usually a sign of autoimmune haemolytic anaemia (see Panel 2.7, p. 125).

NUCLEATED RBCs

These are sometimes referred to as rubricytes, normoblasts or erythroblasts, with appropriate prefixes. When larger than usual (e.g. in folate deficiency), these cells are called megaloblasts.

These are immature developmental RBCs, preceding reticulocytes in development, released from the bone marrow. One or two may be present in the blood of normal healthy dogs and cats.

Increased numbers usually appear in severe regenerative anaemia (haemorrhagic or haemolytic) accompanied by much larger numbers of reticulocytes.

They may also be seen in association with *small* numbers of reticulocytes (or even no reticulocytes) in disorders such as myeloproliferative diseases (especially erythroleukaemia and erythraemic myelosis in the cat), haemangiosarcomas, chronic lead poisioning and some types of liver disease (see Panel 2.5, p. 115).

MACROCYTES

Macrocytes (or megalocytes) are large RBCs. When present in significant numbers they will raise the MCV.

Usually they are reticulocytes (associated with regenerative anaemias) that appear polychromasic and hypochromic on Romanowsky-stained smears, and show the characteristic reticulum with supravital staining.

Alternatively they may be:

- Nucleated RBCs (see above).
- Large mature RBCs associated with folate or niacin deficiency – causing, very rarely, megaloblastic anaemia.
- Macrocytes due to an inherited disease (in Poodles, Alaskan Malamutes and Siamese cats).
- Macrocytes resulting from increased RBC differentiation and decreased maturation time (in half the cases of feline hyperthyroidism).
- An artefact – the result of prolonged contact with EDTA giving RBC swelling (see 'Causes of increased MCV', p. 57).

MICROCYTES

These are small RBCs. RBCs which have a smaller diameter *and* a smaller volume (MCV) are usually the result of iron deficiency.
Less common causes are:

- RBCs infected with *Haemobartonella* in cases unresponsive to treatment.
- Pyridoxine (vitamin B$_6$) deficiency.
- An inherited condition in Japanese Akita dogs.

RBCs which have a smaller diameter *but* a normal volume (MCV) are *spherocytes* as described previously (see p. 66).

ANISOCYTES

These are RBCs of different sizes occurring in the blood of the same animal at the same time. Some degree of anisocytosis (variation in RBC size) is normal in cat RBCs.
Anisocytosis is due to the presence of a significant number of macrocytes or, less often, microcytes, among RBCs of normal size (see 'Macrocytes' and 'Microcytes' above).
Most cases will be due to the presence of reticulocytes (slightly larger than mature RBCs) in regenerative anaemia.
(Some electronic RBC counters will provide a measure of the variability of RBC size (i.e. anisocytosis) termed 'red cell size distribution width' (RDW); normal values are 8–10.)

POLYCHROMASIC RBCs

Also called polychromic, polychromatic or polychromatophilic RBCs, these are RBCs which, when stained with Romanowsky stains, appear bluish but show some variation in colour within the cell, due to the presence of residual RNA. When stained with supravital stains a reticulum becomes apparent within each cell allowing them to be recognized as reticulocytes.
Consequently, polychromasia is seen most often in the regenerative anaemias (haemorrhagic and haemolytic) including the mild (dilutional) anaemia in late pregnancy and immediately post partum.

HYPOCHROMIC RBCs (HYPOCHROMASIC RBCs)

Hypochromic RBCs are poorly pigmented RBCs, with very pale central areas, i.e. having a reduced haemoglobin content and giving a decreased MCHC.
Mild hypochromasia is a feature of reticulocytosis (i.e. with regenerative anaemia). It is also seen in the uncommon condition of iron deficiency anaemia and, rarely, with severe protein deficiency.

Red blood cell inclusions

HEINZ BODIES (ERYTHROCYTE REFRACTILE BODIES = ER BODIES = SCHMAUCH BODIES)

These are round or oval bodies ($0.5–3\,\mu m$), a single one of which may occur at the periphery of, or protrude from, an RBC. They result from the oxidative denaturation of haemoglobin – first to methaemoglobin.

Heinz bodies stain best (dark blue) using supravital staining on an unfixed blood smear; with Romanowsky staining of fixed smears they appear as circular pale areas.

Heinz bodies are unusual in healthy dogs but occur in up to 10% of the RBCs of apparently healthy cats (even up to 50% in some cats).

Abnormal numbers are caused primarily by oxidative poisons and their resultant removal by phagocytes (in the spleen) can produce haemolytic anaemia (see 'Causes of haemolytic anaemia', p. 101).

Increased numbers are also associated with:

1. In cats:
   (a) intestinal diseases,
   (b) feline dysautonomia (Key–Gaskell syndrome), although without anaemia.
2. In dogs:
   (a) regular prednisolone therapy,
   (b) splenectomy (reducing Heinz body removal from the blood).

Large numbers will *falsely increase* the value for haemoglobin concentration and, therefore, for MCHC (and MCH).

HOWELL–JOLLY BODIES

These are round inclusions (dark blue on Romanowsky-stained smears) which represent nuclear remnants and appear singly in immature RBCs, i.e. one per cell (see Panel 2.5, p. 115).

They are rarely present in normal dogs but appear in up to 1% of the RBCs of apparently healthy cats.

Increased numbers are associated primarily with degenerative anaemia (haemolytic or haemorrhagic) but they also occur:

- With reduced splenic function, e.g. splenectomy and splenic tumours.
- Following administration of glucocorticoids to dogs.
- In the condition of macrocytosis in Poodles.

PAPPENHEIMER BODIES (SIDEROTIC GRANULES OR INCLUSIONS)

These are iron-containing granules (staining blue-black on Romanowsky-stained smears) found in the RBCs called siderocytes (see p. 68).

In regenerative anaemia (especially haemolytic) they may be found in an occasional young RBC.

They are also recorded in lead poisoning.

BASOPHILIC STIPPLING

This appears as multiple, dark-blue dots (on Romanowsky-stained smears) and is seen best *without* the use of anticoagulants or previous fixing.

It represents the aggregated ribosomal RNA found in reticulocytes and, therefore, basophilic stippling is associated primarily with regenerative anaemias (haemorrhagic and haemolytic, e.g. with autoimmune haemolytic anaemia).

It is *also* classically associated with the exaggerated regenerative response seen in many cases of lead poisoning in dogs (due to the effect of lead on bone marrow, even when there is no obvious anaemia (see Panel 2.5, p. 115)).

Note

In the dog basophilic stippling of mature (and nucleated) RBCs without severe anaemia strongly suggests lead poisoning.

DISTEMPER INCLUSION BODIES

These aggregations of viral nucleocapsids are seen in very small numbers of RBCs and neutrophils, and rather more commonly in lymphocytes, of dogs with canine distemper.

With Romanowsky staining they appear light blue and are generally larger than Howell–Jolly bodies (up to 3 µm).

PROTOZOAL PARASITES

Babesia spp. in dogs and cats (appearing as annular or piriform bodies) and *Cytauxzoon* spp. in cats (looking like round or oval bodies, or as dots) may be seen in parasitized RBCs in stained blood smears, although not in the UK.

Babesia spp. stain better with Giemsa stain and even better with Stévenel's blue stain.

HAEMOBARTONELLA

To find these bacterial inclusions it *is important* to examine fresh, unpreserved blood.

H. felis

This is relatively common in cats and on Romanowsky staining appears as purple/blue cocci, rods or rings, usually attached to the surface of RBCs but sometimes free (in *thick* areas of blood smears the organisms almost invariably appear as cocci).

They are stained most effectively by acridine orange, although Giemsa stain can be used successfully. With new methylene blue staining affected RBCs can be confused with punctate reticulocytes. Often *H. felis* appears secondary to other infectious diseases, e.g. chronic bacterial infections, FeLV infection and FIV (feline immunodeficiency virus) infection.

H. canis

This is uncommon in dogs and may have the same appearance as *H. felis*, but more usually the bacteria form chains across the surface of the RBCs.

They are usually associated with normocytic/normochromic anaemia, appearing particularly after splenectomy.

HAEMOGLOBIN CRYSTALLOIDS

Up to 5% of RBCs from apparently normal cats contain crystalloid haemoglobin granules.

Note

Other substances in the smear, lying adjacent to or overlying one or more RBCs may be *mistaken* for the inclusions listed above, particularly platelets, specks of dust, granules of precipitated stain and contaminating bacteria. Contaminants of a stain can be excluded by prior filtration.

Erythrocyte sedimentation rate (ESR)

ESR is the *rate* at which the RBCs in a blood sample contained in a glass (or plastic) tube settle (i.e. sediment) under the force of gravity. It is expressed in millimetres per 1 hour (the standard time taken for measurement), i.e. mm per 1 h.

It is a non-specific test used to indicate the existence of disease. The test is of limited usefulness and certainly not essential. It has been used chiefly in the dog, and not in the cat, because:

- It requires a comparatively large amount of blood.
- The ESR needs to be corrected for changes in the PCV and appropriate correction factors have not been devised for the cat.

In both dog and cat the test needs to be performed as soon as possible, ideally within 6 hours. It may be measured using the Wintrobe or Westergren tubes, or commercial variants of these, but the correction factors currently available apply only to the Wintrobe tube.

The ESR is influenced by changes in both the RBCs and the plasma. It increases:

- Either as the PCV falls.
- Or as the concentration in the plasma of fibrinogen and α_2- and γ-globulins increases.

ESR decreases:

- Either as the proportion of reticulocytes and other leptocytes increases.
- Or as the concentration of albumin in the plasma increases.

Note

The presence of large numbers of reticulocytes (and other leptocytes) becomes evident because they impart a reddish tinge to the lower part of the plasma layer, owing to their slower rate of sedimentation ('streaming').

NORMAL REFERENCE RANGE

Experience shows that the *majority* of ESRs in animals with normal PCVs fall within the ranges:

- Dog: 0–5 mm/h.
- Cat: 0–12 mm/h (Aliakbari, 1975).

However, for accuracy interpretation is best based on a *corrected* rather than an observed ESR value.

CORRECTION

Ideally interpretation of the ESR should be based on the *corrected ESR*, which is obtained by correcting the *observed ESR* (i.e. the actual reading) for the effects of the PCV. These corrections are applicable only to dogs and only to measurements made using a Wintrobe tube, and are made as follows:

- At a PCV above 50% (= >0.5 l/l) the *corrected* ESR=observed ESR.
- At a PCV between 37% and 50% (= 0.37–0.5 l/l) the *corrected* ESR=observed ESR − 50 + PCV (as %).
- At a PCV between 23% and 36% (= 0.23–0.36 l/l), the *corrected* ESR = observed ESR − 86 + (2 × PCV (as %)).
- At a PCV less than 23% (= <0.23 l/l), the corrected ESR = observed ESR − 109 + (3 × PCV (as %)).

Example

Observed ESR of 15 mm/ h at a PCV of 0.30 l/l (30%) produces a *corrected* ESR of 15 − 86 + (2 × 30) = 15 − 86 + 60 = 15 − 26 = − 11 mm/1 h.
   Corrected ESRs may therefore be negative or positive values.

Causes of an elevated corrected ESR (i.e. a high positive ESR)

The correction to establish conclusively that there is a high positive ESR can only be applied to an ESR from canine blood in a Wintrobe tube. Nevertheless, any *excessive increase* in the ESR relative to the PCV (i.e. especially when the PCV is within the 'normal' range) in either dog or cat, could be attributable to one of the following causes:

- Acute generalized infection, e.g. a normal ESR would tend to rule out a diagnosis of bacterial endocarditis.
- Acute localized inflamation of serous membranes, e.g. pleuritis, pericarditis or peritonitis.
- Dermatitis.
- Rheumatoid arthritis.
- Chronic localized infection, e.g. abscess formation before encapsulation, or pyometra.
- Extensive trauma, including surgery, burns and fractures.
- Widespread structural changes in the skin, e.g. hypothyroidism and Cushing's syndrome.
- Malignant neoplasia.
- Pregnancy (related to haemodilution effects). In bitches ESR increases from the second to third week of pregnancy to a maximum at parturition and then returns to normal in about 8–9 weeks.
- End-stage renal disease (possibly due to increased fibrinogen and/or decreased albumin levels).

- Hyperproteinaemia (although this depends on the proportions of individual proteins).

Where successive samples show a declining positive ESR it suggests healing, and an increasing positive value suggests that the disease process has become uncontrolled.

Causes of a negative corrected ESR

It can be difficult to establish that there is a negative corrected ESR unless the observed ESR is measured on canine blood in a Wintrobe tube. However, all possible known causes would be readily apparent from the history and/or routine tests, and there would be no real need for performance of the ESR.

- Young growing animals – this is a *normal* finding, because of low total protein and fibrinogen levels and a relatively high albumin level.
- Hypoproteinaemia – although the result depends on the proportions of individual proteins.
- Haemorrhagic anaemia, due to increased numbers of reticulocytes and hypo-proteinaemia. If there is evidence of haemorrhage and a *positive* ESR, it suggests that there is bleeding at a site where the plasma proteins that are lost can be readily recirculated, principally in the gut.

Panel 2.1 Diagnosis and differentiation of anaemia

Anaemia is a reduction in red cell mass and oxygen-carrying capacity, having many different causes.

Summary

Diagnose anaemia on PCV $\pm$ clinical signs (especially pallor)

Differentiate type of anaemia by:

- Clinical signs and speed of onset
- Evidence of regeneration (reticulocytosis $\pm$ nucleated RBCs)
- Routine tests, i.e. MCV and MCHC (from RBC count and haemoglobin concentration); total and differential WBC count; RBC and WBC appearance; urea; ALT and ALP; FeLV test and FIV test
- Specific tests as necessary, e.g. platelet count and appearance; liver function tests; urinalysis; tests of haemostasis; autoimmune testing; bilirubin; iron; other serology; hormone assays; occult blood in faeces; radiography; aspiration and biopsy; endoscopy etc.

The tests required to estabish the type of anaemia are mostly routine haematological and biochemical tests that form a small group of generally useful tests that could be described as a 'small animal profile' (see p. 8), with the exception of the reticulocyte count. This might need to be specially requested but a good laboratory will often perform, or suggest, it in cases of anaemia. The other tests would be PCV (plus RBC count and haemoglobin concentration to calculate the MCV and MCHC), total and differential WBC counts, total protein, albumin, urea, alanine aminotransferase (ALT = SGPT), and alkaline phosphatase (ALP = SAP), plus an FeLV test and FIV test in the cat.

Diagnosis of anaemia

Anaemia is, in general, best diagnosed on an abnormally low PCV provided it is measured by the spun haematocrit method. In 'human' laboratories the PCV is a *calculated* value, and then anaemia is best assessed on the haemoglobin concentration.

The PCV value will indicate the degree of severity of the anaemia. Anaemia exists when the PCV is:

Dog: <0.37 l/l (<37%).
Cat: <0.30 l/l (<30%).

But note: the normal range varies in some breeds and under certain conditions (see p. 35).

Remember that

1. PCV could be falsely low due to:
   (a) haemolysis, during collection and/or sample handling (if evident rely on haemoglobin concn for diagnosis, or preferably re-sample) **CHECK** – MCHC will be high } falsely *very* low values possible
   (b) collecting blood sample from *cannula or cannulated vein* during intravenous fluid administration
   (c) *serious under-filling* of the EDTA tube } falsely *very* low values unlikely
   (d) *overhydration* of the patient with intravenous fluid
2. PCV could be within the *normal range even though anaemia is present*:
   (a) if there is *dehydration* of the *patient* concurrently
   (b) there is *dehydration* of the *sample* (leaving sample uncapped for a long period allows water loss)
   (c) soon after *acute haemorrhage* – haemodilution occurs slowly and makes little difference to the PCV for (1–)2 hours (although it continues for 2–3 days). In acute haemolytic anaemia and hypoproliferative anaemia there is *no* fall in blood volume and therefore this problem does not arise
   (d) immediately after *acute haemorrhage* because *splenic contraction* infuses RBCs into the circulation and can temporarily elevate the PCV
   (e) with *fear and excitement* during blood collection splenic contraction occurs which temporarily increases the PCV

Also in compensated haemolytic anaemia the PCV will have returned to normal. In this disorder RBC destruction continues but RBC production has increased sufficiently to keep pace with it. (See pp. 35–42 for further information on factors affecting PCV.)

Measurement of PCV

This is generally simpler and more accurate than either haemoglobin concentration or RBC count (error using microhaematocrit = ± 1%, but error in *haemoglobin concentration* = ± 5%, and *in RBC count* with correctly adjusted electronic counter = ± 3% or with manual count = ± 20%).

The factors listed above as affecting PCV will also affect haemoglobin concentration and RBC count, *except* that increased EDTA concentration affects neither, and haemolysis does not affect haemoglobin concentration. This is another reason why some haematologists prefer to diagnose anaemia on the haemoglobin value. But, of course, haemolysis occurring intravascularly will reduce the oxygen-carrying capacity of the blood and *will* be reflected in a low PCV but *not* in the haemoglobin value, i.e. the haemolysis may not be detected.

CONFIRM DIAGNOSIS

Confirm the diagnosis by major clinical signs, wherever possible:

- Pale mucous membranes.
- Weakness and poor exercise tolerance.
- Rapid heart beat and respiratory rate (i.e. panting) – with severe anaemia, even at rest.
- Haemic murmur – soft mid-systolic murmur in the aortic region.

Note

1. These *signs are not evident in mild anaemia* but become more pronounced as its severity increases, e.g. in dogs anaemia is severe enough for marked signs to appear in only 10% of cases.
2. All these *signs (except the murmur) could occur with severe shock* (i.e. other than shock due to severe haemorrhage – which happens when a third of total blood volume is lost over a short period, or half of it is lost during a day).

CHECK – in shock the capillary refill time (CRT), using gums or tongue, will be prolonged (more than 2 seconds).

3. In many *non-anaemic cats* mucous membranes appear pale.
4. With anaemia of comparable severity signs are more pronounced:
   (a) in dog than in cat;
   (b) if onset is rapid, i.e. more pronounced in acute anaemia than in chronic anaemia of comparable severity, e.g. in *dog* marked signs appear at a PCV of <0.2 l/l (<20%) with acute anaemia and at <0.12–0.15 l/l (<12–15%) with chronic; in cat at <0.12–0.15 l/l (<12–15%) with acute and <0.08–0.1 l/l (<8–10%) with chronic;
   (c) in older than in younger animals, because of decreased ability to compensate;
   (d) in haemolytic than in haemorrhagic anaemia.

Differentiation of the type of anaemia

This is important for correct treatment and prognosis.

Anaemia arises from three main causes:

1. Blood loss = haemorrhagic anaemia.
2. Increased RBC destruction = haemolytic anaemia.
3. Reduced RBC production = hypoproliferative anaemia (if complete = aplastic anaemia).

THE TYPE AND CAUSE OF ANAEMIA

This may often be determined by reference to the clinical signs and speed of onset.

Clinical signs

The clinical signs, e.g. bleeding and jaundice, together with features in the case history are discussed in Panels 2.2, 2.3 and 2.4 (pp. 86, 95 and 107).

Speed of onset

All three types can develop gradually (chronic anaemia) but only haemorrhagic and haemolytic can arise suddenly (acute anaemia). Because of the long lifespan of the RBCs (110 days in the dog, 70 days in the cat), even a sudden, complete stoppage of RBC production would take several days to produce a discernible fall in the PCV. Therefore, hypoproliferative anaemia is always chronic.

REGENERATIVE OR NON-REGENERATIVE ANAEMIA

It is important to know if the anaemia is *regenerative* or *non-regenerative.*

In regenerative anaemias (responsive anaemias), i.e. *haemorrhagic and haemolytic,* immature RBCs are released into the circulation to correct the deficiency. These cells are *not* released in a *hypoproliferative* anaemia unless the cause has been corrected i.e. unless it is in remission (although sometimes there is a *slight* regenerative response).

These cells will be principally *reticulocytes* (i.e. there will be a reticulocytosis), *plus*, in severe cases, nucleated cells as well. The more severe the anaemia the less mature are the cells that are released. (A reticulocyte is the stage in RBC development immediately preceding the mature RBC and a small number are normally present in the circulating blood.)

Detection of increased reticulocyte number

The best way to detect the increased number of reticulocytes is to perform a *reticulocyte* count, which requires a blood smear stained with supravital stain. It provides a definite numerical result. From this can be calculated the *absolute reticulocyte count* and/or the *reticulocyte production index* (see p. 120), which increases the reliability of the diagnosis.

	Normal reticulocyte count	*Count indicative of regenerative anaemia*
Dog	approx. 1%	3–5%
Cat	(aggregate alone) approx. 0.5%	>1.5–2%
	(aggregate plus punctate) approx. 1.5–11%	

A significant absolute reticulocyte count in the dog or cat, i.e. indicative of regenerative anaemia, is $>60 \times 10^9/l$ (i.e. >60 000/µl).

Reticulocyte production index (RPI)
In non-regenerative anaemia RPI <2
In regenerative anaemia   RPI >2
In haemolytic anaemia   RPI >3

Otherwise it is necessary to depend on *less satisfactory evidence* of *reticulocytosis*, namely finding:

- RBCs showing polychromasia, on the normal Romanowsky-stained smear, although these *may* not be clearly reported by a laboratory.
- An increased MCV with a normal or decreased MCHC.

Note

It takes 3 days for reticulocytes, the usual immature RBCs, to appear in the circulation.

CHECK – to distinguish a regenerative anaemia where there is no, or little, reticulocyte production because the sample was collected too early, from a non-regenerative anaemia, examine another blood sample after at least 3 days.

Note

The release of immature RBCs is *more* marked where blood is lost from the body (external haemorrhage and gastrointestinal haemorrhage) than in cases of haemorrhage into body cavities, because in the latter types two-thirds of the RBCs return to the circulation, effectively reducing the loss.

To summarize:

- Reticulocytosis characterizes a regenerative anaemia.
- The greater the degree of reticulocytosis, the more severe is the regenerative anaemia.
- The absence of reticulocytosis after 3–4 days of anaemia (although not necessarily the absence of all reticulocytes) denotes a non-regenerative anaemia.

Severe regenerative anaemia

In severe regenerative anaemia RBCs of even greater immaturity are released by the bone marrow. These are:

- RBCs still possessing nuclear remnants that are termed 'Howell–Jolly' bodies. (Normally there are no Howell–Jolly bodies in canine RBCs, but they can appear in a few (<1%) of feline RBCs.)
- *Nucleated RBCs* – if present these should be evident on a normal Romanowsky-stained smear and *should* be reported by the laboratory.

In normal circumstances these nucleated cells are seldom seen outside the bone marrow, but with *increasingly severe anaemia* a number appear in the blood, in addition to the reticulocytosis. The nucleated RBCs form a succession of developmental stages in the bone marrow, before losing their nuclei to become reticulocytes (see Figure 2.2); usually it is the later stages which appear in the blood. The earlier the RBC stage that is present, the more severe is the anaemia.

Although the stages of development are given different names by different authors they will be described in laboratory reports as *rubricytes, normoblasts* or *erythroblasts*, with appropriate prefixes denoting the stage of development.

For the best estimate of the severity of the anaemia the *nucleated RBCs should be counted*. Their number is usually expressed per 100 WBCs (which are also nucleated cells), e.g. 9 nucleated RBCs/100 WBCs.

In general then, reticulocytosis denotes a regenerative anaemia, and nucleated RBCs plus a reticulocytosis denote a severe regenerative anaemia, provided that these changes are accompanied by a corresponding fall in the PCV.

Note

Also note that reticulocytosis and/or nucleated RBCs can appear in the blood in conditions other than regenerative anaemia.

1. Reticulocytosis with a PCV in the normal range (i.e. without anaemia) suggests poor oxygenation of the blood, e.g. chronic lung disease.
2. Nucleated RBCs, possibly with a reticulocytosis, but without a *corresponding* fall in the PCV (although anaemia can be present) might indicate chronic lead poisoning (for diagnostic features see Panel 2.5, p. 118).
3. Nucleated RBCs with no reticulocytes, or a disproportionately small number, occur in the blood in most myeloproliferative disorders and may appear, in smaller numbers, in other myelophthistic disorders (i.e. disorders in which the bone marrow is infiltrated and replaced by abnormal tissue, e.g. leukaemic cells, metastatic tumours or granulomatous lesions), and with reduced splenic function (including splenic tumour), severe infection, and extramedullary haematopoiesis (i.e. RBC formation outside the bone marrow).
4. Nucleated RBCs without reticulocytosis but with immature (band form) neutrophils (a shift-to-the-left) constitute a *leucoerythroblastic reaction*, which may occur in:
   (a) severe haemorrhagic or haemolytic anaemia (as an intense response);
   (b) disseminated haemangiosarcoma;
   (c) myeloproliferative disorders (see Panel 3.2, p. 189).

The anaemia associated with (2), (3) and (4) above (except (4a)) will be a non-regenerative anaemia – see Panel 2.4, p. 107.

Nucleated RBCs without reticulocytosis are potentially sinister.

Note

In late pregnancy and for a time after giving birth, females show a mild–moderate regenerative anaemia, *not* due to haemorrhage or haemolysis. It is a dilutional anaemia, the RBCs being diluted by an increased plasma volume.

REGENERATIVE AND NON-REGENERATIVE CATEGORIES OF ANAEMIA

These are not always rigid.

Regenerative anaemia may become non-regenerative

Prolonged RBC losses which produce a chronic haemorrhagic anaemia will also result in a significant loss of iron. If this iron is not replaced in the diet, *iron deficiency anaemia* can develop. This is essentially non-regenerative anaemia (characterized in its later stage by microcytosis, hypochromasia and poikilocytosis) although *some* degree of reticulocytosis may occur.

It is especially likely to arise in:

- Young growing animals, particularly those on a solely milk diet because of its low iron content.
- Blood donor animals bled repeatedly.

CHECK for signs of iron deficiency.
1. Find a low MCV and MCHC (in its later stages).
2. Examine RBCs on a blood smear and find microcytosis, hypochromasia and poikilocytosis.
3. Find a low serum iron level, despite a normal total iron binding capacity.
4. Find that a bone marrow biopsy shows that there is no longer an erythroid response.

Non-regenerative anaemia may become regenerative

This can occur when the underlying cause of a hypoproliferative anaemia is corrected, assuming that to be possible. A regenerative response (i.e. *reticulocytosis*, with or without some nucleated RBCs) would become evident in the blood, and this response could be confirmed by bone marrow biopsy.

Non-regenerative anaemia may show features suggestive of a regenerative anaemia

- Haemorrhage may be the *result* of a platelet deficiency (thrombocytopenia) associated with a non-regenerative anaemia (e.g. in a myeloproliferative disorder) and this might give the superficial impression that the anaemia is haemorrhagic in origin.

CHECK with a *non-regenerative* cause of platelet deficiency:
1. Multiple haemorrhages are usual.
2. A reticulocytosis (i.e. a regenerative response) is absent.
3. Platelet count is low (whereas with primary haemorrhage, unless persistent, it is usually increased).
4. Large, bizarre platelets (and possibly the bone marrow cells, megakaryocytes, from which they arise) may be seen.

- Extravascular haemolysis may occur in some types of hypoproliferative anaemia (e.g. possibly with chronic renal failure, and in myeloproliferative disorders).

In summary: Non-regenerative anaemia may be associated with haemorrhage or haemolysis

OTHER DIAGNOSTIC TESTS

Other commonly performed tests can help to diagnose the type of anaemia – see Table 2.2, p. 86.

Haematological indices

These indices, i.e. the MCV and MCHC, are calculated from the PCV in combination with the RBC count and haemoglobin concentration respectively (see p. 54). *Remember errors in these tests* can produce *misleading* values.

1. Severe regenerative anaemias are macrocytic and hypochromic; if less severe, macrocytic and normochromic, although:
   (a) immediately after haemorrhage (before reticulocytes appear) anaemia will be normocytic and normochromic;
   (b) immediately after severe intravascular haemolysis the free haemoglobin in the blood plus the loss of cells will give the impression of a normocytic/hyperchromic anaemia (see p. 65).
2. Nutritional anaemias (uncommon) generally produce changes in RBC size:
   (a) folic acid and niacin deficiencies result in a macrocytic/normochromic anaemia;
   (b) pyridoxine deficiency results in a microcytic/hypochromic anaemia;
   (c) severe protein deficiency results in a normocytic/hypochromic anaemia;
   (d) iron deficiency starts as a normocytic/normochromic anaemia and progresses through reductions in size and pigmentation to become microcytic/hypochromic.
3. Apart from the nutritional anaemias most hypoproliferative anaemias are normocytic/normochromic.
4. Changes in size and pigmentation are also associated with anaemia in some hereditary disorders.

Total and differential WBC count

The total WBC count increases in severe, acute regenerative anaemia due primarily to an increase in neutrophils (with a shift-to-the-left) as an associated bone marrow response. Where anaemia is due to bone marrow depression or destruction involving all cell types the numbers of WBCs will be lower, but in other types of anaemia, WBC numbers are usually normal.

Also examination of the Romanowsky-stained smear, used for the differential WBC count, allows detection not only of nucleated RBCs and RBCs containing Howell–Jolly bodies but other abnormalities of the WBCs and RBCs, including inclusions which may indicate the cause of the anaemia.

Total plasma protein and albumin levels

These will be decreased in severe acute haemorrhage, but not in other types, except in rare cases due to hypoproteinaemia.

The total protein level may appear to be increased in haemolytic anaemia due to the inclusion of the free haemoglobin.

Urea

Uraemia can give rise to a depression anaemia.

ALT and ALP

High levels of ALT and ALP may be associated with chronic liver damage associated with bone marrow depression.

FeLV test

In cats this test is important since FeLV infection can be responsible for all three types of anaemia.

FURTHER CONFIRMATORY FEATURES

CHECK – the *features* of the type of anaemia provisionally diagnosed by reference to the appropriate later panel (i.e. on the features of haemorrhagic, haemolytic and hypoproliferative anaemia respectively, pp. 86, 95 and 107) to see whether they fit with the case, and to decide which other investigations are necessary to provide the required degree of diagnostic detail.

Platelet count

Platelet numbers *increase* within 3 hours of acute haemorrhage although decreased numbers can be the cause of haemorrhage. Platelet numbers may *decrease* if anaemia is due to bone marrow destruction or depression, and tend to be variable in other types.

Other liver function tests

These can confirm the cause of a depression anaemia.

Urinalysis

In haemolytic anaemia especially, urinalysis may be helpful, e.g. in detecting haemoglobinuria and urinary bilirubin.

Tests of haemostasis

These are valuable in haemorrhagic anaemia.

Tests for autoimmunity

Tests, such as Coombs' test, the ANA test and the LE cell test, may help in haemolytic anaemia.

Plasma bilirubin and van den Bergh test

These can assist in diagnosing intravascular haemolytic anaemia.

Plasma iron concentration and total iron-binding capacity

These may be helpful in haemorrhagic (and, rarely, in nutritional) anaemia.

Table 2.2 Distinctive features of each type of anaemia

	Haemorrhage	Haemolysis		Bone marrow destruction or depression		Hypoproliferation — Nutritional deficiency	
		Intravascular	Extravascular	Affecting RBCs alone	Affecting all cells	Iron/vitamin B_6/protein	Folate (or antagonist)
PCV	↓ (Acute – only after 2–3 hours)	↓ Rapid	↓ Slow[a]	↓[n]	↓[o]	→	→
Total protein	Acute – ↓ after 2–3 hours; Chronic – slight ↓ (but with internal haemorrhage usually N)[q]	N or ↑[f]	N (or ↑)[q]	N usually	N usually	N if iron or vitamin B_6 ↓ if protein	N
RBC polychromasia and reticulocytosis	Yes – after 2–3 days[b,g]	Yes – after 2–3 days[g]	Yes[g]	No (occasionally slight)	No	No (may be slight)	No
Reticulocyte production index	>2	>3	>3	2 or <2	2 or <2	2 or <2	2 or <2
Nucleated RBCs	Yes – if severe	Yes – if severe	Yes – if severe	No	Usually no[j]	No	No
MCV	Slight ↑ (transient)[d]	Slight ↑	Slight ↑	N	N (or ↑)[j]	↓ – late iron/vitamin B_6; N – early iron/protein	↑
MCHC	(N or) ↓	May appear ↑ – essentially (N or) ↓[f]	(N or) ↓	N	N	→	N
Total WBC count	↑ About 3 hours after if severe and acute	↑	↑	N (occasionally ↑ or ↓)	Usually ↓[j]	Usually N, although variable	
Neutrophil count	↑ If acute[h]	↑	↑ (Common[h])	N (occasionally ↑)	Usually ↓[l]		
Shift-to-the-left	Yes	Yes	Yes	No	Usually		
Monocyte count	N	N or ↑	↑	N	Usually ↓[p]		

Platelet count	↑ (Within 3 hours if acute)[c]	Variable	Variable	N (may be slight ↑)	Variable	Variable
Myeloid:erythroid ratio (bone marrow)	N for 2–3 days (acute) – then ↓[d]	↓ After 2–3 days	↓	↑	Variable: often difficult to assess[j]	Usually ↓
Plasma bilirubin	N[e]	↑ After 8–10 hours if severe (essentially unconjugated)	N	N	N (or ↑)[k]	N
Other features	Anisocytosis Howell–Jolly bodies	Haemoglobinaemia (if severe) Anisocytosis and Howell–Jolly bodies Specific cells and inclusions depending on cause, see Panel 2.3	N	May be anisocytosis	[m]	Large hypersegmented neutrophils Howell–Jolly bodies

N = normal, ↑ = increased, ↓ = decreased.

a PCV may be *normal* in compensated haemolytic anaemia.

b In *acute haemorrhage* – polychromasia and reticulocytosis appear after 2–3 days and maximize after 7 days. Usually disappear after 1–2 weeks; persistence for >2–3 weeks suggests continuing haemorrhage.

c Increased platelet count for >2–3 weeks implies continuing haemorrhage. Decreased platelet count could arise due to massive acute haemorrhage, disseminated intravascular coagulation, bone marrow suppression *or* immune destruction (autoimmune thrombocytopenia or systemic lupus erythematosus).
Note: Platelet deficiency could be the CAUSE of the haemorrhage.

d Persistent blood loss *may* lead to iron-deficiency anaemia (non-regenerative), with *decreased* MCV and an increased myeloid:erythroid ratio in the bone marrow.

e Bilirubin can be increased with liver damage or an extensive haematoma.

f Large amounts of free haemoglobin will falsely elevate the MCHC, and the level of total protein.

g A poor regenerative response *may* occur if there is bone marrow damage or a lack of nutrients.

h Leucopenia can arise in autoimmune disorders where there are antibodies against neutrophils.

i Rarely cases due to chronic inflammation or neoplasia develop iron deficiency with reduced MCV and MCH. There are slight falls in the levels of both serum iron *and* total iron-binding capacity.

j In different types of myeloproliferative disorder (see Panel 3.2) there *may* be such features as nucleated RBCs which may raise the MCV (generally unaccompanied by reticulocytosis), an increased number of WBCs, or an increased number of platelets. In lymphoproliferative disorders the number of WBCs may be elevated.

k Hyperbilirubinaemia may (rarely) occur in myeloproliferative disorders due to atrophy of liver cells and/or increased phagocytosis of the RBCs.

l A neutrophilia is seen with early oestrogen toxicity, with granulocytic and myelomonocytic leukaemias, and in the recovery stage of feline infectious enteritis.

m In iron deficiency there is a significantly low level of serum iron but *normal* total iron-binding capacity.

n Includes pure RBC aplasia (possibly immune mediated or due to FeLV infection), anaemia due to chronic inflammation and neoplasia (but not of the bone marrow) and anaemia due to a deficiency of erythropoietin.

o Includes bone marrow damage due to infectious diseases, chemicals, drugs and myelophthisis (i.e. neoplasia arising in the bone marrow [myeloproliferative and lymphoproliferative disorders], neoplastic metastases from elsewhere and the deposition of fibrous tissue or bone).

p Monocytosis occurs in monocytic and myelomonocytic leukaemias.

q Anaemia due to pregnancy (last third) being only moderately regenerative and without changes in plasma protein levels *might* be confused with chronic haemorrhage or extravascular haemolytic anaemia.

Hormone assays

These can establish a hormonal cause of a non-regenerative anaemia.

Other serology

Serology may confirm infectious causes of the anaemia.

Faecal examination

Examination for occult blood may help in cases of haemorrhagic anaemia.

Other procedures

Other procedures of value in diagnosis are:

- *Radiography* in the diagnosis of splenomegaly, hepatomegaly and tumours elsewhere.
- *Aspiration and biopsy* of the bone marrow, lymph nodes or spleen.
- *Endoscopy* in cases of gastric and colonic ulcers.

Panel 2.2 Features of haemorrhagic anaemia

This is the most common cause of anaemia in small animals.

ACUTE OR CHRONIC

Blood loss may be:

- Either acute (short term and therefore necessarily severe).
- Or chronic (long term and therefore a much less rapid loss).

EVIDENCE OF BLOOD LOSS

Evidence of blood loss (frequently present) includes:

- External – haemorrhage from visible wounds and lesions or from body openings (e.g. nostrils, anus); usually associated with signs of trauma.
- Internal – blood seen in excreted material: urine, faeces, vomit. It may appear as 'fresh' blood (i.e. pink/red), or haemoglobin may have been converted to methaemoglobin (dark-brown/black).

A very small amount of blood in such excretions may produce no discernible colouration and therefore not be apparent. This is termed 'occult blood' (i.e. hidden blood). It can still be detected by chemical testing or by microscopic examination.

Chemical testing

Tests are performed, e.g. on urine and faeces to detect breakdown products. Such tests are very sensitive and normal dog and cat faeces will contain sufficient haemoglobin products to almost *always* give a positive result, even using commercial tests that in human patients discriminate satisfactorily between those with gastrointestinal haemorrhage and those without (unless a commercial test is used which is *specific* for human haemoglobin) which will give no meaningful result in the dog or cat. Therefore, in order to establish that there really is gastrointestinal haemorrhage it is necessary to deprive the patient of blood-containing foods (meat and offal, though not fish, eggs or cheese) for at least 3 days before collection of the faecal sample. Even then a *false positive* result may be obtained if the patient is:

- Either licking blood from external lesions.
- Or swallowing blood that reaches the pharynx from a nasal lesion or is coughed up from the lower respiratory tract.

CHECK – a *false negative* result may be obtained if a commercial test is used which is *specific* for human haemoglobin.

Microscopic examination

Microscopic examination of urinary sediment or faeces may detect large numbers of intact RBCs.

Circumstantial evidence

Where there are *no signs* of blood loss circumstantial evidence includes:

- Finding *large numbers* of blood-sucking parasites, e.g. fleas, ticks (and in some parts of the world other parasites such as the tropical hookworm *Ancylostoma*).
- A history of recent trauma or surgery.

Confirmation

Haemorrhage into body cavities can be confirmed by paracentesis, i.e. withdrawing a fluid containing many RBCs. In uncomplicated haemorrhage the PCV of this fluid will be the same or greater than that of the circulating blood, but it might be diluted by an exudate or transudate giving difficulty in distinguishing it from a blood-stained transudate.

Significant haemorrhage into the thoracic and pericardial cavities will impair the action of the lungs and heart, respectively, producing clinical signs.

MULTIPLE HAEMORRHAGES

Without obvious trauma multiple haemorrhages indicate defects in the mechanisms to prevent blood loss (haemostatic defects) (see p. 207). These may be either congenital clotting defects or acquired defects, e.g. the result of anticoagulant poisoning, disseminated intravascular coagulation (DIC) or increased destruction of platelets. Defective clotting may also be due to deficient platelet production by hypoproliferative bone marrow associated with a non-regenerative anaemia, i.e. haemorrhage can be the *result* of a hypoproliferative anaemia. (See 'Causes of haemorrhagic anaemia', p. 91.)

DELAYED ONSET IN ACUTE CASES

1. For the first 2–3 hours after severe acute haemorrhage, PCV and other RBC parameters remain relatively normal, because:
   (a) Haemodilution (the transfer of fluid into the blood to maintain the blood volume) is slow to start. (Immediately after haemorrhage the total blood volume is reduced but the *concentration* of RBCs and haemoglobin in the remaining blood is the same.) After 2–3 hours haemodilution takes place and continues for up to 2–3 days.
   (b) Splenic contraction pushes a stored mass of RBCs into the circulation, which temporarily slightly elevates the PCV.
2. Plasma protein level remains relatively normal for the first 2–3 hours after severe acute haemorrhage because of delayed haemodilution (as above).

AFTER THE FIRST 2–3 HOURS

Two to three hours following severe acute haemorrhage, as *haemodilution* takes place, there are reductions in:

- RBC parameters (PCV, RBC count, haemoglobin concentration).
- Plasma protein concentrations (both total protein and individual proteins, e.g. albumin).

These values continue to fall for 12–24 hours.

The decreases are less where there is haemorrhage into body cavities (internal haemorrhage) than with external haemorrhage or gastrointestinal haemorrhage. This is because two-thirds of the RBCs shed into body cavities can be 're-absorbed' and re-enter the circulation, and the plasma proteins and iron from the rest of the cells still remain in the body and can be used for further RBC production. (In gastrointestinal haemorrhage RBCs cannot be retained, but if it is sufficiently severe some protein and iron resulting from digestion of the blood may be absorbed.)

REGENERATIVE RESPONSE

Three days (2–4 days) after severe acute haemorrhage, signs of regeneration become obvious, i.e. an increased number of reticulocytes, (only a few are normally present), an increased number of RBCs containing Howell–Jolly bodies (a few of which are normally present) *plus*, if the haemorrhage is very severe, some nucleated RBCs (virtually none of which are normally present).

After 4–5 days the reticulocyte production index (RPI) is more than 2 (see p. 120), *unless* the haemorrhage has occurred into a body cavity (when that is the case, the absorption of intact RBCs that takes place means there is less need for new RBC production).

By the time *chronic haemorrhage* causes signs of anaemia regeneration will already be under way, but the regenerative response is more marked in acute, than in chronic anaemia (see Panel 2.5, p. 115).

Regeneration is most marked 7 days after a single severe haemorrhage. If reticulocytosis and thrombocytosis, accompanied by a continuously depressed plasma protein level, persist for more than 2–3 weeks continuing haemorrhage should be suspected.

But the regenerative response may be poor or absent if the bone marrow is damaged or its activity suppressed, e.g. by neoplasia or infection (see 'Causes of hypoproliferative anaemia', p. 111).

CHANGES IN MCV AND MCHC

Reticulocytes and nucleated RBCs are larger than normal mature RBCs and in significant numbers will increase the MCV (and in really large numbers decrease the MCHC).

The reticulocytosis:

- Creates anisocytosis (differences in size of RBCs, evident from a stained smear).
- Gives a reddish colour to the lower *plasma* layer when performing the haematocrit or ESR.

If iron deficiency anaemia develops (see Panel 2.4, p. 109), decreases in both MCV and MCHC will gradually arise, as a non-regenerative microcytic/hypochromic anaemia supervenes.

LEUCOCYTOSIS, NEUTROPHILIA AND A SHIFT-TO-THE-LEFT

These are usually evident around 3 hours after a severe acute haemorrhage, due to increased neutrophil production as part of a generalized regenerative response by the bone marrow. This has nothing to do with infection.

PLATELET NUMBERS

Platelet numbers generally increase within the first 3 hours following acute haemorrhage (and the platelets are large and granulated), reflecting the bone marrow's response to increased demand.

Where the platelet numbers remain increased for more than 2–3 weeks, it suggests continuing haemorrhage, i.e. chronic demand for large numbers of platelets.

Where platelets numbers are *low* (thrombocytopenia) it indicates either excessive platelet consumption or a primary platelet deficiency.

Splenic sequestration of platelets might, rarely, be responsible (see p. 203).

Excessive platelet consumption

This could arise from:

- A massive acute haemorrhage (functional thrombocytopenia); this is most likely to be the cause when platelet numbers are between $20 \times 10^9/l$ and $200 \times 10^9/l$).
- Disseminated intravascular coagulation (see Panel 4.2, p. 216).

A primary platelet deficiency

This could exaggerate the effects of haemorrhage and may arise from:

- Either bone marrow suppression.
- Or increased platelet destruction in autoimmune thrombocytopenia or systemic lupus erythematosus (see Panel 2.7, p. 125).

IRON DEFICIENCY ANAEMIA

The persistent demand for new RBCs to replace those lost can result in iron deficiency anaemia, i.e. a non-regenerative anaemia develops. It is more likely with *external* haemorrhage than with haemorrhage into body cavities.

It is most often seen:

1. In young rapidly growing animals, especially around the first month of life and particularly where there is a heavy infestation with blood-sucking parasites, such as fleas.
2. Where the diet is iron deficient (e.g. mainly or solely milk).
3. Where there is chronic blood loss, for instance:
   (a) gastrointestinal, or urinary tract haemorrhage from ulcers or neoplasms,
   (b) blood donors repeatedly bled *or*,
   (c) heavy infection with the tropical hookworm (*Ancylostoma*) – but not in the UK.

However, bone marrow exhaustion (i.e. with no erythroid response) can arise at times, even with internal haemorrhage if prolonged.

The features of iron deficiency anaemia are summarized on p. 84.

URAEMIA

With gastric and high intestinal haemorrhage, protein digestion and absorption lead to a marginally increased urea level in the plasma but without a rise in the level of creatinine.

Severe acute blood loss can be the cause of prerenal acute renal failure causing increases in both urea *and* creatinine levels, although the increase in urea will be greater (see 'Causes of increased plasma urea', p. 227).

In contrast, anaemia *caused by* uraemia is non-regenerative, with no immature RBCs, normal MCV and MCHC values, and with elevation of the creatinine as well as the urea level.

ABNORMAL CELLS

These are not a feature of haemorrhagic anaemia apart from:

- The reticulocytes, RBCs with Howell–Jolly bodies and nucleated RBCs that constitute the regenerative responses.
- Poikilocytes (irregularly shaped cells) and microcytic/hypochromic RBCs seen when iron deficiency has developed.

PLASMA BILIRUBIN LEVEL

This is not increased unless:

- Either haemoglobin in an extensive haematoma is being broken down.
- Or the haemorrhage is associated with liver damage – there may be a deficiency of clotting factors.

Causes of haemorrhagic anaemia

Summary

Trauma [most common]
Haemostatic defects
● Anticoagulant poisoning [common]
● Inherited disorders
● Low platelet count
● Platelet defects
● Severe liver disease
Neoplasia
Infection
Internal lesions, ulcers etc.

General diagnostic features

● Reticulocyte production index of more than 2 (except in cases of haemorrhage into body cavities).
● A low plasma protein concentration.

The *most common cause of blood loss* is trauma, especially road traffic accidents, and the next most common cause is some defect in haemostasis, particularly anticoagulant poisoning.

TRAUMA [MOST COMMON]

Any haemorrhage caused is usually acute.

● Road traffic accidents, cuts (broken glass, jagged metal, knives, wire nooses in animal traps) and puncture wounds (bites involving major blood vessels, impaling on spikes).
● Gunshot wounds.
● Internal haemorrhage often due to falls on to hard surfaces, crush injuries and kicks.
● Surgical wounds (especially when ligatures slip).

Specific diagnostic features of assistance: history, lesions, at times paracentesis or radiography.

HAEMOSTATIC DEFECTS

These often manifest as difficulty in preventing blood loss and usually result in multiple haemorrhages. Bleeding can then follow very slight trauma, e.g. grooming.

Anticoagulant poisoning

This includes poisoning with warfarin, coumarin, coumachlor, coumatetralyl, difenacoum, indanedione, bromadiolone etc. which are widely used as rodenticides (often coloured blue for identification). Dogs and cats are poisoned either by eating the bait or eating rodents that have been poisoned (secondary poisoning). These substances antagonize vitamin K and interfere with the synthesis of prothrombin.

They also impair the synthesis of clotting factors VII, IX and X, and prothrombin, and cause direct damage to the capillary endothelium.

Specific diagnostic features of assistance: history, detection of metabolites in urine for up to 10 days, initially in the disorder there is a prolonged one-stage prothrombin time; later there is also a less marked prolongation of activated partial thromboplastin time and activated coagulation time.

Note

- Sulphaquinoxaline (used as a coccidiostat in poultry) is also a potent vitamin K antagonist that interferes with coagulation, and for this reason has been used in rat poisons.
- A lack of vitamin K could, although rarely, develop due to nutritional lack, malabsorption (a deficiency of bile salts in obstructive jaundice), failure of the liver to utilize the vitamin and antagonism by antibiotic or sulphonamide therapy.
- Vitamin K antagonists (e.g. rodenticides that are anticoagulants) produce more serious haemorrhages than vitamin K *deficiency* alone, because they *also* cause damage to the blood vessels. Their effect may be potentiated by other drugs, e.g. phenylbutazone, aspirin or chloramphenicol.

Inherited disorders of coagulation (congenital coagulopathies)

Inherited deficiencies of clotting factors are less frequent than acquired disorders in dogs and cats. The most common are haemophilia A (factor VIII deficiency), haemophilia B (factor IX deficiency) and von Willebrand's disease (deficiency of an essential clotting factor, VIII-vWF).

Specific diagnostic features of assistance: measurement of bleeding time, one-stage thrombin time, activated partial thromboplastin time, activated coagulation time and activity of specific clotting factors – see p. 210.

Low platelet count (thrombocytopenia)

Specific diagnostic features: by definition platelet count is low; bone marrow biopsy may distinguish the cause.

Spontaneous bleeding does not arise until platelet numbers are below 50×10^9/l and usually below 20×10^9/l ($20\,000$/µl), although the lower limit of normal is approximately 200×10^9/l ($200\,000$/µl). Even then stress on blood vessels is important – rest may avoid haemorrhage whereas exercise can provoke it.

Bone marrow suppression
Bone marrow suppression of platelet formation is caused by:

- Drugs, e.g. oestrogens, phenylbutazone, chloramphenicol (in cats) and chemotherapeutic agents for cancer – also levamisole and the antiviral drug ribavirin in cats.
- Chemicals, e.g. dapsone.
- Radiation.
- Infection (with viruses), or neoplasia, simply because functional tissue is squeezed out by non-functional tissue (i.e. myeloproliferative disorders (see Panel 3.2, p. 189), lymphoproliferative disorders (see Panel 3.1, p. 183) and metastatic neoplasms).
- The low level of cortisol in hypoadrenocorticism (chiefly *primary* – Addison's disease); this also causes thrombocytopenia due to bone marrow suppression.

Increased destruction of platelets

- *Immune-mediated destruction*: in autoimmune thrombocytopenia, and often in systemic lupus erythematosus, antibodies against the platelet membrane result in increased phagocytosis in the spleen and liver. In these disorders there *may also* be antibodies against the megakaryocytes reducing platelet *production* (see Panel 2.7, p. 125). In myasthenia gravis, there may be antibodies against platelets.

  Specific diagnostic features: platelet factor 3 (PF-3) test, large platelets showing clumping on blood smear.

- *Infectious diseases*: in the early stage of many viral and bacterial diseases, platelets are damaged, but numbers can be reduced by disseminated intravascular coagulation (DIC) and bone marrow suppression as well as by direct damage, and it is not easy to distinguish the cause, e.g. in feline infectious peritonitis, feline infectious enteritis, canine parvovirus infection, infectious canine hepatitis, neonatal canine herpes virus infection, leptospirosis, salmonellosis and other endotoxaemias, ehrlichiosis etc. Also in histoplasmosis.

  Specific diagnostic features: serological tests.

(The reduction in platelet numbers following infection with the rickettsiae, *Ehrlichia canis*, *Ehrlichia platys* or *Rickettsia rickettsii* may, in whole or part, be due to direct platelet injury inflicted by the replicating organisms.)

Splenic sequestration (hiding) of platelets

Splenic sequestration of platelets occurs in cases of splenomegaly (hypersplenism), e.g. splenic tumours. This is a rare cause. Usually a third of the platelets are in the spleen: if the size of the spleen increases so does the number of platelets contained within it. (Conversely, when the spleen is removed, the number of platelets in the circulation increases.)

Sequestration of platelets can also occur in the liver and, in cases of hypothermia, in cold areas of the body (usually the extremities).

Disseminated intravascular coagulation (DIC)

In DIC, defective haemostasis is the consequence of a severe reduction in the quantities of platelets and clotting factors in the blood, following their utilization in extensive intravascular coagulation. The tendency for bleeding not to be arrested will be enhanced if there is an accumulation of fibrinogen degradation products (FDPs) from the breakdown of clots (fibrinolysis) – see Panel 4.2, p. 216.

Specific diagnostic features of assistance: poikilocytes and schistocytes on blood smear, decreased number of platelets, increased prothrombin time, decreased level of fibrinogen, increased level of fibrinogen degradation products, possible haemoglobin-aemia and haemoglobinuria.

DIC is initiated by tissue damage (inflammation and necrosis) and major causes are:

- Malignant neoplasia (especially haemangiosarcomas, metastatic carcinomas and lymphosarcoma).
- Acute pancreatitis.
- Chronic active hepatitis.
- Heat stroke.
- Sepsis, due to Gram-negative bacteria, in particular salmonellosis.
- Aortic thromboembolism (in cats).

Note

Haemolysis is another feature of DIC and, with DIC, the anaemia may be both haemolytic and haemorrhagic.

Anaphylaxis

'Rebound' thrombocytopenia

This may follow a thrombocytosis produced by a blood transfusion that supplies a large number of platelets.

Defective thrombopoietin production [very rare]

Idiopathic

Essentially the cause is unknown – some cases may be due to abnormal megakaryocytic production.

Functional defects of platelets

Such defects, e.g. reduced adhesiveness, can result in failure of haemostasis.

Specific diagnostic feature of assistance: prolonged bleeding time despite normal platelet numbers.

These defects are associated with uraemia (renal failure), severe liver disease, myeloproliferative disorders and lymphoproliferative disorders, myeloma, auto-immune disease and arise as a result of therapy with certain drugs, e.g. aspirin, penicillin and phenylbutazone. There are also rare hereditary platelet dysfunctions (Glanzmann's thromboasthenia and the hereditary thrombopathia of Bassett Hounds).

Severe liver disease (hepatic failure)

Specific diagnostic features of assistance: if *acute* – prolonged one-stage prothrombin time and activated partial thromboplastin time; if *chronic* – normal one-stage prothrombin time but prolonged activated partial thromboplastin time. A low fibrinogen level in the absence of DIC denotes a poor prognosis.

A number of factors contribute to the tendency to bleed:

- Diminished synthesis of clotting factors V, VII, IX and X, prothrombin and, in the later stages, of fibrinogen also (a poor prognostic sign).
- Reduced clearance of fibrinogen degradation products which have an anticoagulant effect (see Panel 4.2, p. 216).
- Reduced clearance of gastrin-stimulated hydrochloric acid secreted in the stomach provoking gastric inflammation and ulceration.
- Reduced bile production or outflow decreases vitamin K absorption and, consequently, the production of clotting factors II (prothrombin), VIII, IX and X.
- A reduction in platelet numbers (thrombocytopenia) resulting from (1) increased usage (with DIC), (2) reduced production in the bone marrow (due to abnormal liver metabolism of vitamin B_{12} and folic acid) and (3) splenic sequestration (due to portal hypertension).
- In cirrhosis increased pressure in the portal vein and/or inability to detoxify histamine in the liver may contribute to intestinal haemorrhage.

NEOPLASIA

Haemorrhage can be due to rupture (especially with haemangiosarcomas and haemangiomas) of spleen, liver and lungs, or erosion (especially with duodenal leiomyomas in dogs).

Chronic haemorrhage is common with neoplasms of the gastrointestinal tract, urinary tract (especially bladder) and prostate gland.

There can be intermittent acute haemorrhage into the abdominal cavity producing 'episodes' of severe clinical signs of anaemia followed by rapid improvement, as the majority of the RBCs are taken into the circulation. Blood can be drained from the abdominal cavity. If untreated, such cases terminate fatally.

INFECTION

Parasites

This is an improbable cause in the UK. It is associated with blood-suckers, chiefly ticks and fleas in heavy burdens, mainly in young animals.

Abroad, this may be associated with mosquitos and other ectoparasites, and with hookworm and coccidia.

Micro-organisms

Sufficient haemorrhage to produce anaemia is unlikely to arise *except* in association with disseminated intravascular coagulation (see above), although haemorrhage will occur due to bacterial toxins (e.g. in cystitis, metritis and prostatitis etc.) and with the fungus *Aspergillus* (causing nose bleeds).

INTERNAL LESIONS

Gastrointestinal ulcers

These ulcers, especially of the stomach, duodenum and colon, can cause considerable chronic blood loss.

Specific diagnostic features of assistance: endoscopy, radiography.

There may be an increased anaesthetic risk where there is reduced clearance of gastrin due to liver failure.

Other lesions

With other lesions, there is seldom sufficient haemorrhage to cause anaemia, e.g.

- Intussuception (due to intestinal irritation and chiefly in the region of the ileocaecal valve).
- Foreign bodies, especially gastrointestinal.
- Urinary calculi.
- Prostatic hyperplasia and hypertrophy.

Panel 2.3 Features of haemolytic anaemia

HAEMOLYTIC ANAEMIA

This is the *least common* form of anaemia in small animals. The majority of cases in dogs are due to autoimmune haemolytic anaemia caused by IgG autoantibodies (see Panel 2.7, p. 125).

THE SITE OF HAEMOLYSIS

The site may be:

- Intravascular, i.e. while the RBCs are in the circulation. Haemolysis generally happens suddenly as a result of damage to the RBC membrane – as an acute or peracute episode.
- Extravascular, i.e. in the tissues, due to phagocytosis (chiefly in the spleen, but also the liver). Phagocytosis is the normal method of removing old or damaged RBCs, but there are more 'damaged' RBCs than usual. However, *anaemia* only develops when the rate of RBC destruction exceeds the rate of replacement. Consequently, extravascular haemolytic anaemia arises insidiously and runs a chronic course.

EXTRA-/INTRAVASCULAR HAEMOLYSIS

Extravascular

Most cases of haemolytic anaemia in small animals are extravascular (Harvey, 1980). There is increased phagocytosis of RBCs that are:

- Coated with antibody – chiefly IgG.
- Fragmented or distorted, e.g. by DIC.
- Unable to deform themselves and squeeze through small spaces because they carry Heinz bodies (as a result of oxidant poisoning) or parasites, *or* because they are ATP deficient (e.g. pyruvate kinase deficiency).

Even when *intravascular* haemolysis occurs there is a degree of extravascular haemolysis as well.

Intravascular haemolysis

Intravascular haemolysis is associated primarily with:

- Certain cases of autoimmune haemolytic anaemia, e.g. severe warm autoimmune haemolytic anaemia (complement-mediated lysis) and cold agglutinin disease.
- Disseminated intravascular coagulation (DIC) and splenic torsion.
- Certain types of toxicity, e.g. oxidant drugs (causing Heinz body anaemia), or snake venom.
- Physical lysis, e.g. due to heat, i.e. severe burns, radiation *or* intravenous injection of a hypotonic solution, especially water (osmotic lysis).
- Incompatible blood transfusion.
- Haemolytic disease of the newborn.
- Feline haemobartonellosis (rarely).

FREE HAEMOGLOBIN IN THE PLASMA AND URINE

These are signs specifically associated with haemolytic anaemia, *but* they depend on a large amount of haemoglobin being released from RBCs at the same time. This seldom happens with extravascular haemolysis so these signs generally appear *only in severe intravascular haemolysis*, and since this is uncommon it means that they are *absent* from *most* cases of haemolytic anaemia.

Free haemoglobin in the plasma (haemoglobinaemia)

This is visible as a pink/red colour:

- In the plasma layer when performing the haematocrit or ESR.
- In the plasma or serum when separating it for biochemical tests.

It takes only a few hours to clear the haemoglobin from plasma.

Note

A far more common cause of haemolysis is trauma to the RBCs during the collection or handling of the blood sample.

Free haemoglobin in the urine (haemoglobinuria)

This may be visible as an obvious pink/red colour in the urine, and it can only *follow* haemoglobinaemia. It appears when the renal threshold for haemoglobin reabsorption (0.8–1.5 g/l in the dog) is exceeded.

Note

Urine-test strips will distinguish between haemoglobinuria and haematuria (i.e. *intact* RBCs in the urine, denoting haemorrhage in the urinary or reproductive tracts). However, intact RBCs will lyse in the urine, after a time, due to the abnormal conditions present (pH, specific gravity etc.), and then the test result will appear as haemoglobinuria. Also any myoglobin present (e.g. in cases of muscle damage) will react as if there were haemoglobinuria.

INCREASED BILIRUBIN LEVEL IN PLASMA (HYPERBILIRUBINAEMIA)

This is a sign generally seen only with *intravascular* haemolysis, and therefore it is not a feature of most cases of haemolytic anaemia in small animals.

Bilirubin is formed from haemoglobin and its derivatives (haem, methaemalbumin) by macrophages of the mononuclear phagocyte system (or reticuloendothelial system) and is then bound to albumin. This initial 'unconjugated' and protein-bound bilirubin cannot be excreted by the liver or kidney. It is transported to the liver and there conjugated with glucuronic acid, to form 'conjugated bilirubin' which *can* be excreted in the bile and, if plasma levels are exceptionally high, in the urine. (See 'Plasma bilirubin', p. 254 and 'Urinary bilirubin', p. 440.)

- Following haemolysis there will be increased formation of conjugated bilirubin but a significantly increased total bilirubin level in the plasma ($>5\,\mu mol/l$ in the cat (>0.3 mg/dl), $>10\,\mu mol/l$ (>0.6 mg/dl) in the dog) will arise *only* if bilirubin is being formed *faster* than it can be conjugated and excreted. This is much more likely to occur in intravascular haemolysis because generally more haemoglobin is liberated all at once. In any case it will take about 8–10 hours after the haemolysis for an appreciable amount of bilirubin to form. Consequently, a plasma sample collected too soon will *not* show this change.
- A van den Bergh test will confirm that most bilirubin is unconjugated (or 'indirect-reacting'). But where very marked haemolysis results in severe anaemia, the consequent lack of oxygen to the liver cells causes cellular swelling and partial closure of the bile canals. This partial obstruction interferes with bile excretion, and

therefore with the removal of conjugated bilirubin. This means that a higher proportion of the bilirubin retained in the blood will be conjugated (or 'direct-reacting').
- Hyperbilirubinaemia gives rise to jaundice (icterus). Unless the plasma (or serum) sample is visibly yellow there is little point in estimating the bilirubin level.

REGENERATIVE RESPONSE (RETICULOCYTOSIS)

Three days (2–4 days) after severe acute haemolysis, signs of regeneration become obvious, i.e. *increased numbers of reticulocytes* (only a few are normally present) *plus*, if very severe, some nucleated RBCs (none of which are usually present). This response will already be evident by the time *chronic* (extravascular) haemolysis produces obvious clinical signs of anaemia.

Marked reticulocytosis will also result in:

- Anisocytosis (differences in the size of RBCs), especially if spherocytes are also present.
- A reddish 'streaming' in the lower part of the plasma layer when performing the haematocrit or ESR (see Panel 2.5, p. 115).

The reticulocyte production index (RPI) is more than 3 (see p. 120). This regenerative response is more marked than with haemorrhagic anaemia of comparable severity, because iron and protein are retained in the body, and is *more marked* with intravascular (acute) than extravascular (chronic) haemolysis.

But a poor regenerative response, or none at all, occurs in cases where:

- There is also bone marrow damage, e.g. by disseminated lymphosarcoma or infection,
- There are also specific antibodies against RBC stem cells in the bone marrow, i.e. in immune-mediated cases (e.g. autoimmune haemolytic anaemia).
- There is a lack of nutrients (e.g. folic acid).
- Not enough time has elapsed (3 days) for numbers of reticulocytes to appear.
- A blood transfusion has recently been given. This temporarily reduces the regenerative response.

CHANGES IN MCV AND MCHC

Since reticulocytes (and nucleated RBCs) are larger than normal mature RBCs, when they are present in significant numbers there is an *increase in MCV*, and in even larger numbers a *decrease in MCHC*.

- In immune-mediated haemolysis the agglutination of RBCs or the increased fragility of RBCs can reduce their numbers on electronic counting, *increasing the MCV*.
- Large numbers of spherocytes, usually present in immune-mediated haemolysis, will tend to *reduce the MCV*, and the overall effect may be that it remains in the normal range.
- The sudden release of a large amount of free haemoglobin into the plasma will result in an *erroneously high MCHC*, because the PCV will be lower than normal but the total haemoglobin concentration stays the same.
- A large number of Heinz bodies (in oxidant poisoning) will *raise the MCHC*.

(See 'Haematological indices', p. 54.)

ABNORMAL RBCs AND RBC INCLUSIONS INDICATIVE OF HAEMOLYTIC ANAEMIA

These consist of the following (see p. 66).

- Reticulocytes, RBCs with Howell–Jolly bodies and nucleated RBCs indicating RBC regeneration.
- Spherocytes, which strongly suggest immune-mediated haemolysis (primarily in the dog; difficult to detect in the cat).
- Poikilocytes, i.e. abnormally shaped RBCs, and cells with pieces missing, which usually precede RBC fragmentation, and schistocytes (fragmented RBCs) are *both* seen, especially with *intravascular* haemolysis, and suggest disseminated intravascular coagulation (DIC) or uraemia as a cause.
- Acanthocytes or spur cells, with blunt projections, can arise in hyperbilirubinaemia (associated with severe liver disease), uraemia or with a haemangiosarcoma.
- Echinocytes or burr cells – with spicules – are a feature of ATP deficiency and arise especially in pyruvate kinase deficiency.
- Stomatocytes, which occur in stomatocytosis (see p. 68).
- Sometimes a blood smear may show evidence of *phagocytosis*, suggesting immune-mediated haemolytic anaemia, e.g. erythrophagocytosis (an RBC being ingested by a neutrophil or monocyte), or (rarely) LE cells, indicative of systemic lupus erythematosus (SLE). An LE cell is a neutrophil which has ingested the nucleus from a dead or dying cell, and appears to have two nuclei.
- Agglutination (clumping) of RBCs which indicates an immune-mediated haemolytic anaemia. Agglutination may be confused with rouleaux formation. It can be distinguished by examining a blood smear but not necessarily by the addition of saline (see p. 127).
- A number of RBCs containing Heinz bodies indicating poisoning with oxidants.
- RBCs bearing parasites, especially *Haemobartonella felis*, less commonly *Haemobartonella canis*, *Babesia* spp. and *Cytauxzoon*, and in imported dogs the microfilariae of *Dirofilaria immitis* – the heartworm. (To see *H. felis*, smears should be made using freshly collected blood since the organism often detaches in blood containing EDTA and/or in blood which has been refrigerated.)

PLATELET NUMBERS

These can be below, within or above the normal range.

- Increased numbers are due to increased platelet production stimulated by increased utilization.
- Decreased numbers are more commonly found due either to increased destruction (as in half the immune-mediated cases of haemolytic anaemia in dogs), *or* to excessive consumption (as in disseminated intravascular coagulation).

WHITE BLOOD CELL NUMBERS

These vary depending on the underlying cause.

- Leucocytosis, neutrophilia and a shift-to-the-left frequently accompany a marked reticulocyte response, especially in the dog. They are seen most consistently in autoimmune haemolytic anaemia.

- Monocytosis commonly occurs, especially with immune-mediated haemolytic anaemia in the dog.
- Leucopenia can arise in immune-mediated conditions if there are also antibodies against neutrophils (e.g. as in systemic lupus erythematosus).

PLASMA PROTEIN LEVELS

These do *not* fall as with haemorrhagic anaemia and, in fact, the total plasma protein level may *rise* due to inclusion of liberated haemoglobin and, in immune-mediated disorders, increased antibody production. (The albumin level, however, does not rise.)

PROTEINURIA

This will inevitably accompany haemoglobinuria. If that is absent, proteinuria is suggestive of systemic lupus erythematosus as a cause of haemolytic anaemia, particularly if there is an increased plasma level of globulin (especially a polyclonal hypergammaglobulinaemia, see p. 296).

COMPENSATION

If the degree of extravascular haemolysis is only slight, the bone marrow may be able to continue to replace RBCs at the same rate as they are destroyed so that the PCV stays in the normal range. This is termed 'compensated haemolytic anaemia'.

INCREASED ACTIVITY OF LACTIC DEHYDROGENASE (LDH)

Increased LDH activity in plasma or serum occurs in haemolytic anaemia, because there is an isoenzyme of LDH (LDH_1) released from the RBCs.

SPLENOMEGALY

In extravascular haemolysis (usually immune-mediated), splenomegaly (sometimes accompanied by hepatomegaly) is often present due to both:

- Increased phagocytic activity.
- Extramedullary haemopoiesis in the spleen.

IRON CONCENTRATION

The level of iron in serum is generally elevated, especially in intravascular haemolysis, i.e. $>42\,\mu mol/l$ ($>233\,\mu g/dl$) although the total iron-binding capacity in serum is unaltered ($51–103\,\mu mol/l = 284–572\,\mu g/dl$).

LOW CREATININE VALUE

In association with haemolysis a low plasma creatinine value may be found due to interference with the test.

LESS COMMON TESTS FOR INTRAVASCULAR HAEMOLYSIS

Decreased haptoglobin concentration in plasma

Free haemoglobin in the blood binds to haptoglobin (an α_2-globulin) and the resulting complex is removed by phagocytes in the liver. The level of haptoglobin is reduced for a short period after haemolysis (12–24 hours in dogs and up to 48 hours in cats) so that samples *must* be collected within that time. Unfortunately, it may not be as reliable a test of intravascular haemolysis as once thought because the haptoglobin level can vary for other reasons, e.g. increasing in association with inflammation.

Haemosiderinuria and haemosiderin-containing cells in urine

Excess free haemoglobin (i.e. when the haptoglobin is saturated) is filtered (as dimers) through the kidney, reabsorbed in the proximal tubules and there catabolized to bilirubin. (Only when the renal threshold for haemoglobin is exceeded does haemoglobin appear in the urine.) Liberated iron can be detected as haemosiderin – both free in the urine and contained in any renal tubule cells that are sloughed off and passed in the urine.

Decreased haemopexin concentration and increased methaemalbumin concentration in plasma

Free haemoglobin in the circulation is also converted (via methaemoglobin) to haem, which binds to haemopexin, a glycoprotein in plasma. The complex which forms is removed by phagocytes in the liver and, therefore, the concentration of haemopexin falls. Any surplus haem remaining after this has occurred combines with albumin to form methaemalbumin and therefore the level of this compound *increases*.

Causes of haemolytic anaemia

Summary

- Immune-mediated [most common]
- Disseminated intravascular coagulation
- Poisoning, *especially* with oxidants
- Inherited disorders
- Infectious organisms, especially *Haemobartonella felis* and leptospires
- Physical lysis (water, burns, radiation)
- Hypophosphataemia
- Malignant tumours

Causes that produce *intravascular haemolysis* will result in haemoglobinuria, haemoglobinaemia and the other features mentioned in 'Features of haemolytic anaemias' (p. 95).

General diagnostic features include a reticulocyte production index of more than 3, fragmentation and, although seldom measured, increased LDH activity and increased iron concentration (especially in intravascular haemolysis).

IMMUNE MEDIATED

Specific diagnostic features: spherocytes and, sometimes, intravascular signs. See Panel 2.7, p. 125.

Autoimmune haemolytic anaemia (AIHA)

This is the *most common* cause of haemolytic anaemia in dogs (see p. 125). Autoantibodies against RBCs produce haemolysis, mainly extravascular. AIHA may be primary (not in the cat) or secondary, i.e. associated with another disease, such as:

- Infectious diseases (especially FeLV infection and also haemobartonellosis).
- Neoplasia, especially lymphoproliferative and myeloproliferative disorders and haemangiosarcomas.
- Other autoimmune conditions, such as immune-mediated thrombocytopenia or systemic lupus erythematosus.

Diagnosis is based on finding one or more of the following:

- Spherocytes.
- In some cases, intravascular signs.
- Autoagglutination (at blood heat or lower temperatures – optimally 4°C).
- Increased osmotic fragility.
- Positive Coombs' antiglobulin test (at blood heat or at lower temperatures).
- Positive enzyme-treated RBC test (e.g. papain test).

Together with specific tests (and signs) for other diseases in secondary cases, e.g.:

- FeLV infection – positive FeLV test.
- Systemic lupus erythematosus – polyarthritis, skin lesions, fever, decreased number of platelets, proteinuria, positive ANA test, positive LE cell test.
- Immune-mediated thrombocytopenia – decreased number of platelets, positive platelet factor 3 test.

Drug-induced immune haemolytic anaemia

The drug, or drug metabolite, attaches to the RBC membrane and an antibody forms against the drug or metabolite, *or* the membrane antigens are altered and antibodies form against these new antigens. This is suspected to occur with penicillin in dogs, and possibly with other drugs.

Specific diagnostic features of assistance: history of drug use, spherocytes, increased osmotic fragility, specialized serological tests.

Alloantibody-induced haemolytic anaemia

Specific diagnostic features of assistance: history very important, spherocytes, increased osmotic fragility, cross-matching of blood, intravascular signs.

Incompatible blood transfusion

This results in a *transfusion reaction* with agglutination, haemolysis and phagocytosis of the donor RBCs, i.e. both intravascular and extravascular haemolysis.
The alloantibodies may be:

- Either naturally present – such as the anti-A antibodies present in most cats that have B antigens on their RBCs (dogs either possess no, or no significant amounts of, *natural* alloantibodies).
- Or produced in response to a previous incompatible transfusion (e.g. in dogs, 8–12 days later).

Haemolytic disease of the newborn (neonatal (iso)erythrolysis)
This is very rare in dogs and cats. Maternal antibodies against the antigens on the offspring's RBCs are transferred, in the colostrum, from a mother previously sensitized by blood transfusion, vaccination or the leakage of fetal RBCs. Intravascular and extravascular haemolysis results.

MICROANGIOPATHIC HAEMOLYSIS DUE TO DISSEMINATED INTRAVASCULAR COAGULATION (DIC)

In DIC, fibrin strands are deposited in small blood vessels, mainly arterioles, and damage the RBCs. Haemolysis is both intravascular (due to shearing of the RBC membranes) and extravascular (phagocytosis of RBCs that are mis-shapen (poikilocytes) and fragmented (schistocytes).

Specific diagnostic features of assistance: poikilocytes and schistocytes on blood smear, decreased number of platelets, increased prothrombin time, decrease in fibrinogen, increase in fibrinogen products, intravascular signs.

DIC is initiated by tissue damage (inflammation and necrosis) and major causes are:

- Malignant neoplasia (especially haemangiosarcoma, metastatic carcinoma and lymphosarcoma).
- Acute pancreatitis.
- Chronic active hepatitis.
- Heat stroke.
- Sepsis, due to Gram-negative bacteria, in particular salmonellosis.
- Aortic thromboembolism.

For a full list of the causes see Panel 4.2 (p. 216).
Similar RBC damage may result from vasculitis initiated by infectious canine hepatitis, infection with *Angiostrongylus vasorum* or immune polyarteritis.

Note

Multiple haemorrhages are also a feature of DIC and therefore anaemia may be haemorrhagic *as well* as haemolytic.

POISONING

Oxidant poisons

These can cause intravascular haemolysis. Methaemoglobin is formed by the action of mild/moderate oxidants (i.e. causing methaemoglobinaemia). Stronger oxidative poisons also denature and precipitate haemoglobin to form Heinz bodies which find it difficult to squeeze through small spaces. The affected RBCs are then phagocytosed in the spleen (extravascular haemolysis).

Specific diagnostic features of assistance: increased number of Heinz bodies, muddy colour of mucous membranes due to methaemoglobin, level of methaemoglobin in blood usually more than 2%.

Examples of oxidant poisons:

- Raw onions (*N*-propyl disulphide)
- Chlorate
- Nitrate (fertilizer, converted to toxic nit*rite* in the alimentary tract)
- Methylene blue (urinary antiseptic)
- Paracetamol (acetaminophen) – analgesic

- Phenazopyridine (urinary analgesic)
- Benzocaine (topically as local analgesic)
- Propylthiouracil in cat (antithyroid drug)
- Phenacetin
- Ketamine anaesthesia (in cats)
- Sulphonamides
- Dapsone

Other poisons and toxins

These primarily attack the RBC membrane.
  Examples include:

- Lead (in dog) – specific diagnostic features: basophilic stippling, nucleated RBCs, high blood/urine level – see p. 118
- Benzene and related compounds
- Phenol compounds (disinfectants etc.)
- Naphthalene (mothballs)
- Acetohydroxamic acid (to dissolve struvite calculi)
- Dimethylsulphoxide (DMSO)
- Snake venom (specific diagnostic features: RBC fragments, spherocytes)
- Bacterial toxins – in severe infections
- Copper (see 'Copper-storage disease' in Bedlingon Terriers, under 'Inherited disorders' below)

INHERITED DISORDERS (INTRINSIC RBC FACTORS)

Pyruvate kinase (PK) deficiency

- In Basenjis and Beagles, usually <1½ year old.
- An autosomal recessive trait.
- The ATP deficiency and accumulation of calcium ions causes spiculated RBCs and echinocytes (burr cells), later losing their deformability and becoming spherical with spicules (spheroechinocytes).

Specific diagnostic features of assistance: echinocytes, spheroechinocytes, reticulocytes, low RBC PK concentration; low PK levels can identify carriers.

Stomatocytosis

- In Alaskan Malamutes with chondrodysplasia (short-limbed dwarfism).
- Adults are *not* anaemic.
- RBC membrane defects cause RBCs to be bowl shaped (stomatocytes).

Specific diagnostic features of assistance: stomatocytes.

Congenital porphyria (Siamese cats)

- Increased concentrations of porphyrins in plasma, and uroporphyrins in urine.
- Associated with photosensitivity and renal disease.

Specific diagnostic features: macrocytic/hypochromic RBCs, pink/brown colour to teeth, bones and urine which fluoresce in ultraviolet light.

'Haemoglobin C' disease (Siamese cats)

Specific diagnostic features of assistance: square or rectangular RBCs containing crystalloid bodies.

Copper-associated liver disease

This is seen in Bedlington Terriers (one-third of those in the UK), also Dobermanns, West Highland White Terriers and Cocker Spaniels. (Also known as Bedlington Terrier disease or copper-storage disease.)

- Acute form occurs in young animals (2–5 years old) giving intravascular haemolysis (rare).
- Chronic form is seen in older dogs.
- Also there is an asymptomatic form.
- Causes hepatitis progressing to cirrhosis.

Specific diagnostic features of assistance: intravascular signs in acute cases, increased copper levels in liver (biopsy), i.e. >300 μg/g dry weight, decreased albumin level, increased activities of ALT, ALP and GGT, reduced BSP clearance.

INFECTIOUS ORGANISMS

RBC parasites

In the UK chiefly those causing haemobartonellosis in cats and leptospirosis in dogs.

Haemobartonella felis[fairly common]
This occurs mainly in young males and is responsible for feline haemobartonellosis (feline infectious anaemia).

Pleomorphic bacteria (rods, rings or cocci) are attached to the surface of RBCs, most likely to be discovered in smears of fresh blood (uncoagulated and unrefrigerated).

Acridine orange demonstrates them better than Romanowsky stains – otherwise stain as described in Appendix I (p. 468). Affected RBCs are phagocytosed.

Specific diagnostic feature of assistance: *H. felis* on RBCs.

The absence of a regenerative response in association with FIA suggests concurrent FeLV infection causing both immunosuppression (allowing FIA to develop) and bone marrow suppression.

Haemobartonella canis[rare]
This causes canine haemobartonellosis and results in anaemia only in splenectomized dogs.

Specific diagnostic feature of assistance: *H. canis* as rods, dots and, most commonly, chains on RBC surface.

Cytauxzoon felis
This does not occur in the UK – it is a protozoan parasite causing feline cytauxzoonosis, e.g. in mid-western and southern USA.

Specific diagnostic feature of assistance: *C. felis* as rings, dots or 'safety-pin' shapes in RBCs.

Babesia felis
This causes feline babesiosis (not in the UK).

Specific diagnostic features of assistance: parasites difficult to find, increased lymphocyte count, serology, indirect fluorescent antibody test, may be positive Coombs' antiglobulin test.

Babesia canis, Babesia vogeli or *Babesia gibsoni*

Canine babesiosis is caused by *Babesia canis*, *Babesia vogeli* (large pyriform protozoa in one or more pairs) or *Babesia gibsoni* (small ring-shaped protozoa) – not in the UK.

Special diagnostic features of assistance: parasites (difficult to find), increased lymphocyte count serology, indirect fluorescent antibody test, may be positive Coombs' antiglobulin test.

Leishmania donovani

This causes leishmaniasis – uncommon in the UK.

Other organisms

Leptospira icterohaemorrhagiae

This causes leptospirosis in dogs and may cause haemolytic crises – seldom seen with *L. canicola*.

Specific diagnostic features of assistance: leptospires in urine, serology (rising titres in samples 10–15 days apart in acute infections or high titre with chronic infection), usually increased blood urea, possible proteinuria. May be intravascular signs.

Dirofilaria immitis

This causes heartworm disease in dogs – not in the UK. The venae cavae (or postcaval) syndrome of dogs (large numbers of heartworm in the right atrium and venae cavae) is characterized by intravascular haemolysis due to disseminated intravascular coagulation, along with respiratory problems and liver damage.

Specific diagnostic features of assistance: microfilariae in blood, intravascular signs, laboratory features of DIC, modified Knott's test.

PHYSICAL LYSIS CAUSING INTRAVASCULAR HAEMOLYSIS

Specific diagnostic features of assistance: intravascular signs.

Hypotonic solutions

Lysis can be caused by solutions equivalent to less than 0.5% saline in dogs or less than 0.6% saline in cats.

Burns

Heat causes lysis of adjacent RBCs.

Radiation

This increases fragility of RBCs.

HYPOPHOSPHATAEMIA

Malabsorption of inorganic phosphate or other disorders (see 'Causes of decreased phosphate', p. 379) can result in hypophosphataemia. The level of ATP in RBCs falls impairing glycolysis and RBCs lose their ability to deform and are removed by the mononuclear phagocyte system (reticuloendothelial system), i.e. extravascular haemolysis occurs.

Specific diagnostic features of assistance: plasma inorganic phosphate of less than 0.3–0.5 mmol/l (1–1.5 mg/dl), spherocytes.

MALIGNANT TUMOURS (PARTICULARLY SPLENIC)

Haemolysis is especially a feature of haemangiosarcomas, and it arises through DIC and other mechanisms as well.

Specific diagnostic features of assistance: fragmented cells (schistocytes) and Howell–Jolly bodies are prominent; also acanthocytes (spur cells) and small numbers of nucleated RBCs – more than expected for the degree of anaemia.

Note

Uraemia, which is known to cause haemolysis in humans, appears to be an unlikely cause in the dog and cat.

Panel 2.4 Features of hypoproliferative anaemia (non-regenerative anaemia)

ABSENCE OF RETICULOCYTOSIS

No marked reticulocytosis is the *essential diagnostic feature* of hypoproliferative anaemia.

Reticulocytes are generally either absent, or not present in any greater number than usual.

The only exception to this rule is that in some nutritional deficiency diseases associated with a moderate anaemia (e.g. iron or protein deficiency) and with some depression anaemias (e.g. those due to malignant neoplasia or liver disease) there may be a *poor* attempt at regeneration resulting in some slight increase in reticulocyte numbers.

However, bear in mind that for the first 2–3 days following haemorrhage or haemolysis there will be no substantial increase in the number of reticulocytes.

SLOW DEVELOPMENT

Hypoproliferative anaemia develops slowly, i.e. it is always chronic, never acute.

MAINLY NORMOCYTIC/NORMOCHROMIC

The hypoproliferative (non-regenerative) anaemias are normocytic and normochromic *apart from* the nutritional anaemias and those associated with:

- Some myeloproliferative disorders (principally erythraemic myelosis and erythroleukaemia in cats)
- Chronic inflammatory disease or neoplasia (at times).

Nutritional anaemias characteristically show variations in the size and pigmentation of the RBCs whereas anaemias due to destruction or suppression of the bone marrow are *in general* characterized by RBCs that are normal in their size and pigmentation on blood smears and have a normal MCV and MCHC, termed 'normocytic/ normochromic anaemia'.

NUTRITIONAL DEFICIENCY ANAEMIAS

Nutritional anaemias are rarely encountered.

Due to folate or niacin deficiency

A nutritional deficiency anaemia can de due to a deficiency of folate or very rarely niacin (or presumably of vitamin B_{12} – although this appears to be unrecorded as a cause of anaemia in the dog or cat). Dosing with a folate antagonist, e.g. phenytoin, trimethoprim, pyrimethamine or methotrexate, produces the same effect, as do drugs which have a long-term effect on folate synthesis, e.g. sulphonamides.

There are macrocytic/normochromic RBCs (it can be called a megaloblastic anaemia), i.e. there is an increased MCV and a normal MCHC. Also there are small numbers of hypersegmented neutrophils.

Care

1. Being macrocytes these RBCs *might* be confused on size alone with reticulocytes, although the latter are hypochromic (i.e. the MCV is decreased) and these cells are not.
2. Slightly macrocytic RBCs (leptocytes, including target cells) may also be seen on blood smears in the non-regenerative anaemia due to liver disease.
3. Macrocytic/normochromic RBCs can occur with non-regenerative anaemia in some myeloproliferative disorders, primarily erythraemic myelosis and erythroleukaemia in cats (sometimes in monocytic leukaemia and myelofibrosis) – see Table 2.1, p. 75.

Due to protein deficiency

Nutritional deficiency anaemia can be due to a protein deficiency, arising from severe malabsorption or protein loss.

Rarely there may be slightly hypochromic RBCs of normal size accompanied by a moderate hypoproteinaemia.

Care

The low plasma protein level may lead to confusion with haemorrhagic anaemia, although generally with haemorrhage the degree of both anaemia and of protein loss would be greater, and reticulocytes would be prominent after 2–3 days.

Due to iron deficiency

This begins as a normocytic/normochromic anaemia but develops through a microcytic/normochromic or normocytic/hypochromic anaemia to a microcytic/hypochromic anaemia.

Iron deficiency anaemia is *rarely* due to a dietary deficiency and is *usually* the consequence of severe haemorrhagic anaemia (and therefore often associated with a thrombocytopenia).

Iron is transported in the blood attached to a protein and, in the diagnosis of iron deficiency, it is necessary not only to measure the concentration of iron (in the plasma) but to check that the blood's *capacity* to carry iron is not the limiting factor. In iron-deficiency anaemia the total iron-binding capacity (TIBC) of plasma remains normal(51–103 µmol/l = 284–572 µg/dl) in the dog, but the concentration of iron falls markedly (<15 µmol/l = <84 µg/dl). In contrast, in anaemia due to inflammation both of these parameters may show a modest decrease (see 'Iron', p. 381).

Care

Rarely a microcytic/hypochromic non-regenerative anaemia (i.e. with decreased MCV and decreased MCHC) is seen where there is chronic inflammatory disease or a neoplastic disorder.

Due to pyridoxine (vitamin B₆) deficiency

Nutritional deficiency anaemia can be due to pyridoxine deficiency (or very rarely to a riboflavin (vitamin B₂) deficiency). The RBCs tend to be microcytic and normochromic.

DESTRUCTIVE OR DEPRESSIVE ANAEMIAS

These are the more common types of hypoproliferative anaemias. Essentially, with one or two exceptions, RBCs are normal in size and haemoglobin content (i.e. normocytic and normochromic).

There may be a reduction:

- Either only, or mainly, in the number of red blood cells, i.e. with normal numbers of WBCs and platelets.
- Or in all (or most) of the cells (and platelets) coming from the bone marrow, i.e. reduced numbers of RBCs, WBCs and platelets.

Reduction only or mainly in the number of RBCs

This is termed 'pure erythroid hypoplasia or aplasia', and bone marrow aspirates and biopsies show reduced erythroid cell activity but normal myeloid and megakaryocytic activity, i.e. there is an increased myeloid:erythroid (M:E) ratio. The major types of this form of anaemia are given below.

Pure RBC aplasia
It is thought that later these cases may show a reduction in WBCs and platelets, i.e. they become cases of pancytopenia (see below).

The interference with RBC production is possibly immune mediated (some cases are Coombs' test positive) and, in the cat, FeLV is a major cause (these cases are FeLV positive).

Anaemia of inflammatory disease
See below.

Anaemia of malignancy
Chronic inflamation, i.e present for a month or longer and either infectious or non-infectious, or neoplasia somewhere in the body *other than* the bone marrow, results in the diversion of iron to macrophages in the bone marrow so that it is not available for RBC formation. There is a modest fall in both the level of serum iron and of total iron-binding capacity (see 'Iron', p. 381). *Rarely* this can result in the microcytic/hypochromic anaemia characteristic of iron deficiency.

Anaemia due to lack of erythropoietin
This can also be due to defective bone marrow response to erythropoietin. It occurs in:

• Chronic renal failure (end-stage renal disease with uraemia).
• Chronic liver disease (e.g.cirrhosis).
• Endocrine disorders, e.g. hypoadrenocorticism, hypothyroidism and hypo-androgenism.

Note

The anaemias of inflammation, malignancy and deficient erythropoietin are termed 'secondary anaemias'.

A clear classification on the basis of cause is difficult because probably all of them are multifactorial, i.e. as well as reduced RBC production there are factors which reduce RBC survival.

At times there may be a poor regenerative response with some reticulocytes appearing, e.g. in neoplasia and liver disease.

At times WBCs and platelet numbers may be altered, e.g.

• In *neoplasia* there may be more granulocytes (neutrophils and eosinophils primarily).
• In *liver disease* the number of WBCs may be increased or decreased.
• In *chronic renal failure* the platelet count may be slightly increased (although platelet function is impaired).

Reduced numbers of RBCs, WBCs and platelets

The bone marrow is so deficient in all cell types (hypocellular) that it can be *difficult to establish the myeloid:erythroid (M:E) ratio*. (If some stage of WBC (myeloid cell) production is stimulated, as in some myelophthistic anaemias, i.e. with myeloproliferative disorders, then the M:E ratio will be *increased*.)

Due to stem cell destruction
When it is due to stem cell destruction, the anaemia is, by long-standing convention, called simply 'aplastic anaemia' (although this name could confuse it with pure RBC aplasia *or* haemopoietic hypoplasia/aplasia).

If *all* cell types are reduced in number the disorder can be called a *pancytopenia*. The deficiency of WBCs and platelets usually becomes evident *before* obvious anaemia because they have a shorter lifespan.

Common causes are infection, neoplasia, toxic agents and, rarely, radiation.

Due to bone marrow invasion and replacement
When anaemia is due to bone marrow invasion and replacement of the functional bone marrow cells by abnormal tissue it is termed 'myelophthistic anaemia'.

This can be caused by:

- Neoplasia arising in the bone marrow (primary haemopoietic tumours), i.e. myeloproliferative disorders and lymphoproliferative disorders. In the cat most of these disorders are linked with FeLV infection (i.e. cases are usually FeLV positive).
- Metastasis to the bone marrow of malignant neoplasms elsewhere (secondary haemopoietic tumours), including lymphosarcomas – two-thirds of which in the cat are linked to FeLV infection (i.e. cases are FeLV positive).
- Granulomatous change in the bone marrow, e.g. due to myelofibrosis or a reaction to chronic marrow infection (e.g. tuberculosis) or bony change (osteoporosis).

Generally the MCV and MCHC are normal, but a raised MCV is seen in cases of erythraemic myelosis and erythroleukaemia in cats, and in some cases monocytic leukaemia and myelofibrosis, due principally to increased numbers of nucleated RBCs.

Reticulocytosis is absent unless there is RBC proliferation in the spleen, liver and lymph nodes, e.g. in myelofibrosis.

The number of WBCs can at times be increased, e.g.:

- In some myeloproliferative and lymphoproliferative disorders, especially chronic (the type of WBC depends upon the cell line affected).
- In early oestrogen toxicity; there is neutrophilia, later followed by neutropenia.

Causes of hypoproliferative anaemia

Summary

Nutritional deficiencies [uncommon]
- Folate, niacin (?vitamin B_{12})
- Protein
- Iron, pyridoxine, riboflavin

Bone marrow destruction or depression
- Affecting RBCs primarily
  1. Pure RBC aplasia (idiopathic, immune-mediated, FeLV)
  2. Chronic inflammation
  3. Malignant neoplasia
  4. Erythropoietin lack, or poor response
- Affecting RBCs, WBCs and platelets
  1. Stem cell destruction (aplastic anaemia) – infection/ toxins/radiation
  2. Bone marrow invasion (myelophthistic anaemia) – neoplasia (primary, secondary)/fibrous tissue

Some agents cause anaemia by more than one means (especially FeLV infection).

NUTRITIONAL DEFICIENCIES [UNCOMMON]

These usually cause a mild to moderate anaemia.
There may be a dietary deficiency *but* deficiencies can also arise from:

- Antagonists, e.g. drugs antagonistic to folate.
- Exceptional losses, e.g. of iron or protein.

Folate, niacin and vitamin B₁₂ deficiencies

Folate deficiency can be due to dosing with a folate antagonist (e.g. phenytoin, methotrexate, pyrimethamine or trimethoprim, or drugs which long term reduce folate production by bacteria in the gut, e.g. sulphonamides).
A vitamin B_{12} deficiency anaemia has not been recorded in dogs or cats.
Deficiencies result in macrocytic/normochromic RBCs.

Protein deficiency

Protein deficiency can be due to exceptional losses through the kidneys or gastrointestinal tract (rarely through burns). Long term this leads to normocytic/ hypochromic RBCs.

Iron, pyridoxine (vitamin B₆) and riboflavin (vitamin B₂) deficiencies

Iron deficiency is usually due to chronic haemorrhage and consequent increased loss of iron, but it could be due to a solely milk diet in young animals.
Pyridoxine and riboflavin deficiencies are very rare.
All these deficiencies can lead to microcytic/hypochromic RBCs (although in iron deficiency anaemia the RBCs start as normocytic/normochromic – see p. 109).

DESTRUCTION OR DEPRESSION OF BONE MARROW

Primarily affecting RBCs

Bone marrow shows an increased myeloid:erythroid (M:E) ratio.

Pure RBC aplasia (true RBC aplasia)
- Idiopathic (i.e. cause unknown).
- Immune-mediated (positive Coombs' test).
- FeLV infection (FeLV test is positive).

Despite normal WBC and platelet numbers, the platelets may be large and bizarre. Later, WBC and platelet numbers may also show a fall, i.e. this may be the first indication of a developing pancytopenia.

Anaemia of inflammation
Chronic inflammation (i.e. lasting 1 month or more), which may or may not be associated with infection, e.g. rheumatoid arthritis, generalized demodicosis (in over 50% of canine cases), chronic liver disease and chronic pyometra. (PCV may be as low as 15 l/l, leucocytosis, monocytosis, neutrophilia, shift-to-the-left.)

Anaemia of malignancy

Malignant neoplasia somewhere in the body *other than* the bone marrow (i.e. non-haemopoietic neoplasia).

Lack of erythropoietin or poor response

Lack of erythropoietin, or failure of the bone marrow to respond to it is seen in:

- Chronic renal failure (which may terminate with end-stage kidneys).
- Chronic liver disease (thin macrocytes, target cells, acanthocytes).
- Endocrine disorders: hypoadrenocorticism, hypothyroidism, pituitary dwarfism and hypoandrogenism.

Note

In hypoadrenocorticism (Addison's disease) anaemia is often masked by dehydration. In hypothyroidism there is a reduced demand for oxygen and therefore for RBCs to carry it.

Usually in anaemias of malignancy and inflammation and from lack of erythropoietin, there is mild/moderate anaemia. With these secondary anaemias there is no obvious intrinsic bone marrow damage (it can also be termed 'anaemia of systemic disease').

Primarily reducing the numbers of all bone marrow elements

This bone marrow destruction/depression primarily reduces RBCs, WBCs and platelets, resulting in pancytopenia. Many of these are secondary anaemias but there is often serious bone marrow damage.

Aplastic anaemia

Aplastic anaemia (haemopoietic aplasia/hypoplasia) is due to bone marrow stem cell destruction.

Infectious causes include:

1. Viral
   (a) feline panleucopenia (FPL), otherwise feline infectious enteritis (FIE) (reduced numbers of RBCs, WBCs and platelets);

Note

FPL in recovery shows neutrophilia.

   (b) feline infectious peritonitis (FIP) (reduced numbers of WBCs and platelets);
   (c) feline immunodeficiency virus (FIV) infection, previously known as feline T-lymphotrophic lentivirus (FTLV) infection – non-regenerative anaemia has been noted in about a third of cases;
   (d) feline leukaemia virus (FeLV) infection;
   (e) canine distemper;
   (f) canine parvovirus infection.
2. Bacterial
   (a) bacteraemia, septicaemia and especially toxaemia (as with chronic abscessation and sometimes other problems, e.g. foreign bodies);
   (b) ehrlichiasis (not in the UK).

> **Note**
>
> The finding of *Haemobartonella felis* on blood smears *and* a non-regenerative anaemia (when usually *H. felis* provokes a regenerative anaemia, i.e. haemolytic anaemia) suggests that there could be concurrent FeLV or FIV infection (which by immunosuppression allows haemobartonellosis to develop) and bone marrow suppression.

3. Protozoal:
    (a) leishmaniasis (not in the UK); anaemia may be regenerative or non-regenerative;
    (b) hepatozoonosis (not in the UK);
    (c) trypanosomiasis (not in the UK);
4. Fungal: histoplasmosis (?not in the UK).

Drug and chemical toxicity – effects may be transient:

- Oestrogens (although in early stages these produce neutrophilia) – both administered (exogenous), especially oestradiol cyprionate but also stilboestrol, and endogenous, e.g. oestrogens from Sertoli cell tumours and granulosa cell tumours.
- Phenylbutazone (although neutropenia is more common than anaemia).
- Chemotherapeutic (i.e. anti-neoplastic) agents, e.g. cyclophosphamide.
- Alkylating agents.
- Chloramphenicol; in the cat it reduces numbers of neutrophils, lymphocytes, platelets and reticulocytes.
- Aspirin.
- Amphotericin B.
- Benzene and other organic chemicals, e.g. organic arsenicals.
- Methylene blue (as well as giving rise to haemolysis).
- Lead poisioning.
- Mercury poisioning.

Radiation: in excessive levels whole body gamma radiation affects all bone marrow elements.

Myelophthistic anaemia

Due to bone marrow invasion and replacement of functional bone marrow cells by abnormal tissue.

- Neoplasia arising in the bone marrow, i.e. myeloproliferative disorders and lymphoproliferative disorders; in the cat these are largely associated with FeLV infection.

    Specific diagnostic features: large numbers of mature/immature cells of the WBC line affected, M:E ratio increased with proliferation of WBC lines.

    Macrocytic, normochromic RBCs (giving an increased MCV) are a feature of certain myeloproliferative disorders (see Panel 3.2, p. 189) and/or nucleated RBCs, *without* increased numbers of reticulocytes.

- Metastasis to the bone marrow of a primary malignant neoplasm elsewhere – including lymphosarcomas, two-thirds of which in the cat are due to FeLV infection.
- Granulomatous change – due to deposition of fibrous tissue, e.g. due to myelofibrosis as a sequel to a myeloproliferative disorder or chronic bone marrow infection (e.g. with tuberculosis) or bony change (osteoporosis).

Also rare congenital bone marrow aplasias have been recorded in the dog.

Note

Aspiration or biopsy of the bone marrow is valuable in all hypoproliferative anaemias in shedding light upon the cause.

Panel 2.5 Immature red blood cells

RBCs are formed and mature in the red bone marrow before being released into the blood. The sequence of development is shown in Figure 2.2 (p. 45). Throughout the maturation process, from the pluripotential haemopoietic stem cell, through the nucleated stages and the reticulocytes, to the mature RBC (erythrocyte or normocyte), the cells become progressively smaller. Normally there is a small number of reticulocytes in the blood but no earlier cells, which collectively are referred to as nucleated RBCs.

Release of large numbers of immature RBCs

Large numbers of immature RBCs are released into the circulation in two main situations.

HAEMORRHAGIC AND HAEMOLYTIC ANAEMIAS

In haemorrhagic and haemolytic anaemias (but not in hypoproliferative anaemia), regeneration of RBCs by the bone marrow is stimulated by the reduced oxygenation of the tissues, i.e. these are *regenerative anaemias* (responsive anaemias). To replace the missing RBCs quickly the bone marrow releases younger, immature forms into the circulation, and the more severe the anaemia the younger are the forms that are released. Most of these cells are reticulocytes plus, in severe anaemia, some nucleated RBCs. Increased numbers of reticulocytes constitute a *reticulocytosis*.

Reticulocytosis is also a response to the mild (dilutional) anaemia of pregnancy. This is seen during late pregnancy and immediately post partum and is especially marked in the cat. It is also prominent in newborn animals.

MYELOPROLIFERATIVE DISORDERS

In myeloproliferative disorders there is neoplastic proliferation of the nucleated RBCs in the bone marrow which spill over into the blood, and in some of these disorders considerable numbers of these cells appear (see Panel 3.2, p. 189). In these conditions there is *no reticulocytosis*.

Types of immature RBCs seen in a stained smear

NUCLEATED RBCs

These form a succession of developmental stages in the bone marrow and, under normal circumstances, eventually lose their nuclei before becoming reticulocytes and passing into the circulation. The stages of development are given different names by different authors, but will be described in laboratory reports as *rubricytes, normoblasts* or *erythroblasts*, with appropriate prefixes (see Figure 2.2, p. 45).

Normally only occasional nucleated RBCs are found in the blood (except in some Miniature Schnauzers where there can be a small number).

RBCs STILL POSSESSING NUCLEAR REMNANTS

These inclusions are termed 'Howell–Jolly bodies'. Normally they are absent from the blood of dogs but may appear in a small number (<1%) of feline RBCs.

RETICULOCYTES

All, or most, of the immature RBCs which appear in regenerative anaemias are reticulocytes. Reticulocytes are best identified on a supravitally stained smear.

When released into the circulation a reticulocyte contains an aggregation of ribosomal RNA and is termed an 'aggregate reticulocyte'. With time the amount of ribosomal RNA decreases to a few specks or threads, and this older cell is described as a *punctate reticulocyte*.

- In the dog aggregate reticulocytes are the type usually seen in the blood, accounting for around 1% of the total RBCs.
- In the cat aggregate reticulocytes account for about 0.5% of the total RBCs. However, the disappearance of the RNA is slower in this species, so that in normal health a further 1–10% of the RBCs are punctate reticulocytes, i.e. punctate reticulocytes are more numerous and persist longer. (In the cat *total* reticulocytes, including punctate = 1.5–11% of all RBCs.)

Recognition of immature RBCs on a stained blood smear

ON A ROUTINELY STAINED SMEAR

The following can be looked for on a smear stained for the differential WBC count with a Romanowsky stain (such as Leishman's, Wright's or May–Grünwald–Giemsa).

Nucleated RBCs

These can be clearly recognized. They are larger cells, and therefore may be reported as *macrocytes*, with prominent nuclei.

Howell–Jolly bodies

These also show up clearly.

Reticulocytes

However, reticulocytes are not so easily distinguished. They will appear, and therefore may be reported, as:

- Slightly larger RBCs (i.e. macrocytes or macrocytic RBCs).
- Having some variation in the staining within each cell, termed 'polychromasia' (polychromia, polychromatophilia), due to residual RNA (>3–5 such cells per oil immersion field suggests a moderate to marked reticulocytosis).
- Generally appearing bluish (basophilic) due to this residual RNA (sometimes reticulocytes are termed 'basophilic erythrocytes'). There may be diffuse basophilia or basophilic stippling (the latter seen especially in the cat).

In addition:

- Their slightly larger size means that when reticulocytes are present in significant numbers there is an obvious variation in the size of the RBCs (anisocytosis).
- They are discernibly thinner (i.e. have a large surface area in relation to the volume of their contents). Such thin cells are termed 'leptocytes'.

CHECK – reticulocytes that appear as leptocytes will always be polychromic (polychromasic, polychromatic, polychromatophilic, i.e. they will show variable staining). This is important since *orthochromic* (i.e. normal staining) leptocytes can occur in certain chronic debilitating diseases, liver diseases etc. – see 'Abnormal RBCs and RBC inclusions', p. 66.

- These thin cells have a tendency to become folded in different ways and consequently *may* be reported as – target cells (codocytes), looking like a shooting target; folded cells (knizocytes), looking like the head of a screw; bowl-shaped cells (resembling, although not as pronounced as, stomatocytes).

ON A SUPRAVITALLY STAINED SMEAR

The supravital stain commonly employed is *new methylene blue stain*. The RNA 'reticulum' of the reticulocytes shows up allowing them to be easily counted; therefore, this is the staining required for a *reticulocyte count*.

Note

Many laboratories will not routinely perform either supravital staining or a reticulocyte count as part of a haematological examination. Consequently, they may need to be specially requested. However, some laboratories *do* include a reticulocyte count in their usual 'haematological profile' or, if there is evidence of anaemia, will either perform it routinely or recommend that it be performed.

Counting the immature cells and the significance of abnormal numbers (usually increased numbers)

NUCLEATED RBCs

The Romanowsky-stained smear is used, and the number of nucleated RBCs is usually expressed as a percentage of the WBCs, e.g. 9 nucleated RBCs/100 WBCs, or 9%. Knowing the total WBC count would then allow the *absolute* number of nucleated RBCs to be calculated, although this is not done routinely. Since there are usually none in the blood the finding of more than an occasional cell is significant.

Increased numbers of nucleated RBCs can appear in the blood in a variety of disorders.

Severe regenerative anaemia

In most cases an increase in nucleated RBCs will be due to severe regenerative anaemia (i.e. haemorrhagic or haemolytic) in which some are released from the bone marrow and appear in the circulation together with a much greater number of reticulocytes. The reticulocytosis is the main (i.e. primary) response.

Inappropriate release

Nucleated RBCs with a non-regenerative anaemia
Nucleated RBCs (i.e. with no reticulocytes, or a disproportionately small number) occur in the blood in most myeloproliferative disorders. They are especially numerous in erythroleukaemia and erythraemic myelosis in the cat (see Panel 3.2, p. 189).

Primitive cells that *resemble* nucleated RBCs are a feature of the rare myeloproliferative disorder – reticuloendotheliosis.

Small numbers of nucleated RBCs with an apparent non-regenerative anaemia
Nucleated RBCs without an obvious reticulocytosis may also appear in the blood in:

- Hyposplenism (i.e. reduced splenic function) due to a splenic tumour, usually haemangiosarcoma.
- Severe acute infection causing bone marrow damage (i.e. in bacteraemia, septicaemia, toxaemia (endotoxic shock) and viral diseases).
- Extramedullary haemopoiesis (i.e. RBC formation outside the bone marrow) as can occur in myeloproliferative disorders and other myelophthistic disorders (in which the bone marrow is infiltrated, and replaced, by leukaemic cells, metastatic tumours or granulomatous lesions).
- Some cases of liver disease where there is an impaired bone marrow response.

Nucleated RBCs, with or without reticulocytosis, but without a corresponding (i.e. proportionate) fall in the PCV
These might indicate *chronic lead poisoning* (usually in dogs, and generally young). Any anaemia is essentially a combination of haemolytic anaemia and, especially in cats, non-regenerative anaemia, but it is not always present. Even if it is the PCV is usually >0.28 l/l (>28%).

CHECK for:
- Characteristic basophilic stippling of RBCs on a Romanowsky-stained blood smear: >1.5 stippled cells/1000 RBCs is suggestive, >4/1000 RBCs is virtually diagnostic of lead poisoning (although stippled cells, usually fewer in number, can appear as part of an intense regenerative response for other reasons, primarily immune-mediated haemolytic anaemia). When supravitally stained these stippled cells appear as reticulocytes. (Stippling shows up best on smears made from fresh blood, i.e. not anticoagulated with EDTA etc.)
- Other features on a blood smear, e.g. siderocytes (i.e. showing Pappenheimer bodies – see p. 68), leucocytosis in dogs or leucopenia in cats, neutrophilia, shift-to-the-left, and sometimes hypochromic cells and poikilocytes.

- Clinical signs of chronic lead poisoning (vomiting, diarrhoea, abdominal pain, CNS signs including blindness, weight loss).
- Raised lead levels in the plasma (dog >2.9 μmol/l (>0.06 mg/dl), cat >1.9 μmol/l (>0.4 mg/dl)) and/or a raised δ-aminolaevulinic acid level in the urine. (In the cat *urinary* lead levels are believed to be a better guide to toxic damage than blood lead levels).

Nucleated RBCs without any reticulocytes
Nucleated RBCs without reticulocytes but plus immature (band form) neutrophils (a shift-to-the-left) constitute a leucoerythroblastic reaction, which *may* occur in:

- Severe haemorrhagic or haemolytic anaemia (as an intense response).
- Disseminated haemangiosarcoma.
- Myeloproliferative disorders.

Nucleated RBCs in 'normal' animals

In small numbers, they may appear in the blood of some apparently normal Miniature Schnauzers.

HOWELL–JOLLY BODIES

If numerous these could be counted in the same way as the nucleated RBCs.
    Their numbers increase:

- In regenerative anaemia.
- With reduced splenic function, e.g. splenectomy and splenic tumour.
- Following administration of glucocorticoids in dogs.
- In macrocytosis in Poodles (see p. 59).

RETICULOCYTES

Aggregate reticulocytes *only* are counted on a supravitally stained smear. The number of reticulocytes may be expressed as:

- The reticulocyte count (most common).
- The absolute reticulocyte count.
- The reticulocyte production index (RPI).

The reticulocyte count

The reticulocytes are recorded as a *percentage of all the RBCs*.

	Normal reticulocyte count	*Count indicative of regenerative anaemia*
Dog	approx. 1%	>3–5%
Cat	(aggregate alone) approx. 0.5% (aggregate plus punctate) approx. 1.5–11%	>1.5–2%

    Increased reticulocyte counts (i.e. higher percentages) suggest the increased production of reticulocytes, *but* of course the percentage of reticulocytes will also increase as the number of mature RBCs decreases (e.g. if the number of mature RBCs is halved the percentage of reticulocytes will double). To avoid reticulocyte production *appearing* to increase faster than it really is, the absolute reticulocyte count can be used instead.

The absolute reticulocyte count

This is obtained by multiplying the percentage of reticulocytes (i.e. the reticulocyte count) by the RBC count and dividing by 100 (in the same way as absolute counts are obtained for the different types of WBC).

A significant absolute reticulocyte count in the *dog* or *cat* indicative of regenerative anaemia is $>60 \times 10^9/l$ (i.e. $>60\,000/\mu l$).

However, even this measurement may overstate the rate of reticulocyte production, since in regenerative anaemia reticulocytes are released from the bone marrow earlier and then stay longer in the blood becoming mature cells. At any one time more are in the blood. Consequently, to correct for this it is possible in the dog (but *not* in the cat in which reticulocyte kinetics are different) to calculate the reticulocyte production index.

The reticulocyte production index (RPI)

$$RPI = \frac{\text{Patient's reticulocyte count (as \%)} \times \text{Patient's PCV}}{\text{Reticulocyte maturation time (days)} \times \text{Mean normal canine PCV}}$$

The mean normal canine PCV is taken as 0.45 l/l or 45%, and the patient's PCV should be in the same units. (For Greyhounds and other breeds with a high normal PCV use 60 l/l or 60%.)

The reticulocyte maturation time, in days, varies with the patient's PCV; for a PCV of 0.45 l/l (45%) the time = 1, for 0.35 l/l (35%) = 1.5, for 0.25 l/l (25%) = 2 and for 0.15 l/l (15%) = 2.5. The RPI represents the increase in RBC production, i.e. an RPI of 4 indicates that RBCs are being produced at four times the normal rate.

- In non-regenerative anaemia RPI ≤ 2.
- In regenerative anaemia RPI >2.
- In haemolytic anaemia RPI >3.

Causes of increased reticulocyte counts

RETICULOCYTOSIS IN REGENERATIVE ANAEMIA

Reticulocytosis occurs almost solely in cases of regenerative (i.e. haemorrhagic or haemolytic) anaemia. The number of aggregate reticulocytes increases significantly in haemorrhagic and haemolytic anaemias. (Furthermore, in the cat there is a considerable increase in punctate reticulocytes in regenerative anaemias – and their numbers stay elevated for 2–4 weeks.)

> **Note**
>
> - This reticulocyte (regenerative) response is not apparent for 3 days (2–4 days) after sudden haemorrhage or haemolysis, because it takes time for increased numbers to be produced, so that a regenerative anaemia may *initially* appear to be non-regenerative.
>
> **CHECK** – to confirm the type of anaemia, repeat the reticulocyte count after at least 3 days.
>
> - Reticulocytosis reaches a peak after a week; if it persists beyond 2–3 weeks it implies further haemorrhage or haemolysis, usually the former. With continuing reticulocytosis and continuing thrombocytosis (more than 2–3 weeks), plus a continuing low total plasma protein level, suspect continuing haemorrhage.
> - Reticulocyte counts are higher in haemolytic anaemias than in haemorrhagic anaemias of comparable severity, because iron (from the haemolysed RBCs) is more readily available. Only in haemolytic anaemias is the reticulocyte production index more than 3.
> - The reticulocyte response is usually less marked in chronic anaemia, although it will be evident as soon as anaemia is detectable – i.e. there is no waiting for reticulocytes to appear as in acute anaemia.
> - The reticulocyte response is greater in the dog than in the cat.
> - The existence of a regenerative response can also be established by a bone marrow biopsy (looking for erythroid hyperplasia). Usually this is unnecessary, but in critical cases a response will be apparent there before it is seen in the blood. (See Panel 2.1, p. 75.)

RETICULOCYTOSIS IN HYPOPROLIFERATIVE ANAEMIA

A reticulocytosis *may* be seen in cases of hyproproliferative (non-regenerative) anaemia:

- If the underlying cause is corrected (assuming that to be possible).
- At times as a *poor* response (i.e. the reticulocyte count is not increased as much as would be expected for the fall in PCV), e.g. in iron deficiency anaemia, and anaemia associated with chronic liver disease or malignant neoplasia (so-called secondary anaemia).

RETICULOCYTOSIS AS A PHYSIOLOGICAL RESPONSE

This arises in:

- Pregnancy (associated with a fall in PCV), e.g. the last 3 weeks in the cat.
- The newborn: cells resembling punctate reticulocytes account for up to 50% of the RBCs in newborn kittens. In newborn puppies the reticulocyte count = 7%, falling to the adult level in the next 2–3 months.

RETICULOCYTOSIS WITH A PCV IN THE NORMAL RANGE

This reticulocytosis (i.e. without anaemia) suggests poor oxygenation of the blood, e.g. chronic lung disease.

RETICULOCYTOSIS AS RESPONSE IN LEAD POISONING

Reticulocytosis as part of an exaggerated regenerative response occurs in many cases of lead poisoning in dogs (due to the effect of lead on the bone marrow), even without obvious anaemia. Numbers of RBCs show basophilic stippling (with the usual Romanowsky staining) and, when supravitally stained, these RBCs are seen to be reticulocytes. Among other features nucleated RBCs are often present.

RETICULOCYTOSIS IN BREED-RELATED HAEMATOLOGICAL DISORDERS

Reticulocytosis also occurs in breed-related haematological disorders:.

- Cyclic haemopoiesis (Grey Collie syndrome) in Collies and Collie/Beagle cross-breds. Reticulocytosis appears approximately every 11 days, accompanied by deficiencies of neutrophils and platelets.
- Pyruvate kinase deficiency in Basenjis and Beagles.
- Stomatocytosis in *adult* Alaskan Malamutes.
- Erythropoietic porphyria in Siamese cats.

Indications of immature RBC production (chiefly reticulocytosis) from other routine haematological tests

HAEMATOCRIT (i.e. WHEN MEASURING THE PCV)

This test gives no accurate indication of the number of reticulocytes, but it can provide evidence of regeneration in that reticulocytes, being less dense than mature RBCs, mix with the lower part of the buffy coat (WBCs and platelets) and can give it a red tinge ('streaming').

When present in large numbers the reticulocytes can colour all, or most, of the buffy coat so that on superficial examination it appears to be absent or very thin. This *could* result in it being included in the RBC layer so that the PCV is read as higher than it actually is.

This effect can also be produced by abnormally high numbers of nucleated RBCs, e.g. in myeloproliferative disorders.

ESR

Again this procedure provides no accurate count of reticulocytes, but it can give evidence of regeneration, because the reticulocytes (being slow to sediment as they do not form rouleaux) produce a reddish tinge in the plasma above the main column of blood.

This effect may also be produced by large numbers of nucleated RBCs in myeloproliferative disorders.

HAEMATOLOGICAL INDICES, MCV AND MCHC

MCV

Since immature RBCs (reticulocytes and nucleated RBCs) are larger than mature RBCs (i.e. macrocytes), an appreciable increase in their numbers will raise the MCV. But if there are also large numbers of small cells, e.g. spherocytes in haemolytic anaemia or microcytic RBCs in the later stage of iron deficiency (or in Akita dogs), the MCV may be in the normal range *despite* a reticulocytosis.

MCHC

Because immature RBCs (reticulocytes and nucleated RBCs) contain relatively less haemoglobin an appreciable increase in their numbers, at the peak of a regenerative response, could slightly lower the MCHC. *But* if there is acute haemolysis the MCHC will at first *increase* (because haemoglobin free in the plasma will be included in the haemoglobin value, and will be assumed to be contained in the smaller number of intact RBCs remaining).

However, both these indices are unfortunately very subject to error (see pp. 57–66), and even to diurnal variation, and this may conceal any changes.

Neither index is as reliable as examining a stained smear, which will allow many other features to be recognized. But they do have the merit that they can be calculated when a smear has not been prepared, examined or commented on.

Hb ESTIMATION AND/OR RBC COUNT

Neither of these will provide any direct evidence of regeneration but, with the PCV, can be used to calculate the MCV and MCHC, which may show changes (see above).

Panel 2.6 Polycythaemia

Polycythaemia is an increase in the number of red blood cells. It may be either absolute or, far more commonly, merely relative.

Absolute polycythaemia

This is due to a genuine increase in the number of red blood cells, which increases the PCV and also expands the total volume of the blood. This excessive concentration of RBCs makes the mucous membranes appear markedly redder, and increases the blood viscosity causing a sluggish flow of blood with consequent tissue hypoxia. It may appear paradoxical that tissue oxygenation should be less than normal, with regard to the increased number of RBCs, but it is attributable to the greater difficulty in moving this 'thicker' blood around the body.

Absolute polycythaemia is a rare condition, recorded in only a few dogs and even fewer cats. There are two forms.

PRIMARY (POLYCYTHAEMIA VERA OR TRUE POLYCYTHAEMIA)

The underlying defect is in the bone marrow. It is considered to be an unusual 'malignancy' of the haemopoietic stem cell in the bone marrow which results in excessive and uncontrolled production of mature RBCs, i.e. it is a chronic myeloproliferative disorder (see Panel 3.2, p. 189). In at least two-thirds of cases it is accompanied by increased production of white blood cells and platelets, i.e. there is leucocytosis (especially a neutrophilia with a shift-to-the-left) and thrombocytosis.

The degree of oxygenation of the blood is normal, and erythropoietin production is either normal or, more often, reduced.

SECONDARY

RBC production by the bone marrow is stimulated by increased levels of erythropoietin, and immature RBCs may be present in the circulation. Increased numbers of white blood cells and platelets seldom arise. There are two causes:

1. The excess erythropoietin is produced by the renal tubular epithelium, as a physiological response to reduced oxygenation.
   (a) The oxygen lack can be the result of chronic pulmonary (alveolar) disease or a right-to-left cardiac shunt (principally the tetralogy of Fallot) and usually cyanosis is evident.
   (b) Polycythaemia also occurs, *without cyanosis*, at high altitudes and when the local blood flow to the kidney(s) is impaired (i.e. the renal epithelium responds to its own poor oxygenation). Mild polycythaemia without cyanosis *may also* be noted in cats with hyperthyroidism and in dogs with acromegaly, and (occasionally) with hyperadrenocorticism (Cushing's syndrome), e.g. where a bitch has excess androgen production or there is poor alveolar ventilation (however this last-named complication usually *will* result in cyanosis).
2. A neoplasm of the kidney, e.g. a renal carcinoma, autonomously secretes erythropoietin. (Possibly, as in humans, there can also be autonomous secretion by non-neoplastic renal tissue cysts and hydronephrotic kidneys, and by neoplasms of other organs.) In this type cyanosis is *not* seen.

Table 2.3 Differentiation of polycythaemia

Incidence	Type	Total protein or albumin concn (serum or plasma)	Erythropoietin concn (serum or urine)	Arterial oxygen saturation	RBC mass	Plasma volume
Rare	*Primary polycythaemia* (↑ RBC count + usually ↑ WBC count and ↑ platelet count)	N	↓ (or N)	N	↑	N (or no significant ↓)
	Secondary polycythaemia 1. Reduced oxygenation	N	↑	↓	↑	N (or no significant ↓)
	2. Inappropriate erythropoietin secretion	N	↑	N	↑	N (or no significant ↓)
Common	*Relative polycythaemia* 1. Dehydration	↑	N	N	N	↓
Common, though transient	2. Splenic contraction	N	N	N	↑	N

N = value within 'normal' reference range.
↑ = value above 'normal' reference range.
↓ = value below 'normal' reference range.

Relative polycythaemia

This is a term which can be used to describe the far more common increases in PCV that are due to either dehydration or splenic contraction.

DEHYDRATION

Dehydration reduces the plasma volume and increases the concentration of plasma protein(s) and RBCs.

SPLENIC CONTRACTION

In animals under stress, especially cats and excitable dogs, splenic contraction causes the *transient* appearance of large numbers of RBCs in the blood. However, the plasma protein levels are unchanged.

Panel 2.7 Immune-mediated blood disorders

Immune-mediated haemolytic anaemia

AUTOIMMUNE HAEMOLYTIC ANAEMIA (AIHA)

Autoantibodies, produced by an animal against its own RBCs, cause increased RBC destruction.

Autoimmune haemolytic anaemia is much more common in dogs than in cats, especially German Shepherd Dogs, Miniature Dachshunds, Irish Setters, Cocker Spaniels, Scottish Terriers, Poodles, Old English Sheepdogs and Vizslas. It is twice as common in bitches. Autoimmune haemolytic anaemia may be either primary or secondary.

Primary

Primary cases arise because of a defect in the immune mechanisms which normally allow an animal to 'tolerate' its own tissues. This type has not been proven to exist in cats; in dogs it may be initiated by a viral infection or hormonal imbalance.

Secondary

Secondary cases are associated with diseases or infectious agents which cause 'new' antigens to appear on the RBC membrane (by revealing antigens that were previously concealed, by binding haptens to the RBC membrane *or* by depositing antigen–antibody complexes on it). This is followed by the formation of an antibody to attack them. Some infectious organisms have antigens *in common* with the RBC membrane, so that antibodies formed against these organisms *also* damage the RBCs.

Diseases that are associated with autoimmune haemolytic anaemia in dogs and cats include:

- Infection with FeLV (responsible for 50–70% of feline cases of AIHA), *Haemobartonella, Babesia, Ehrlichia, Leishmania* and heartworm.
- Neoplasia, especially of lymphoid tissue (leukaemia and lymphosarcomas) and bone marrow (myeloproliferative disorders), and also haemangiosarcomas.
- Other autoimmune conditions, especially immune-mediated thrombocytopenia and systemic lupus erythematosus (SLE).

Most autoantibodies are of the IgG fraction, less commonly of IgM and very rarely of IgA (IgA antibodies are usually accompanied by IgG antibodies). These autoantibodies may cause the following changes in RBCs:

- Agglutination of RBCs in the circulation – chiefly IgM antibodies, but occasionally IgG, are responsible. RBCs are negatively charged and repel each other, but the IgM molecules are large enough to connect up adjacent RBCs. However, in albumin this negative charge is less, so the RBCs come closer together and even the smaller IgG molecules, if they are present in a high concentration, may be able to connect the RBCs producing agglutination.
- Lysis of RBCs in the circulation following the activation of complement (intravascular haemolysis). IgM antibodies are the most efficient at fixing complement.
- Phagocytosis of the RBCs by macrophages of the mononuclear phagocyte system (reticuloendothelial system), i.e. *extravascular haemolysis*. This happens primarily in the spleen but also in the liver giving rise to splenomegaly and hepatomegaly, usually with an associated lymphadenopathy. Phagocytosis happens when the RBCs are coated with an immunoglobulin that is insufficient in quantity or avidity to cause direct agglutination or lysis, and is the usual fate of RBCs when IgG is present alone.

Mostly the reaction between antigen and antibody takes place at blood heat, but with some antibodies, especially IgM, it only happens at lower temperatures (such as exist at the body's extremities in cold weather), i.e. below 30–34°C, and optimally at 4°C. Possibly this is because the relevant RBC antigen only becomes exposed at these lower temperatures. Agglutination which occurs at lower temperatures disperses again at blood heat. The antibodies involved are referred to as *warm-acting* or *cold-acting* (or simply 'warm' and 'cold') antibodies respectively, depending upon the temperature at which they act.

Most AIHA in dogs is due to IgG antibodies that bring about extravascular haemolysis (i.e. phagocytosis) at blood heat. At times more than one type of antibody is present so that there is more than one type of response.

Laboratory diagnosis of AIHA

This is based on finding one or more of the following.

Autoagglutination
Autoagglutination is the spontaneous clumping of RBCs in freshly collected blood. A drop of blood on a slide or other clean surface has a flocculent appearance. Usually this happens at blood heat, sometimes at a lower temperature. Autoagglutination occurs more often in cats than in dogs.

False positives can occur:

• What looks like agglutination *may* in fact be due to massive rouleaux formation. The best way to distinguish the two is to examine the blood microscopically; the RBCs in rouleaux are arranged like a pile of pennies that has fallen over. It is often suggested that the distinction can be made by adding physiological saline to the blood which will cause any clumping due to rouleaux to disperse. However, agglutination due to warm IgG antibodies will also disappear upon the addition of physiological saline (Slappendel, 1986).
• Some normal dogs without any other sign of haemolytic anaemia show spontaneous RBC agglutination.

Spherocytes (in a Romanowsky-stained blood smear)
Damage to the RBC membrane by complement or phagocytes allows water to pass into the RBCs and they swell, becoming more spherical. Compared with normal these RBCs appear smaller (because of their reduced diameter) and denser (i.e. without the central pallor caused by the biconcave shape). Recognition of spherocytes in cats is virtually impossible because their RBCs are normally small and dense (but they can be distinguished by testing osmotic fragility).
   Spherocytes also appear in haemolytic anaemia caused by other immune disorders (i.e. not just autoimmune), pyruvate kinase deficiency, some toxic disorders and hypophosphataemia. They are not invariably present in AIHA (Werner, 1980).

Increased osmotic fragility of RBCs
This is seen in 85% of dogs with AIHA.
   Spherocytes will rupture when suspended in a hypotonic saline solution that is not sufficiently hypotonic to rupture normal RBCs, because they are unable to take up as much water as normal cells.

Positive result to Coombs' antiglobulin test
This is also known as Coombs' test *or* antiglobulin test.
   Coombs' antiglobulin test detects the presence of antibodies against the RBCs.

• The *direct* Coombs' test (direct antiglobulin test) is the most useful test and the one that is *performed routinely*. It detects immunoglobulins or complement attached to the patient's RBCs. The blood sample must be collected in EDTA (or acid citrate dextrose=ACD) to remove, i.e. to bind, the calcium in the plasma and thereby prevent complement becoming bound to the RBCs in vitro.
• The *indirect* Coombs' test (indirect antiglobulin test) detects free antibody in the plasma but is much less sensitive and *only* used if a sample of the patient's RBCs is unavailable. The test requires a plasma or serum sample.

   To detect 'cold' antibody the tests must be performed at lower temperatures (usually 4°C).
   A positive result denotes the presence of autoantibodies; *on the RBCs* in the case of the direct test, *in the plasma/serum* in the case of the indirect test.
   False positive and false negative results can occur for a variety of reasons (the presence of * in the lists below indicate that the veterinary surgeon can help eliminate the problem):

1. *False positive reactions* are *largely* due to the presence in the test antisera of antibodies against other constituents of the patient's RBCs or plasma (i.e. in

addition to antibodies against IgG, IgM and complement), such as those against transferrin, albumin or blood group antigens etc. Such antibodies *should* be removed from the antisera (by absorption, performed by the manufacturer and/or the testing laboratory) prior to their use.

Damaged RBCs, or RBC fragments, can adsorb serum proteins onto their membranes. False positive reactions will *also* arise:

(a) following an incompatible but non-fatal blood transfusion (i.e. the first transfusion in a dog) when donor RBCs are present to which are attached the recipient's antibodies against them;*

(b) due to inadequate washing of the patient's RBCs in the test procedure to remove non-specifically bound immunoproteins;

(c) because of failure to collect blood in EDTA or ACD and thereby to avoid the binding of complement to the RBCs;*

(d) because of the presence of complement on the RBCs for other reasons, i.e. due to infections, neoplastic disease and drugs (following the formation of circulating immune complexes) – usually there is no other evidence of haemolytic anaemia;

(e) due to particulate matter, or bacterial contamination, in the antisera or sample.*

2. *False negative reactions* are probably *in the main* the result of using a single, fixed dilution of a commercial 'broad-spectrum' antiserum, i.e. one that has activity against IgG, complement *and* IgM (although often the activity against the last two is poor). Even though these immunoproteins *are* present on the patient's RBCs, too low a concentration of antiserum, or too high a concentration of antiserum ('prozone phenomenon'), will fail to produce a positive reaction. It is therefore far preferable to use *serial dilutions* of *separate specific antisera*. False negative reactions will *also* occur:

(a) where the amount of autoantibody coating the RBCs is too small to be detected;

(b) where 'cold' antibodies are present but the test has only been performed at blood heat;

(c) where IgA alone is responsible (testing for IgA is not routine);

(d) where the disease has gone into remission;

(e) where immunosuppressive drugs are used before collecting the sample – although there is evidence that corticosteroid therapy does *not* result in a negative result unless given for a long time (if ever);*

(f) where antisera are inactive, e.g. outdated or poorly stored;

(g) where antisera are not species specific, i.e. not intended for use in the dog or cat respectively.

Positive enzyme-treated RBC test (e.g. papain test)
This is stated to be more sensitive than Coombs' test, but little is known about false positive results. Where there are autoantibodies on the RBCs and in the patient's serum, but in amounts too low to cause autoagglutination or even result in a positive Coombs' antiglobulin test, they may be detected by pre-treating the RBCs with an enzyme (usually papain) to reveal more antigen sites and enhance the antigen–antibody reaction. Usually this is combined with the use of a low ionic strength solution to reduce the ionic forces around the RBCs.

RBC agglutination following incubation is a *positive* result.

DRUG-INDUCED IMMUNE-MEDIATED HAEMOLYTIC ANAEMIA

Drugs may be responsible for some cases of immune-mediated haemolytic anaemia. It is believed that, in most of these, the RBCs are damaged as 'innocent bystanders' when a reaction between a drug (or a drug metabolite) and an antibody formed against it takes place on the RBC surface. Alternatively, the drug may chemically alter the antigens of the RBC membrane, or expose previously hidden antigens, with the result that antibodies form against, and then attack, these new antigens. Such instances can only be distinguished from cases of AIHA by sophisticated tests that demonstrate the drug's involvement.

ALLOANTIBODY-INDUCED HAEMOLYTIC ANAEMIA

The blood of some individuals contains antibodies against antigens present on the RBCs of others. These alloantibodies may be either naturally present or formed as a result of previous contact with those antigens. If the antibodies are introduced into an animal possessing RBCs with those antigens the result is agglutination, haemolysis and phagocytosis of the cells.

The two main ways in which the transfer of antibodies could occur are by:

1. A blood transfusion, referred to as *incompatible* when this antibody–antigen reaction is the result.
2. The suckling of colostrum, resulting in haemolytic disease of the newborn (otherwise termed 'neonatal (iso)erythrolysis').

A significant number of cats possess natural alloantibodies (e.g. most cats with B antigens on their RBCs already possess anti-A antibodies) but dogs do not. The practical implication of this is that a dog that has not previously had a blood transfusion can probably safely receive one from any canine donor. However, dogs and cats alike will produce alloantibodies in response to:

- A previous blood transfusion (given 8–12 days beforehand).
- A vaccination which transmits the antigens.
- In the case of a pregnant animal, leakage of fetal RBCs into the mother's circulation.

An incompatible blood transfusion is the most *likely* cause of alloantibody-induced haemolytic anaemia; haemolytic disease of the newborn is very rare in small animals.

The presence of alloantibodies can be determined by cross-matching plasma and RBCs or by a direct Coombs' test, although to detect low titres (e.g. after a long interval) an indirect Coombs' test is required.

Immune-mediated thrombocytopenia (IMT)

This was previously known as idiopathic thrombocytopenic purpura (ITP). This condition is generally regarded as being synonymous with autoimmune thrombocytopenia (or autoimmune thrombocytopenic purpura) since most cases are due to *auto*antibodies.

*Allo*antibodies are insignificant as a cause in transfusion reactions and unknown in the newborn. *Drug-induced* IMT in dogs has been suspected, due to sulphonamides, phenylbutazone, digoxin and chlorpromazine.

Autoimmune thrombocytopenia is rare in cats, but is a common cause of a haemorrhagic diathesis (i.e. a tendency to bleed) in dogs. A quarter of canine cases are primary, and the remainder are associated with viral and rickettsial infections, neoplasia or other autoimmune disorders, such as systemic lupus erythematosus and autoimmune haemolytic anaemia. It appears to be twice as common in bitches, and occurs frequently in Poodles.

Autoantibody (IgG) against antigens of the platelet membrane usually provokes phagocytosis in the spleen and liver, but occasionally intravascular lysis.

Platelet loss can be exacerbated by *diminished production* resulting from autoantibodies against antigens in the membrane of the megakaryocytes within the bone marrow. With low levels of platelets ($<50 \times 10^9$/l, and especially <20–25×10^9/l), petechial haemorrhages and ecchymoses (haemorrhages more than 1 cm in diameter) can arise spontaneously.

LABORATORY DIAGNOSIS

Confirmation of autoantibodies against platelets is obtained from a positive platelet factor 3 (PF-3) test.

Platelets from a normal dog are incubated with globulin from the patient (plasma sample) and, separately, with globulin from a normal dog. A modified activated partial thromboplastin time (APTT) for both samples is compared and, if that of the patient's sample is appreciably shorter, this constitutes a positive result. This shorter time is due to platelet factor 3 (PF-3) being exposed on platelets by the autoantibodies. Thirty to 40% of cases give a false negative result.

The existence of antibodies against megakaryocytes can be established by immunofluorescent techniques on bone marrow biopsy samples.

Systemic lupus erythematosus (SLE)

This is a generalized immunological disorder and an affected animal produces antibodies (autoantibodies) against a large number of its own tissues. These vary but can include skin, muscle, myocardium and thyroid gland, as well as the RBCs, WBCs and platelets.

Damage to these blood constituents results in autoimmune haemolytic anaemia, immune-mediated leucopenia (an ill-defined disorder but one which is strongly suspected to arise as part of this disorder, even if not on its own) and immune-mediated thrombocytopenia. These three disorders arise respectively in slightly more than a third, a quarter and 10% of dogs with SLE.

Viruses are believed to be responsible for initiating the disorder, which occurs in both cats and dogs, especially Collies and Shetland Sheepdogs. Three-quarters of canine cases occur in bitches.

Among the multiple autoantibodies, antibodies against nucleic acids (especially DNA), i.e. antinuclear antibodies, are consistently present. These can result in antigen–antibody complexes being deposited in the kidney, arterioles and synovial membranes, causing respectively glomerulonephritis (with an associated proteinuria), arteritis (vasculitis) and arthritis.

LABORATORY DIAGNOSIS

Confirmation of AIHA can be obtained by the tests previously described (see pp. 126–128) especially Coombs' test, and of immune-mediated thrombocytopenia by the platelet factor 3 (PF-3) test (see p. 470).

The presence of antinuclear antibodies can be demonstrated by a positive antinuclear antibody test or finding LE cells.

Positive antinuclear antibody test (ANA test)

Sometimes, confusingly, this is called an LE test or SLE test (see below).

This is an immunofluorescent test that involves incubating dilutions of the patient's serum with sections of mouse or rat liver (as a source of DNA) and then detecting antibody binding by adding a fluorescein-labelled antiserum.

However, false positive results due to detectable levels of antinuclear antibodies may occur in:

- Some normal dogs.
- Dogs under treatment with certain drugs, such as griseofulvin, penicillin, tetracyclines, sulphonamides, procainamide and phenytoin.
- Some dogs with liver disease.
- Some dogs with lymphosarcoma.

Finding lupus erythematosus (LE) cells

The antinuclear antibodies bind to the nuclei of degenerating cells and, in the circulation, such nuclei are phagocytosed by neutrophils which in consequence appear as if they had two nuclei. These neutrophils are termed 'LE cells'.

The test involves incubating clotted blood from the patient, disrupting the clot and looking for LE cells in the buffy coat. However, 40% of canine SLE cases produce a false positive result.

In addition cases of SLE show a polyclonal hypergammaglobulinaemia, i.e. an increase in all constituents of the γ-globulin fraction of the plasma, evident on plasma electrophoresis, associated with enlargement of the lymph nodes and thymus.

Common clinical signs of SLE include polyarthritis, skin lesions (especially at mucocutaneous junctions) and pyrexia.

Chapter 3

White blood cells (WBCs)

Total white blood cell count (total WBC count)

The total WBC count is the number of WBCs of *all* types in a stated volume of blood, which in SI units is one litre.

The recommended SI units are thousand millions per litre written as $10^9/l$ (e.g. $10.4 \times 10^9/l$). Previously the total WBC count was reported in terms of $10^3/\mu l$, $10^3/mm^3$, thousand/μl or thousand/mm^3, which are all numerically equivalent to $10^9/l$ and to each other (e.g. $10.4 \times 10^3/\mu l$).

NORMAL REFERENCE RANGE (ADULTS)

Dog: $6{-}17 \times 10^9/l$ $(= 6{-}17 \times 10^3/\mu l)$. This range is lower in Greyhounds $(3.5{-}10.5 \times 10^9/l)$.
Cat: $5.5{-}19.5 \times 10^9/l$ $(= 5.5{-}19.5 \times 10^3/\mu l)$.

- An abnormally high total number of WBCs is termed 'leucocytosis'.
- An abnormally low total number of WBCs is termed 'leucopenia'.
- Panleucopenia is an abnormally low number of *all* types of WBCs (i.e. an across-the-board reduction) *but* its existence cannot be established unless *both* the total WBC count *and* the differential WBC count are performed.
- Total WBC counts outside the normal reference range are due to a change in the numbers of neutrophils and/or lymphocytes, the WBC types that contribute most to the total count (although abnormal numbers of other WBCs can accentuate the change).
- An abnormal number of the other WBCs (eosinophils, basophils or monocytes) *without* an increase or decrease in neutrophil or lymphocyte numbers will be insufficient in almost all cases to move the *total* WBC count outside the normal range.
- In general then, *leucocytosis* is due to an increased number of neutrophils and/or lymphocytes, and *leucopenia* is due to a decreased number of neutrophils (even a complete absence of lymphocytes is unlikely to reduce the total WBC count below the normal range).

AGE

Despite slight variations with age, the total WBC count value remains within the normal range. In young dogs values increase gradually as activity increases, i.e. throughout the day.

SEX

Overall there are few consistent differences; in the *cat* total counts tend to be slightly lower in females and in the *bitch* there is an increase in WBC numbers during pregnancy, e.g. to $20 \times 10^9/l$ at parturition, with a return to normal values after weaning.

COUNTING

There are three main methods of counting WBCs.

Manual haemocytometer counting

The blood is diluted and the WBCs counted on the grid of a haemocytometer counting chamber.

The accuracy is $\pm 20\%$. Dust particles and other debris, e.g. of lysed RBCs, may be counted as WBCs.

Do not use Thoma pipettes which are extremely inaccurate.

Electronic counting systems

These are used by commercial laboratories. After dilution of the blood the WBCs can be counted automatically by an electronic counter (e.g. a Coulter counter).

Usually the accuracy is $\pm 3\text{--}5\%$. Used correctly the counts are more accurate and reproducible than manual counts.

Total WBC counts on blood (usually cat blood) containing numerous (1) large platelets, (2) clumps of platelets, and/or (3) Heinz bodies clumped together, may be *falsely elevated* to an unpredictable degree because all of these features will be counted as WBCs. Similarly, dust particles in the blood may be included.

Conversely any WBC clumping or WBC fragility will result in a *falsely low* count.

Both the above methods require the use of a diluting fluid which will also lyse the RBCs; if an incorrect concentration of the chemical producing lysis is used it is possible that:

- Either RBCs could persist and falsely raise the total 'WBC' count (unlikely).
- Or WBCs could also be destroyed decreasing the total WBC count.

Destruction of WBCs can occur (despite a correct concentration of lysing agent) if they are neoplastic.

Also with both methods above, nucleated RBCs will be counted as if they were WBCs. (A correction can be made by determining the ratio of nucleated RBCs to WBCs (from examining the stained smear used for the differential WBC count) and subtracting the appropriate percentage of nucleated RBCs to obtain the *true* total WBC count.)

The QBC-V Hematology System

Essentially this sensitive method of measuring the components of the buffy coat provides an acceptable measurement of the total WBC count (see Appendix I, p. 470).

It is also possible to distinguish, and make counts of, the WBCs that comprise:

- The granulocytes (i.e. neutrophils and eosinophils).
- The non-granulocytes (i.e. lymphocytes and monocytes).

In addition it is possible to measure the platelet count and the PCV.

Note

It is important for the *correct species* to be registered on the instrument before counting so that the appropriate species coefficient is used for converting the length of tube occupied by each group of cells into the *number* of cells. If this is *not* done inaccuracies will result.

Causes of leucocytosis

Summary

- Bacterial infection
- Effect of steroids
- Lymphoproliferative disorders (lymphosarcoma and lymphoid leukaemia)
- Feline infectious peritonitis
- Tissue necrosis and severe inflammation (without infection)
- Pregnancy/parturition (bitch)
- Myeloproliferative disorders [rare]
- Systemic lupus erythematosus [rare]
- Hyperthyroidism in cats

In all cases, leucocytosis is due to neutrophilia *except* in lymphoid leukaemia (due chiefly to lymphocytosis).

Much greater diagnostic discrimination can be achieved by performing the differential WBC count as well as the total WBC count on the *same* blood sample; this allows the absolute numbers of each WBC type to be calculated. The same blood sample should be used for both counts, since WBC numbers can change rapidly. Reference can then be made to the sections between pp. 145 and 180, dealing with each WBC type in turn, for interpretation of the significance of those absolute numbers. Many conditions which increase the number of one type of WBC do not produce an overall leucocytosis. Those which *often* do include the following.

BACTERIAL INFECTION (INCREASE IN NEUTROPHILS)

Leucocytosis occurs especially if it is a localized purulent bacterial infection *but not* if there is septicaemia or toxaemia.

EFFECT OF STEROIDS

Leucocytosis is an effect of exogenous (i.e. administered) or endogenous steroids and is due to an increase in neutrophils.

The increase in the total WBC count may be slight, but a quarter of canine Cushing's syndrome cases show a leucocytosis.

LYMPHOPROLIFERATIVE DISORDERS

Lymphosarcoma

This causes an increased WBC count in 25% of cats and 40% of dogs, due primarily to neutrophils.

Lymphocytic leukaemia

This leucocytosis is due to an almost invariable increase in lymphocytes – except for most cases of acute lymphoblastic leukaemia in cats.

FELINE INFECTIOUS PERITONITIS

The leucocytosis is due to an increase in neutrophils.

TISSUE NECROSIS AND SEVERE INFLAMMATION NOT ASSOCIATED WITH INFECTION

The increased WBC count is due to an increase in neutrophils, e.g. acute pancreatitis, rheumatoid arthritis, burns, invading foreign bodies, steatitis etc. (see p. 153).

PREGNANCY/PARTURITION

In the bitch WBC numbers steadily increase from the third to the seventh week of pregnancy before declining, and then sharply increase again just before parturition to give a second short-lasting peak. Both these increases are due to mature neutrophils and, at their peaks, especially that at parturition, the numbers of total WBCs and of neutrophils may exceed the normal reference ranges (Doxey, 1966). No similar increases occur in the cat (Berman, 1974).

MYELOPROLIFERATIVE DISORDERS [RARE]

This is due to an increase in neutrophils, e.g. chronic granulocytic leukaemia and primary polycythaemia.

SYSTEMIC LUPUS ERYTHEMATOSUS

Leucocytosis can arise from a neutrophilia, although *leucopenia* is more common.

HYPERTHYROIDISM IN CATS

Any increase is due to neutrophilia.

Note

Strenuous exercise will raise the total WBC count temporarily, but certainly not enough to put it outside the normal range.

Causes of leucopenia

Summary

- Viral diseases
- Overwhelming bacterial infection
- Anaphylaxis
- Toxic drugs and chemicals
- Neoplasia of bone marrow – lymphoproliferative and myeloproliferative disorders/metastasis
- Systemic lupus erythematosus
- Acute toxoplasmosis
- Leishmaniasis (uncommon in the UK)
- Endogenous toxaemia, e.g. uraemia

Generally, leucopenia is due to neutropenia. *But*, in acute bacterial toxaemia and septicaemia, some viral diseases, acute toxoplasmosis and leishmaniasis, there is also (and occasionally *only*) lymphopenia.

Much greater diagnostic discrimination can be achieved by performing the differential WBC count as well as the total WBC count on the *same* blood sample; this allows the absolute numbers of each WBC type to be calculated. The same blood sample should be used for both counts since WBC numbers can change rapidly. Reference can then be made to the sections between pp. 145 and 180, dealing with each WBC type in turn, for interpretation of the significance of those absolute numbers.

VIRAL DISEASES

Leucopenia can be caused by viral diseases that are uncomplicated by secondary bacterial infection, for example:

- Feline infectious enteritis (FIE) (feline panleucopenia (FPL)) – decrease is in neutrophils, less often in lymphocytes.
- Feline leukaemia virus (FeLV) infection – decrease is in lymphocytes and neutrophils.
- Feline immunodeficiency virus (FIV) infection, previously known as feline T-lymphotrophic lentivirus (FTLV) infection – the decrease is slightly more common in neutrophils than in lympocytes.
- Canine distemper – often there is a decrease in lymphocytes and neutrophils.
- Infectious canine hepatitis – often a decrease in lymphocytes and neutrophils.
- Canine parvovirus infection – decrease is in lymphocytes and neutrophils.

OVERWHELMING BACTERIAL INFECTION, i.e. EARLY STAGES

Bacterial toxaemia

Endotoxins result in a decrease in lymphocytes and neutrophils (and in platelets); later there is an increase in neutrophil numbers.

Bacterial septicaemia (e.g. salmonellosis)

Toxic changes cause decreases in neutrophils and lymphocytes, together with a degenerative shift-to-the-left, giving a poor prognosis.

ANAPHYLAXIS

Leucopenia occurs because there is a decrease in neutrophils (and there also a reduction in platelets).

TOXIC DRUGS AND CHEMICALS

There is usually a decrease only in neutrophils; this can occur with oestrogen, methimazole, carbimazole, drugs for cancer therapy etc.

NEOPLASIA OF BONE MARROW

Lymphoproliferative disorders

These cause leucopenia primarily by a decrease in the neutrophils. Leucopenia occurs in 12–15% of lymphosarcomas and up to 50% of acute lymphoblastic leukaemias in the cat (but *not* in chronic lymphocytic leukaemia).

Myeloproliferative disorders

These (e.g. myelofibrosis) can act by decreasing the number of neutrophils.

Metastasis

Metastasis from elsewhere can also decrease the number of neutrophils.

SYSTEMIC LUPUS ERYTHEMATOSUS

Leucopenia is due to neutropenia without lymphopenia.

ACUTE TOXOPLASMOSIS

The effect is due to lymphopenia and (often later) neutropenia.

LEISHMANIASIS (UNCOMMON IN THE UK)

Essentially there is a lymphopenia, although all WBCs *may* be equally reduced in number (i.e. a panleucopenia).

ENDOGENOUS TOXAEMIA

This can be a cause, especially in the cat – although not common, for example, due to uraemia.

Differential white blood cell count (differential WBC count)

The differential WBC count provides information on the *relative* numbers of the different types of WBCs, including their developmental forms in the circulating blood.

In isolation the differential WBC count does not indicate whether the numbers of each type are within normal limits. To establish whether that is so it is necessary also to know the value of the *total* WBC count and to use both counts to calculate the *absolute* numbers of each type of WBC (e.g. neutrophils, lymphocytes etc.).

Absolute count of WBC type (in 10^9/l)

$$= \frac{\text{Differential count of that WBC type } (\%)}{100} \times \text{Total WBC count } (10^9\text{/l})$$

A good laboratory will calculate the absolute numbers for you.

Knowing the absolute values can avoid jumping to the wrong conclusion. For instance the WBCs in a canine blood sample might be 85% neutrophils and 10% lymphocytes. Based on 'normal' percentages (see below) there *appears* to be an increased number of neutrophils and a reduced number of lymphocytes. However, if the total WBC count is found to be 12×10^9/l the absolute numbers of both types are in fact within their respective normal ranges (10.2×10^9/l neutrophils and 1.2×10^9/l lymphocytes). However, if it should transpire that the total WBC count is 20×10^9/l, the neutrophil count is indeed high (17×10^9/l) but the lymphocyte count is within normal limits (2×10^9/l). But if the total WBC count is only 5×10^9/l the neutrophil count would fall within normal limits (4.25×10^9/l) and the low absolute lymphocyte count (0.5×10^9/l) would be the abnormal value.

Table 3.1 Normal reference range of WBCs in adults

WBC	Dog		Cat	
	%	Absolute no. ($\times 10^9$/l)	%	Absolute no. ($\times 10^9$/l)
Neutrophils				
Band forms	0–3	0–0.3	0–3	0–0.3
Adults	60–77	3–11.5	35–75	2.5–12.5
Eosinophils	2–10	0.1–1.35	2–12	0.1–1.5
Basophils	Rare	Rare	Rare	Rare
Lymphocytes	12–30	1–4.8	20–55	1.5–7
Monocytes	3–10	0.15–1.35	1–4	0.1–0.85

NORMAL REFERENCE RANGE (ADULTS)

In Greyhounds, although the total WBC range is lower compared with other breeds the percentage distribution is similar (Lording, 1983).

CHANGES IN THE ABSOLUTE NUMBER OF DIFFERENT WBCs

Expressions used for changes in the numbers of circulating WBCs are as follows.

Neutrophils (see p. 145)

Neutrophilia
This is an increase in the number of circulating neutrophils.

Neutropenia
This is a decrease in the number of circulating neutrophils.

A shift-to-the-left
This is an increase in the number of unsegmented (band form) neutrophils in the circulation (see 'Changes in the number of band form neutrophils', p. 157).

A shift-to-the-right
This is an increase in the number of neutrophils in the circulation showing hypersegmented nuclei. An increase in the number of hypersegmented neutrophils indicates that neutrophils are remaining longer in the circulation. This can be due to:

- The presence of corticosteroids (reducing the movement of neutrophils into tissues).
- A deficiency of folate or vitamin B_{12} causing a reduction in cell division.
- Leucocytosis due to neutrophilia (occasionally).

It may also arise as an *error* due to prolonged storage of a blood sample (i.e. a degenerative change).

Note

In humans, five or more lobes is the critical number, but animal neutrophils are normally less segmented and therefore a comparable shift-to-the-right does not occur.

Eosinophils (see p. 163)

Eosinophilia
This is an increase in the number of circulating eosinophils.

Eosinopenia
This is a decrease in the number of circulating eosinophils.

Basophils (see p. 169)

Basophilia
This is an increase in the number of (in practice, often the presence of *any*) circulating basophils.

Basopenia
This is strictly speaking a decrease in the number of circulating basophils but, in practice (since it is normal for *none* to be present), this term is meaningless.

Lymphocytes (see p. 171)

Lymphocytosis
This is an increase in the number of circulating lymphocytes.

Lymphopenia (or lymphocytopenia)
This is a decrease in the number of circulating lymphocytes.

Monocytes (see p. 177)

Monocytosis
This is an increase in the number of circulating monocytes.

Monocytopenia
This is a decrease in the number of circulating monocytes.

The following terms are also used.

Panleucopenia
This is a reduction in every type of WBC (see 'Causes of panleucopenia', p. 143).

Steroidal blood picture
This refers to a relative (and often absolute) increase in the number of neutrophils and (in the dog, less often in the cat) monocytes, together with a decrease in the number of eosinophils and lymphocytes; it is caused by glucocorticoids or related substances (see 'Steroidal blood picture', p. 141).

METHODS

A differential WBC count is conventionally performed by staining a blood smear with a Romanowsky stain (usually Leishman's in the UK, Wright's in North America and May–Grünwald–Giemsa in continental Europe, or a rapid commercial variant, e.g. Diff-Quick) and then examining and classifying at least 200 WBCs (although for speed often only 100 cells are examined). Larger laboratories may use instruments both to make the blood smears and to stain and dry them.

Haematology analysers are available which can differentiate WBCs (on the basis of size, staining, and the density and shape of their nuclei, e.g. using the diffraction of light and laser light) and count the number of each type. Although used increasingly in human medicine, their cost, and sometimes technical difficulties, have limited their use with canine and feline blood samples.

WBCs are classified into the types described previously with the most immature neutrophils (band neutrophils, i.e. unlobulated = unsegmented) listed independently of the more mature segmented neutrophils.

Numbers of other immature or abnormal WBCs should also be recorded separately, i.e. the *developmental forms* (Figure 3.1, p. 144 and Figure 3.3, p. 171) which are normally confined to the bone marrow, and any of the types mentioned in the section 'Abnormal WBCs and WBC inclusions' (p. 180).

OTHER INFORMATION

Examining the smear *also* gives the opportunity to observe and record the following.

Changes in size, shape and staining of the RBCs

See the section 'Abnormal RBCs and RBC inclusions' (p. 180). Examination of the RBCs will:

- Support the calculated values for the MCV and MCHC.
- Detect anisocytosis (variation in the size of the RBCs).

- Detect developmental or abnormal RBCs or RBC inclusions.
- Detect polychromasia (indicative of reticulocytes) and the formation of rouleaux etc.

Presence of blood parasites

Examination of the smear can spot the presence of blood parasites, e.g. trypanosomes or heartworm microfilariae, although some are within or on the surface of the RBCs, e.g. *Ehrlichia*, *Babesia* and the only one common in the UK, *Haemobartonella felis*.

Estimate the number of blood platelets

Examination of the smear can provide such an estimate (see p. 197–198) and discover any change in size or appearance (see 'Changes in platelet appearance', p. 203).

However, not all laboratories will routinely report these additional findings from the blood smear – this is one feature which will distinguish a good laboratory from the others.

Note

The QBC-V Hematology System, in addition to quickly providing the total WBC count, will at the same time determine the percentage and absolute number of the combined granulocytes (neutrophils plus eosinophils, usually no basophils are present) and the percentage and absolute number of the combined non-granulocytes (i.e. the lymphocytes plus monocytes). It is not possible to enumerate each WBC type entirely separately as is usual, and this rather limits the usefulness of the system. It is, however, possible to estimate the number of eosinophils in the dog when they exceed $0.1 \times 10^9/l$ and therefore, by difference, to estimate the number of neutrophils.

Nevertheless, the speed and relative cheapness of this system may make it useful as a clinical screening technique.

Errors in differential WBC counts

- 'Human' laboratories may overestimate the number of band neutrophils; their criteria of segmentation in human neutrophils is more rigid.
- Problems in staining and identification can result in confusion between eosinophils and basophils. It is as well to be aware of this and to suspect confusion when large numbers of basophils and no, or few, eosinophils are reported. Because of the attraction the basophils exert where they are present there should usually also be eosinophils.
- Mechanical blood-spreading instruments used in highly automated laboratories increase the proportion of large cells in the smear, leading to *higher differential counts for monocytes*.

STEROIDAL BLOOD PICTURE

A number of haematological changes, together constituting a 'steroidal blood picture', are attributable to glucocorticoids which are:

1. Either exogenously administered, i.e. as drugs.
2. Or endogenously *released* as in:

(a) prolonged stress (steroidal stress) which accompanies, for example, severe illness, pain or an abnormal rise or fall in body temperature;
(b) Cushing's syndrome (hyperadrenocorticism) where there is overproduction of cortisol by the adrenal glands.

The major changes in the blood include neutrophilia, eosinopenia, lymphopenia and monocytosis (although this last named is an inconsistent feature, especially in the cat). Also 'classically' the total WBC count and the RBC count are lifted into the upper half of their normal ranges (and occasionally above).

However, other factors, e.g. infection or drug usage, may modify these responses so that the total WBC count, and with it the absolute counts of each WBC type, can vary markedly, i.e. they may be either high or low. Because the absolute numbers can vary so much the presence of a steroidal blood picture is best recognized from the differential WBC count (for example in the cat the absolute number of lymphocytes is usually within the normal range, although the *percentage* of lymphocytes is *low*). This is one of the few cases where the overall blood picture is more evident from the relative, than from the absolute, WBC numbers.

All these effects listed above are most prominent in the early stages; with *long-standing* Cushing's syndrome the only consistent haematological signs in dogs are eosinopenia and lymphopenia. In the cat even these signs are not necessarily evident.

In dogs absolute eosinophil counts (indicative of the effect of steroids) should remain below 0.35×10^9/l and lymphocyte counts below 1×10^9/l. In relative terms the eosinophil count is usually 0%, sometimes 1% and very occasionally 2%. Exceptionally it could rise to 3% but a differential eosinophil count above this generally rules out Cushing's syndrome. This eosinopenia is more consistent than the lymphopenia.

The differential lymphocyte count is usually less than 15%, generally less than 12% and frequently even lower, although at times higher percentages *can* be obtained.

Note

1. The percentage eosinophil and lymphocyte counts in cats are very similar to those in dogs.
2. Drugs that have glucocorticoid effects and give the same blood picture are:
   (a) progestogens, e.g. megestrol acetate in the cat,
   (b) certain mineralocorticoids, e.g. fludrocortisone.

Anabolic steroids do not appear to produce this type of blood picture.

In the long term the effect of glucocorticoids is to increase the plasma activity of alkaline phosphatase (ALP) in 95% of dogs although *not* in cats (see p. 321). Increased cortisol production can be confirmed by finding high levels of cortisol in the blood (especially after ACTH stimulation) in both dogs and cats (see p. 403).

The administered steroid is usually *not* cortisol (e.g. prednisolone or betamethasone), but through the pituitary feedback it will depress cortisol production so that the plasma cortisol level will be abnormally low. Ideally therefore the cortisol assay should be specific for cortisol and unaffected by other steroids.

The laboratory finding of a typical steroidal blood picture can also be used:

• To bring to light steroid therapy which may have been overlooked, especially with long-acting glucocorticoids, or not revealed by the owner.
• To check on the reliability of a laboratory's results in cases where it is *known* that steroid has been given.

Note

Leucocytosis with neutrophilia, monocytosis and lymphopenia could be due to either infection (i.e. purulent inflammation), or steroids, especially where previous steroid therapy has been given. To distinguish between these two CHECK:

- The extent of the shift-to-the-left – a marked shift-to-the-left (i.e. >2% of the differential WBC count) suggests *purulent inflammation* and a high demand for phagocytes.
- The extent of the total leucocytosis – a very high total WBC count (i.e. $>25 \times 10^9/l$) suggests *purulent inflammation*.
- The eosinophil count – a differential count of 4% or more indicates *purulent inflammation*, but it may be low in *both* conditions (with steroid administration it is most often 0%).
- The history, especially evidence of pyrexia suggesting infection.

EFFECTS OF SPLENECTOMY

Following splenectomy, there appear in the blood increased numbers of:

- Leptocytes, particularly in the form of target cells (these may be reported under the blanket heading of poikilocytes (abnormally shaped RBCs)).
- Reticulocytes.
- Nucleated RBCs.
- Inclusion bodies in the RBCs, which would normally be removed by the spleen; these include Howell–Jolly bodies, Pappenheimer bodies, *Haemobartonella* (both *felis* and *canis*) and Heinz bodies (although the increase in Heinz bodies may not be apparent, in the cat, where significant numbers can normally occur).
- Leucocytes, essentially monocytes.
- Platelets due to the loss of an inhibitory factor.

Causes of panleucopenia

Summary

- Feline infectious enteritis
- Feline leukaemia virus infection
- Acute toxoplasmosis
- Leishmaniasis
- Severe acute salmonellosis
- Canine parvovirus infection
- Carbimazole/methimazole therapy (cat)

Panleucopenia refers to a reduction in every type of WBC. There will be a low total WBC count (leucopenia) but a *normal* differential WBC count. The use of the term is, however, sometimes stretched to include cases where the fall in one type is not so marked as in the rest.

Classically it accompanies feline infectious enteritis (otherwise known as feline panleucopenia because of this fact), *but* it occurs in other diseases also.

It is a feature of the following.

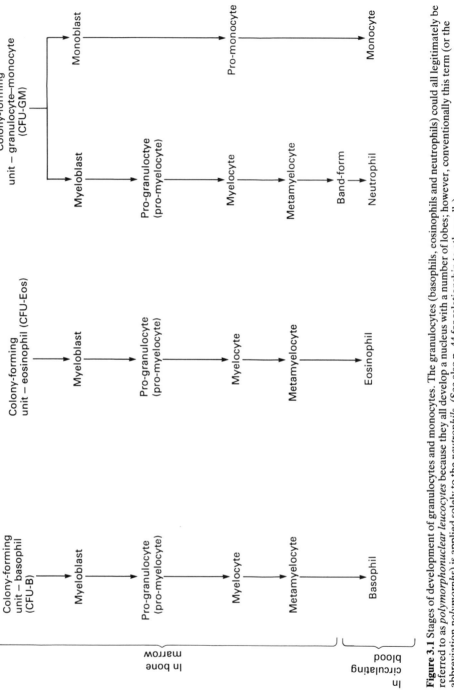

Figure 3.1 Stages of development of granulocytes and monocytes. The granulocytes (basophils, eosinophils and neutrophils) could all legitimately be referred to as *polymorphonuclear leucocytes* because they all develop a nucleus with a number of lobes; however, conventionally this term (or the abbreviation *polymorphs*) is applied solely to the *neutrophils*. (See also p. 44 for relationship to other cells)

FELINE INFECTIOUS ENTERITIS (FIE = FELINE PANLEUCOPENIA OR FPL)

There can be a rapid, extreme fall in all WBC types although a fall in lymphocyte numbers is not as common as a fall in neutrophils.

Twenty-four to 48 hours after finding a leucopenia there is usually a rebound in WBC numbers.

FELINE LEUKAEMIA VIRUS (FeLV) INFECTION

Concurrent neutropenia and lymphopenia are *more* suggestive of FeLV infection than FIE (FPL).

Leucopenia is more persistent with FeLV infection than with FIE (FPL).

ACUTE TOXOPLASMOSIS IN CATS AND DOGS

Absolute neutropenia and lymphopenia (sometimes the latter appears first) with eosinopenia, monocytopenia and a degenerative shift-to-the-left are features that persist until death in severely affected animals, but they give way to leucocytosis in recovery.

LEISHMANIASIS IN DOGS

This is only seen in imported animals in the UK.

Often, especially in severe cases (although not always), there is a leucopenia with a normal differential count; sometimes lymphopenia predominates.

SEVERE ACUTE SALMONELLOSIS IN CATS AND DOGS

This is a Gram-negative septicaemia. There is lymphopenia and neutropenia with a degenerative shift-to-the-left.

CANINE PARVOVIRUS INFECTION

Leucopenia is inconsistent; lymphopenia is more characteristic than neutropenia (the opposite finding to that in FIE) although neither is invariable. Low values may persist to death; those that survive several days tend to show leucocytosis.

CARBIMAZOLE/METHIMAZOLE THERAPY

Treatment of feline hyperthyroidism with these drugs can result in a transient leucopenia with an unaltered differential WBC count.

Neutrophils

Conventionally neutrophils are divided into:

- Adult (mature, lobulated) neutrophils, which normally comprise the vast majority – and often all of them.
- Band form (immature, unlobulated) neutrophils, normally present in very small numbers.

If a laboratory does not report the numbers of adult and band form neutrophils separately, it would generally be assumed that all of them were adult forms.

Table 3.2 White blood cell distribution in various disorders

Cause	Neutrophils		Eosinophil	Lymphocyte	Monocyte	Total WBCs	Other features
	Band	Adult					
Stress and infection							
Fear, excitement, vigorous activity = *acute* stress		±S↑UD / S↑C	Early ↑↓ / Later ↓	↑C			Especially young and healthy cats
Mild (prolonged) stress		↑	N				
Severe stress (due to pain/trauma)		↑	↓	±S↓			
Severe stress with tissue damage (feline hyperthyroidism, malignancy, poisoning, burns etc.)	±↑	↑	↓	±S↓	±↑		
Acute bacterial infection and inflammation	↑	↑			Later ↑	↑	Doesn't occur with infection at *all* body sites
Severe bacterial infection (localized purulent), e.g. pyometra	↑↑	↑↑	±↓ – ↑U	±↓	Later ↑	↑	Toxic neutrophil changes (leukaemoid reaction?)
Overwhelming bacterial infection with toxaemia	Later ↑	↓		↓		↓	Toxic neutrophil changes, ↓ platelets
Septicaemia (widespread infection)	↑ deg	± ↑ – ↓		±↓	±↑	± ↑ – →	Toxic neutrophil changes
Poor prognostic signs	↑ deg						Toxic neutrophil changes
Chronic active bacterial infection							
More chronic	±↑	↑			±↑	↑	? macrophages in blood
More active	↑				↑		Mature monocytes
Chronic infection and post-vaccine (i.e. with antigenic stimulation)				±S↑			Immunocytes
Chronic granulomatous bacterial and mycotic		↑		±↑	↑		

					Variable numbers
Canine distemper	± ↑	↓ – ↑	↓ *		↓ – ↑	
ICH Early		↓	↓		↑	
Late		↑	↑		±	
Canine parvovirus infection	± ↓	↓	± ↓ *		↓	
Canine coronavirus infection			↓		± ↓	
Feline infectious enteritis (FIE = FPL)		↓ *	↓	± ↑	↓	↓ Platelets, n-r an.
Feline infectious peritonitis	± ↑	± ↑	↓ *		↑ (↓ T)	n-r an.
Feline leukaemia virus infection		↓	Early ↓ ↓ Later ± ↑			± n-r an.
Lymphoid atrophy (canine distemper/FIE/FeLV)			↓			
Rebound (postviral infection/toxaemia)	↑	↑	↑			
Hormones and drugs						
Cushing's syndrome {D / C}	±S ↑U	↑ % / ↑ %	↓ %* / ↓ %*	↑ % / ↓ %*	↓ %* / ↓ %	± ↑ PCV / ± ↑
Steroid (glucocorticoid) admin.	±S ↑U	↑ (±C)	↑ (±C)	↓	↑ (±C)	May appear normal picture
Oestrogen toxicity including testicular tumours {Early / Late}	↑	↑ / ↓	↑ / ↑	↓	↑ / ± ↑	↑ Platelets / ↓ Platelets, n-r an.
Cancer therapy drugs	↓	↓	↓		↓	
Hypoadrenocorticism		↑ – ↓ U	± ↑ U	↑		
Megestrol acetate in cat		↓	↓			
Oestrus in bitch		± ↑	↓ %			
Other diseases						
Chronic tissue damage, especially allergic (e.g. skin, lungs etc.)	↑	↑				± ↑ Basophils

Table 3.2 (cont.)

Cause	Neutrophils Band	Neutrophils Adult	Eosinophil	Lymphocyte	Monocyte	Total WBCs	Other features
Parasitism with allergic response	±↑		↑				±↑ Basophils
Heartworm disease	↑ deg		↑				±↑ Basophils
Acute toxoplasmosis		↓		↓			
Anaphylaxis		↓		↓		↓	↓ Platelets
Immune-mediated disorders		±↑		±↓	↑		
Chronic renal failure (CRF)		↑		±↓	±↑	±↑	n-r an.
CRF + suppuration (e.g. abscess)	↑						
Lymphocytic cholangitis		↑		↓			n-r an.
Endogenous toxaemia (e.g. uraemia – long term)		↓		↓		↓	Toxic neutrophil changes, n-r an.
Lymph loss (e.g. chylothorax)				↓			
Tissue damage with phagocytosis (e.g. fractures, burns, malignancy)					↑		
Lymphoproliferative disorders							
Lymphosarcoma		↑–↓ U	↑ UC	±↓		↑–↓	±L-blasts, ±n-r an.
Acute lymphoblastic leukaemia		±↓ C		↑ UC, ↑↑ D		±↓ C, ±↑ D	n-r an., L-blasts
Chronic lymphocytic leukaemia		±↓		↑–↑↑		↑–↑↑	±n-r an.
Plasma cell myeloma		±↓		±↓		±↓	n-r an., ↓ Platelets
Myeloproliferative disorders							
Acute granulocytic leukaemia	↑	↑				↑–↓	↑↑ Dev. Ns

Condition	Changes	Special features
Chronic granulocytic leukaemia	↑ ... ↑	Dev. Ns
Eosinophilic leukaemia	↑	Dev. Es
Basophilic leukaemia	↑	↑ Basophils + Dev. Bs
Monocytic leukaemia	↑	Dev. Ms
Myelomonocytic leukaemia	↑↑ ↑	Dev. Ns and Ms
Primary polycythaemia	±↑ ±↑	↑↑ PCV
Mast cell leukaemia		Mast cells in blood
Myelofibrosis or metastasis to bone marrow	↓ ↓	
Rare disorders		
Canine granulopathy syndrome	↑ ±↑ ↑	
Leucoerythroblastic reaction	↑	
Pelger–Huët anomaly	↑↑	
Autoimmune neutropenia (e.g. in SLE)	↓	
Cyclic haemopoiesis (D)	↓ S↑ – ↓	
Myelokathexis	↓	
Disseminated eosinophilic disease	↑	
Inherited cell-mediated immunodeficiency	↓	
Radiation damage	↓ ↓	

↑ = increase, S ↑ = slight increase.
↑↑ = marked increase, ↑ deg = degenerative shift-to-the-left.
↓ = decrease, S ↓ = slight decrease.
↑% or ↓% = increase or decrease in percentage count.
± = variable sign, U unusual sign, T = terminal case.

* = most consistent feature(s).
C = in cat, D = in dog.
n-r an. = non-regenerative anaemia (= hypoproliferative anaemia).
L-blasts = lymphoblasts.
PCV = packed cell volume.
SLE = systemic lupus erythematosus.

Dev. Ns, Es, Bs and Ms = developmental neutrophils, eosinophils, basophils and monocytes, respectively.

Bear in mind that these basic changes may be modified by other factors.

Earlier developmental forms (e.g. metamyelocytes or earlier; see Figure 3.1, p. 144) are not found in the circulation of healthy individuals and indicate either a profound response to severe infection (leukaemoid response) or a myeloproliferative disorder (see Panel 3.2, p. 189).

NORMAL REFERENCE RANGES

Dog

- Adult neutrophils = $3–11.5 \times 10^9/l$ ($3–11.5$ thousand/µl or mm^3).
- Band neutrophils = $0–0.3 \times 10^9/l$ ($0–0.3$ thousand/µl or mm^3, i.e. $0–300$/µl).

In Greyhounds values are lower:

- Adult neutrophils = $2–6.5 \times 10^9/l$.
- Band neutrophils = $0–0.1 \times 10^9/l$.

Cat

- Adult neutrophils = $2.5–12.5 \times 10^9/l$ ($2.5–12.5$ thousand/µl or mm^3).
- Band neutrophils = $0–0.3 \times 10^9/l$ ($0–0.03$ thousand/µl or mm^3, i.e. $0–300$/µl).

Neutrophils in the body are those:

- In the circulation (circulating pool).
- Marginated along the walls of the capillaries, i.e. adherent to the endothelium, mainly in the lungs and to some extent in the liver and spleen (marginal pool).
- Stored in the bone marrow after production, before their release into the marginal and circulating pools.

There is constant interchange between the first two pools; in the dog each contains roughly equal numbers – in the cat 30% are in the circulating and 70% in the marginal pool (Figure 3.2).

The main function of neutrophils is to destroy and phagocytose invading micro-organisms.

INCREASED NEUTROPHIL NUMBERS

Increased neutrophil numbers in the blood (neutrophilia) occur in the presence of:

- Inflammation (especially due to acute bacterial infection).
- Glucocorticoids (endogenous or exogenous).
- Adrenaline (epinephrine).
- Certain myeloproliferative disorders (unregulated bone marrow production). See 'Causes of neutrophilia', p. 152.

This increased tissue demand for neutrophils is answered by moving cells to the tissues from the marginal and circulating pools and then from the marrow's storage pool. If these responses are inadequate then there occurs increased bone marrow production and release of neutrophils which results in more band form neutrophils being introduced into the circulation (a shift-to-the-left) and, if the high demand persists, it is met by the appearance in the blood of an increasing number of progressively immature neutrophils from the bone marrow. The number of neutrophils in the circulation is dependent on the balance between production and

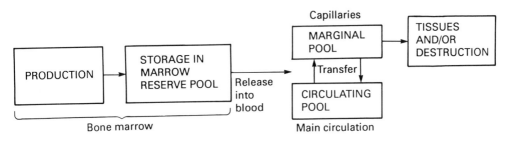

Figure 3.2 Sites of neutrophils

usage. If the production and release from the bone marrow cannot keep pace with utilization by the tissues, neutropenia (not neutrophilia) will result. Associated with this neutropenia, however, there will be an increased proportion of band forms, usually more than 10% of all neutrophils. Consequently in purulent inflammation, the number of neutrophils *can* range from very high to very low.

Increased numbers of *band forms* in the blood (shift-to-the-left) occur when there is a demand for neutrophils, *but* the number in the bone marrow pool is depleted. Band forms then tend to pass straight from the site of production into the circulating and marginal pools. (See 'Changes in the number of band neutrophils', p. 157.)

DECREASED NEUTROPHIL NUMBERS

Decreased neutrophil numbers in the blood (neutropenia) occur principally with:

- Overwhelming tissue demand for neutrophils to combat infection, that cannot be met fast enough.
- Decreased production by bone marrow due to damage by drugs, chemicals, toxins and neoplasia.

Much rarer conditions can also be responsible:

- Destruction of neutrophils in the circulation by antibodies.
- Anaphylactic shock.

See 'Causes of neutropenia', p. 160.

Causes of neutrophilia

Summary

- Physiological – fear/excitement/strenuous exertion (mild neutrophilia)
- Glucocorticoid (or ACTH) administration (moderate neutrophilia)
- Hyperadrenocorticism (Cushing's syndrome)
- Severe chronic stress, necrosis and inflammation *not* due to infection
- Hyperthyroidism (especially cat)
- Infection, principally acute (especially bacterial) but also chronic
- Severe haemolytic or haemorrhagic anaemia
- Rebound neutrophilia
- Chronic granulocytic leukaemia [rare]
- Acute granulocytic leukaemia
- Myelomonocytic leukaemia [rare]
- Primary polycythaemia [rare]
- Oestrogen toxicity
- Canine granulopathy syndrome [very rare]
- Lymphoproliferative disorders
- Systemic lupus erythematosus [rare]
- Pregnancy (bitch)
- Anabolic steroids

Neutrophilia is an increase in the number of circulating neutrophils.

PHYSIOLOGICAL NEUTROPHILIA (PSEUDONEUTROPHILIA) [MILD]

This is the result of adrenaline release which causes a mild, transient redistribution of neutrophils from the marginal pool to the circulating pool, lasting about 30 minutes. There is no increase in neutrophil production or release from the bone marrow and no shift-to-the-left.

It can be triggered by *fear* and *excitement* and by *violent muscular activity*, e.g. in racing Greyhounds. Consequently, it may be associated with the *restraint* and sometimes the struggle involved in collecting a blood sample.

This response is unusual in dogs but common in cats, especially young and healthy individuals. It occurs less often in animals that are ill.

Because adrenaline release occurs with strenuous muscular activity, this effect is seen in association with convulsions and paroxysmal tachycardia. It also follows an injection of adrenaline.

The number of neutrophils rises but not tremendously, and therefore it may be in the upper part of the *normal* range or just above the normal range. In cats, although not in dogs, it is usually accompanied by an increase in the number of lymphocytes which can be *greater*. In making the decision about whether fear/excitement is the cause in cats, therefore look particularly at the lymphocyte count, which will be *elevated*.

ADMINISTRATION OF CORTICOSTEROIDS (i.e. GLUCOCORTICOIDS) OR ACTH [MODERATE]

Their administration causes a moderate neutrophilia, especially in dogs. It is accompanied by an eosinopenia, lymphopenia and monocytosis. This response is seen less often in cats and monocytosis is the effect least likely to occur.

The peak effect is seen 4–6 hours after a single injection, returning to previous WBC levels 24 hours later.

With *short* courses of treatment the effect will persist for longer after the last dose, i.e. 2–3 days or more.

With long-term treatment the neutrophilia persists but is of lesser degree.

The effect on the *total* WBC count is usually to place it in either the upper part of the normal range or just above it. (Generally, total WBC counts are no more than $20–25 \times 10^9/l$ with a maximum figure of $40 \times 10^9/l$ in dogs and $30 \times 10^9/l$ in cats.)

Neutrophils are released from the bone marrow pool at an increased rate and go into the circulation; the number in the marginal pool remains constant. Also the rate at which neutrophils leave the circulation for the tissues is reduced and this increased intravascular survival results in the appearance of neutrophils with hypersegmented nuclei, i.e. with more lobes than normal.

There is usually no shift-to-the-left but a slight shift-to-the-left can occur if the storage pool is depleted at the time and cells need to be replaced directly by the bone marrow.

CUSHING'S SYNDROME (HYPERADRENOCORTICISM)

The same effect as described above is produced by endogenous glucocorticoid, which is chiefly cortisol. Because the disorder is generally present for some long time before the animal is first presented, the neutrophilia is generally less pronounced, although the eosinopenia, lymphopenia and, to a lesser extent, the monocytosis are obvious and very valuable diagnostically (see Panel 8.2, p. 401).

SEVERE CHRONIC STRESS, TISSUE NECROSIS AND INFLAMMATION NOT ASSOCIATED WITH INFECTION

Chronic stress

Chronic stress, e.g. due to pain and extremes of body temperature (very high or very low), stimulates the release of endogenous corticosteroids producing neutrophilia, usually with no, or a very slight, shift-to-the-left. There may be little reduction in eosinophil numbers.

Tissue damage

Such damage, from a variety of causes, results in neutrophilia, often with a modest regenerative shift-to-the-left.

Consequently neutrophilia, usually with a shift-to-the-left, is a feature of conditions where there is significant damage to organs and tissues generally not involving infection, such as:

- Severe burns.
- Acute pancreatitis.
- Foreign bodies invading tissues.
- Feline urological syndrome (FUS).
- Poisoning with a variety of chemicals and drugs, notably lead.
- Steatitis.
- Metabolic toxins, e.g. associated with uraemia (in renal failure) and ketoacidosis in diabetes mellitus.
- Malignant neoplasia, especially of the liver, gastrointestinal tract and bone marrow, and mammary tumours where there is necrosis.
- Tetanus *due to the wounds* rather than the bacterial infection.
- Rheumatoid arthritis.
- Immediately after surgery, i.e. in the first 12–36 hours.

IN HYPERTHYROIDISM

There are varying degrees of neutrophilia and shift-to-the-left, plus lymphopenia and eosinopenia, particularly in the cat. This is almost certainly a 'steroidal' stress response due to the release of endogenous glucocorticoids.

INFECTION [COMMON]

Acute infection chiefly bacterial, causing acute inflammation

Generally it is *acute bacterial infections*, especially with pyogenic bacteria (streptococci, staphylococci, pasteurellae, *E. coli*) which result in neutrophilia, with or without a shift-to-the-left depending on their severity. It is also a feature of acute leptospirosis and sometimes of feline pneumonitis.

The increased demand for neutrophils in the tissues (purulent inflammation) depletes the bone marrow storage (reserve) pool and stimulates increased neutrophil production and replacement, so that numbers of immature (band) neutrophils appear in the circulating blood.

Neutrophilia is *not* a usual feature of uncomplicated acute viral infections, although it is seen with feline infectious peritonitis and some milder cases of neonatal canine herpes virus infection. It is, however, seen when secondary bacterial infection follows viral infection.

A *mild infection* will result in a modest neutrophilia (around $11-12 \times 10^9$/l, i.e. near the upper limit of normal) and *possibly* a slight shift-to-the-left (i.e. band forms slightly above 0.3×10^9/l).

With increasingly severe infection, the magnitude of the neutrophilia and shift-to-the-left increases (i.e. $>1 \times 10^9$/l band forms). As the associated stress becomes more marked, causing cortisol release, eosinophil and lymphocyte numbers are progressively reduced, i.e. the neutrophilia is in part a response to the bacterial infection and in part due to stress.

A severe infection, e.g. in pyometra, can result in a very marked neutrophilia and shift-to-the-left, together with toxic changes in the neutrophils (i.e. vacuolation and basophilia, and occasionally neutrophils with two nuclei signifying failure of cell division). (See 'Abnormal WBCs and WBC inclusions', p. 180).

Prominent toxic changes signify a poor prognosis.

In dogs and cats neutrophil counts usually remain below 30×10^9/l but it is not uncommon for them to reach 50×10^9/l or even higher, especially in the dog.

A greater shift-to-the-left indicates a more severe infection.

Localized bacterial infection with pus formation, especially internally, e.g. in pyometra (especially chronic), pyothorax, empyema, pyelonephritis, endocarditis and abscessation prior to encapsulation, increases the degree of neutrophilia and the shift-to-the-left. Compared to generalized infections neutrophil counts can be extremely high. Certain other points are worth noting:

- After abscesses are encapsulated neutrophil counts fall from these very high levels.
- Surgical removal of the site of localized pus formation produces a temporary rise in neutrophil numbers until the bone marrow stimulus subsides.
- During recovery and convalescence all values are restored to normal, i.e. the number of neutrophils falls from its previously high level, the shift-to-the-left subsides and lymphocyte and eosinophil numbers rise to normal levels.

Note

1. In serious or widespread infection, e.g. septicaemia, there may be neutrophilia *or no rise* in neutrophil numbers. Often a degenerative shift-to-the-left occurs (more band forms than adult neutrophils) which is a poor prognostic sign, especially if associated with a leucopenia.
2. Neutrophilia is *not* a usual feature of bacterial infection and inflammation in certain areas of the body, e.g. it is generally *not* seen in cases of bacterial cystitis, enteritis, dermatitis, or tracheobronchitis.

   Therefore neutrophilia is not usually of any use in diagnosing these conditions.
3. *Developmental neutrophils* may appear in the circulation when the demand for neutrophils is very great and cannot be met by the bone marrow. Consequently, as well as large numbers of adult neutrophils and band forms, there may be metamyelocytes, myelocytes and even progranulocytes and myeloblasts. This is regarded as an extreme form of regenerative left shift.

   This temporary blood picture *resembles* granulocytic leukaemia (see Panel 3.2, p. 189), and is consequently termed a 'leukaemoid reaction'.

   Characteristic distinguishing features indicating it is *not* in fact leukaemia are:
   (a) toxic changes in the neutrophils,
   (b) the absence of anaemia,
   (c) the absence of thrombocytopenia.
   The ultimate distinction can be made by bone marrow biopsy.
4. The number of neutrophils in the circulation is dependent on the balance between production and usage. If the production and release from the bone marrow is unable to keep pace with utilization by the tissues, *neutropenia*, not neutrophilia, will result. Associated with this neutropenia, however, there will be an increased proportion of band forms, usually more than 10% of all the neutrophils. Consequently, in purulent inflammation the number of neutrophils can range from very high to very low.

Chronic infection

With chronic bacterial infection (resulting in chronic purulent inflammation) there are fewer band forms (i.e. less of a shift-to-the-left or even none at all). This is because the bone marrow's production of neutrophils is eventually able to catch up with, and even to exceed, the demand from the tissues. Consequently the number of neutrophils in the bone marrow storage pool is restored to normal and there is no longer any need to release immature neutrophils into the circulation. Leucocytosis persists, however.

The presence of *hypersegmented* neutrophils, often with slightly reduced neutrophil numbers, indicates a long-standing purulent infection. The chronic nature of the condition will invariably be confirmed by an accompanying *monocytosis*, especially if there are some immature monocytes.

Neutrophilia and monocytosis are features of the chronic granulomatous bacterial infections, actinomycosis and nocardiosis, and similar deep mycotic infections – blastomycosis, histoplasmosis, coccidioidomycosis and zygomycosis.

SEVERE HAEMOLYTIC OR HAEMORRHAGIC ANAEMIA

As part of an intense regenerative response to the bone marrow, in these types of anaemia there is often increased WBC production including a neutrophilia with varying degrees of shift-to-the-left.

REBOUND NEUTROPHILIA

Recovery following a *neutropenia* due to viral infection (e.g. feline panleucopenia (feline infectious enteritis) and infectious canine hepatitis) or bacterial endotoxaemia or septicaemia produces a neutrophilia with a shift-to-the-left.

CHRONIC GRANULOCYTIC LEUKAEMIA (CHRONIC MYELOGENOUS LEUKAEMIA, CHRONIC MYELOID LEUKAEMIA) [RARE]

The features of leucocytosis, neutrophilia and a shift-to-the-left, plus small numbers of early developmental forms of neutrophils, strongly resemble the picture that can be found in severe bacterial infection (i.e. they resemble a leukaemoid reaction).

Diagnostically it is useful that this disorder is usually associated with a modest anaemia and a variable number of platelets. In general the shift-to-the-left is uneven, i.e. the most immature forms are not necessarily the least numerous.

Bone marrow biopsy will usually distinguish the disorder.

ACUTE GRANULOCYTIC LEUKAEMIA

This myeloproliferative disorder is unlikely to be confused with other causes of a high neutrophil count because the majority of the 'neutrophils' are early developmental forms, often with myeloblasts or progranulocytes predominating. Although the total WBC count may be increased it may also be normal or decreased. (See Panel 3.2, p. 189).

MYELOMONOCYTIC LEUKAEMIA [RARE]

This shows neutrophilia and monocytosis plus early developmental stages of the granulocyte and monocyte series.

PRIMARY POLYCYTHAEMIA [RARE]

At least two-thirds of cases in the dog show a leucocytosis, particularly a neutrophilia, often with a shift-to-the-left and an accompanying thrombocytosis. This implies a defect in the totipotential stem cell. However, neutrophilia is seldom a feature of secondary polycythaemia.

OESTROGEN TOXICITY

In the dog the continued excessive administration of oestrogen, or excessive oestrogen production (e.g. by a testicular neoplasm – Sertoli cell tumour or interstitial cell tumour), initially stimulates bone marrow production of neutrophils (peaking after 3 weeks and with a shift-to-the-left) and platelets (peaking after 1 week) accompanied by a lymphocytosis and monocytosis.

Then, as the bone marrow is progressively damaged these changes give way to neutropenia, thrombocytopenia and non-regenerative anaemia. Long-term permanent bone marrow damage can result.

In oestrus, in bitches, the WBC count can rise slightly due to neutrophilia but without a shift-to-the-left, and does not go above the upper limit of the normal reference range.

CANINE GRANULOPATHY SYNDROME, e.g. IN IRISH SETTERS [VERY RARE]

Defective phagocytic activity results in significant neutrophilia, regenerative shift-to-the-left and recurrent attacks of pyrexia. There may be an associated monocytosis as the monocytes assume the neutrophils' phagocytic role.

LYMPHOPROLIFERATIVE DISORDERS

Neutrophilia is seen in 25% of cats and 40% of dogs with lymphosarcomas, in association with other typical signs (see Table 3.4, p. 184).

It can also occur in lymphocytic leukaemia, particularly acute lymphoblastic leukaemia in the cat (and accompanied by an overwhelming lymphocytosis) and chronic lymphocytic leukaemia in the dog.

SYSTEMIC LUPUS ERYTHEMATOSUS

However, leucopenia is more usual.

IN PREGNANCY

The number of mature neutrophils (without a shift-to-the-left) rises in pregnancy in the *bitch* from the third week onwards. After the seventh week there is a slight decline which soon reverses to reach a peak around parturition (12–15 × 10^9/l on average).

Neutrophil numbers return to pre-pregnancy levels 2–5 weeks after whelping.

A similar rise does not occur in the cat.

ANABOLIC STEROIDS

These may produce a mild neutrophilia.

Changes in the number of band form (immature) neutrophils

Summary

Regenerative shift-to-the-left
- Infection, chiefly bacterial, usually acute [common]
- Tissue damage and non-infectious inflammation
- Regenerative anaemia (haemorrhagic or haemolytic)
- Rebound neutrophilia
- Primary polycythaemia [very rare]
- Dirofilariasis [variable] (not in the UK)

Degenerative shift-to-the-left
- Septicaemia [common]
- Acute toxoplasmosis

Small numbers of band form neutrophils (<0.3 × 10^9/l) are often found in canine and feline blood. 'Human' laboratories may overestimate the number of band neutrophils; their criteria for segmentation can be more rigid.

The presence of *no band forms* is perfectly normal and therefore has no significance.

Increased numbers of band forms (and other immature forms) constitutes a *shift-to-the-left* (left shift). The term derives from the early convention of recording in a series of columns the number of lobes in each neutrophil counted. The column for recording unlobulated neutrophils was on the left-hand side, with the result that a large number of such cells 'shifted' the count to the left.

A shift-to-the-left reflects an increased demand for neutrophils. If the bone marrow is able to meet that demand a *regenerative* shift-to-the-left occurs, the most usual type, but if it cannot do so a *degenerative* shift-to-the-left results.

REGENERATIVE SHIFT-TO-THE-LEFT (REGENERATIVE LEFT SHIFT = APPROPRIATE SHIFT-TO-THE-LEFT)

Characteristically:

- There is a leucocytosis due to a neutrophilia.
- The number of mature (adult) neutrophils *exceeds* the number of immature forms, unless there are exceptionally large numbers of early developmental forms.
- Earlier developmental forms of neutrophils (metamyelocytes and even myelocytes and progranulocytes; very rarely myeloblasts) may appear in the circulating blood when the demand for neutrophils is very great, e.g. frequently in pyometra. This is termed a 'leukaemoid reaction' (see Panel 3.2, p. 189).
- If there are earlier developmental forms present the number of each type *progressively increases* from the most immature to the most mature, i.e. their numbers increase in the normal sequence of maturation.

Causes

A regenerative shift-to-the-left is seen in association with the following.

Infection [common]
This is chiefly bacterial, *especially* if severe, acute and localized.
The shift-to-the-left subsides in:

- Chronic bacterial infections.
- During recovery and convalescence.

A leukaemoid reaction can occur with exceptionally high demand for neutrophils.

Tissue damage and non-infectious inflammation [common]

Regenerative anaemia (haemorrhagic or haemolytic)

Rebound neutrophilia

Primary polycythaemia (i.e. polycythaemia vera) [very rare]

Heartworm disease (dirofilariasis)
This produces a variable shift-to-the-left.

A regenerative shift-to-the-left should be *distinguished from* the following conditions:

- Chronic granulocytic leukaemia, looking very like a leukaemoid reaction.
- Leucoerythroblastic reaction. A large number of immature neutrophils (including developmental forms) together with nucleated RBCs and only a very small number

of recticulocytes, or none at all, indicates a leucoerythroblastic reaction. The total WBC count can range from low (leucopenia) to slightly raised (leucocytosis). If there is an anaemia present it is referred to as a leucoerythroblastic anaemia. In dogs and cats this condition arises in association with certain myeloproliferative disorders (see Panel 3.2, p. 189).

Note

A left shift with otherwise normal differential and total WBC count may be seen in cases of leishmaniasis.

- Acute granulocytic leukaemia with increased WBCs (a common myeloproliferative disorder).
- Pelger–Huët anomaly – this extremely rare disorder of the dog and cat is an inherited failure of the nuclei of neutrophils (and also eosinophils) to mature to the normal segmented form. Consequently, a left shift *always* appears to be present. An acquired case of Pelger–Huët anomaly was recorded in a dog following chemotherapy.

A shift-to-the-left is usually *not* associated with the neutrophilia due to:

- Physiological leucocytosis associated with adrenaline release (fear, excitement etc.).
- Corticosteroid administration or release, i.e. due to stress or Cushing's syndrome, although a shift-to-the-left may occur at times.

DEGENERATIVE SHIFT-TO-THE-LEFT (DEGENERATIVE SHIFT = INAPPROPRIATE SHIFT-TO-THE-LEFT)

In this type:

- The number of *immature neutrophils exceeds* the number of mature neutrophils.
- Usually there is a leucopenia. At times, however, the number of WBCs is normal, or on rare occasions there is a leucocytosis.

Causes

A degenerative shift-to-the-left is seen in association with the following.

Septicaemia [common]
It is associated with toxic signs, e.g. vacuolation, basophilia and occasionally double nuclei.

In recovery and convalescence a *regenerative* left shift develops and toxic changes are less pronounced.

Acute toxoplasmosis, with neutropenia and lymphopenia

A degenerative shift-to-the-left should be distinguished from:

- A leucoerythroblastic reaction (see above), especially when the total WBC count is low.
- Acute granulocytic leukaemia, especially when the total WBC count is low.
- Pelger–Huët anomaly (see above).

Causes of neutropenia

Summary

Infection [common]
- Overwhelming bacterial, acute and chronic
- Viral
- Protozoal (acute systemic toxoplasmosis)

Autoimmunity – systemic lupus erythematosus
Toxic drugs and chemicals
Radiation
Testicular tumours
Anaphylactic shock
Endogenous toxaemia, e.g. uraemia
Neoplasia/necrosis of bone marrow
Lymphoproliferative disorders [rare]
Cyclic haemopoiesis [rare]
Myelokathexis [highly improbable]

Neutropenia is a decrease in the number of circulating neutrophils.

INFECTION [COMMON]

Infection can cause increased utilization and/or destruction of neutrophils in the tissues and an inability to replace them. This is the most common cause of neutropenia in dogs and cats.

Overwhelming bacterial infection

Neutropenia is often associated with overwhelming bacterial infection.

Acute bacterial infection in the early stages
Neutrophils can leave the circulation for the tissues faster than they can be replaced from the bone marrow storage pool which consequently becomes depleted. This is particularly a feature of purulent infections due to Gram-negative bacteria affecting the lungs (e.g. inhalation pneumonia), thorax (e.g. pyothorax), uterus (e.g. acute metritis) or peritoneal cavity (e.g. intestinal rupture and intussusception); it is also a feature where an abscess ruptures into a body cavity.

It also occurs in association with bacterial endotoxaemia and overwhelming septicaemia, e.g. in acute salmonellosis. Endotoxins of Gram-negative bacteria (*E. coli*, salmonellae) cause a neutropenia (because neutrophils are shifted from the circulating to the marginal pool and adhere to the endothelium for longer), together with a lymphopenia (and consequently a leucopenia) and a thrombocytopenia, followed later by a rebound neutrophilia with a shift-to-the-left.

It is especially likely to occur in individuals that are poorly nourished or have been treated with drugs that depress bone marrow activity.

Bone marrow production is stimulated within 1–2 days and immature neutrophils appear in the circulation, usually showing toxic changes (i.e. vacuolation and basophilia). If, in association with the neutropenia, less than 10% of the neutrophils are immature (band) forms it establishes the high requirement for neutrophils.

Generally neutrophil levels are restored and a *neutrophilia* develops within 3–4 days.

Chronic bacterial infection

Continuing high tissue demands that cannot be met by the bone marrow can result in bone marrow exhaustion.

Neutropenia is seen in chronic ehrlichiosis (not in the UK) – a pancytopenic disease.

Viral infections

Neutropenia commonly occurs due to reduced bone marrow production (i.e. due to damage to bone marrow precursors) especially in:

- Feline panleucopenia (FPL)(feline infectious enteritis (FIE)) as part of the generalized leucopenia.
- Feline leukaemia virus (FeLV) infection. Around half of those cats infected, but without evidence of leukaemia, show neutropenia, often in association with a non-regenerative anaemia and the clinical signs of anorexia, depression and pyrexia. In some the bone marrow is hypoplastic; these cases often show clinical signs that mimic feline panleucopenia. In other cases the bone marrow is hyperplastic and may represent subleukaemic granulocytic leukaemia (or 'pre-leukaemia').
- Feline immunodeficiency virus (FIV) infection (previously termed 'FTLV infection'), in about 40% of cases.
- As a transient feature of canine parvovirus infection.
- Neonatal canine herpes virus infection, where puppies are severely affected.

Often there are also low or *low–normal* neutrophil numbers in uncomplicated cases of canine distemper and infectious canine hepatitis, i.e. those without secondary bacterial infection (e.g. neutropenia occurs in approximately one in eight dogs with canine distemper).

Protozoal infections

In acute systemic toxoplasmosis, neutropenia plus a degenerative shift-to- the-left and lymphopenia is a feature.

AUTOIMMUNE NEUTROPENIA

Destruction of the neutrophils occurs due to the presence of antibodies against them. This disorder is believed to occur as one component of systemic lupus erythematosus, and *possibly* also arises on its own (see Panel 2.7, p. 125).

TOXIC DRUGS AND CHEMICALS

Drugs and chemicals can damage the bone marrow causing neutropenia, usually after repeated/prolonged exposure, and include the following.

Oestrogens

Continued excessive administration initially causes a neutrophilia and shift-to-the-left peaking after approximately 3 weeks, and accompanied by thrombocytosis (peaking after 1 week), lymphocytosis and monocytosis. Then, as the bone marrow is damaged, this blood picture gives way to one of increasingly severe neutropenia, thrombocytopenia and non-regenerative anaemia. In the long term, permanent bone marrow damage is caused.

Cytotoxic drugs

Drugs used in cancer therapy, e.g. vincristine, cause neutropenia. If given for only a short time the bone marrow may recover; long term, there may be irreversible damage.

Phenylbutazone

Neutropenia results if given to dogs in high dosage for a long period – in rare cases it produces agranulocytosis.

Other drugs

A number of other drugs can result in neutropenia in humans, but this ability is not well established in the dog and the cat, although most probably they would produce problems in cats. For example, sulphonamides (and others that compete for folic acid), propylthiouracil, and methimazole and carbimazole (used to treat hyperthyroidism in cats), phenytoin, chlorpromazine and other phenothiazine derivatives, chloramphenicol, ristocetin, novobiocin, nitrofurantoin, metronidazole, ethacrynic acid, procainamide, dapsone and gold salts etc.

RADIATION

Ionizing radiation damages the bone marrow and may produce neutropenia.

TESTICULAR TUMOURS

Testicular tumours secreting excessive amounts of oestrogen (Sertoli cell and interstitial cell tumours) can cause neutropenia as described for oestrogen toxicity above.

ANAPHYLACTIC SHOCK

Neutropenia and thrombocytopenia commonly accompany anaphylaxis.

ENDOGENOUS TOXAEMIA

Neutropenia (due to depression of the bone marrow) *can* result from toxic disorders, particularly in the cat, including long-term uraemia. The production of all WBC types is depressed giving leucopenia. The neutrophils show toxic change (increased size, bizarre nuclear patterns, vacuolation and cytoplasmic basophilia).

NEOPLASIA AND/OR NECROSIS OF THE BONE MARROW

Haemopoietic tissue is replaced by non-functional tissue resulting in reduced granulopoiesis.

Myelofibrosis

In this chronic myeloproliferative disorder, often the end-stage of some *other* myeloproliferative disorder (e.g. erythroleukaemia in cats), there is replacement by fibrous tissue and collagen.

Metastasis

There may be metastasis from a primary malignant neoplasm elsewhere.

LYMPHOPROLIFERATIVE DISORDERS [RARE]

Neutropenia is seen in 12–15% of lymphosarcoma cases in the dog and cat. It is most likely to arise with lymphocytic leukaemia following infiltration of the bone marrow (i.e. see above). It is a feature of up to half the cases of acute lymphoblastic leukaemia in the cat.

CYCLIC HAEMOPOIESIS (CANINE NEUTROPENIA) [RARE]

This autosomal recessive condition occurs in silver–grey Collies. Two-thirds of pups die at birth or within 1 week. In those that survive, recurrent episodes of neutropenia occur throughout life with the first apparent within 2 weeks of birth. They reappear at 10–14 day intervals. Death is usual within the first year due to bacterial infection that is ineffectively combated.

MYELOKATHEXIS [HIGHLY IMPROBABLE]

This disorder, in which neutrophils are retained within the bone marrow and not released, has been recorded in dogs, but in association with the extremely unusual situation of exposure to mustard gas.

Eosinophils

NORMAL REFERENCE RANGE

Dog: $0.1–1.25 \times 10^9/l$ (0.1–1.25 thousand/µl or mm^3).
Cat: $0–1.5 \times 10^9/l$ (0–1.5 thousand/µl or mm^3).

The principal functions of eosinophils are to reduce inflammation and to limit its spread, to regulate allergic responses and to control parasitic infections, i.e. with metazoan parasites rather than with micro-organisms.

Increased numbers of eosinophils are chiefly associated with chronic tissue damage, especially involving allergic reactions (particularly parasitism).

Decreased numbers of eosinophils are due chiefly to the effects of glucocorticoids, both endogenous (stress, Cushing's syndrome) and exogenous (administered).

Also, where an animal is clearly ill, finding an absolute eosinophil count within normal limits could suggest hypoadrenocorticism (and warrant further investigation), since if adrenal function was normal with the stress of illness an eosinopenia would be expected.

Only a small proportion of the body's eosinophils are present in the blood. The majority are in the tissues, particularly the loose connective tissue beneath the epithelial surfaces of the skin, lung, gastrointestinal tract and uterus – sites where foreign materials may enter the body.

After production in the bone marrow (and possibly in small numbers in the spleen, thymus, lymph nodes and small intestine), eosinophils pass into the blood and from there to the tissues.

The blood:tissue ratio is approximately 1:300.

Causes of eosinophilia

Summary

- Chronic tissue damage, especially allergic reactions
- Disseminated eosinophilic disease of cats [rare]
- Eosinophilic leukaemia [very rare]
- Parasitism – migrating/respiratory/cutaneous hypersensitivity/ heartworm
- Eosinophilic leukaemoid reaction in cats [very rare]
- Hypoadrenocorticism
- Drug therapy
- Oestrus (bitch)
- Breed predisposition
- Purulent disorders
- Rebound eosinophilia

Eosinophilia is an increase in the number of circulating eosinophils, i.e. in the dog $>1.25 \times 10^9/l$ (or thousand/µl or thousand/mm^3) and in the cat $>1.5 \times 10^9/l$ (or thousand/µl or thousand/mm^3).

Eosinophilia is often construed as denoting parasitism, although *parasitism does not invariably result in eosinophilia*, and there are also several other causes of eosinophilia. Classification of disorders can be difficult because of an overlap between the mechanisms involved.

CHRONIC TISSUE DAMAGE, ESPECIALLY INVOLVING ALLERGIC REACTION

Damage to tissues that contain large numbers of mast cells (principally the skin, lungs, gastrointestinal tract and uterus) results in mast cell release of histamine and other factors, which attract more eosinophils than usual into the injured area. This results in a temporary circulatory eosinopenia as eosinophils are drained from the blood, but if the injury persists this is frequently followed after a few days by a circulatory *eosinophilia* as the bone marrow responds by stepping up eosinophil production and release.

A frequent cause of the underlying injury is an *allergic reaction* (i.e. immediate hypersensitivity reaction). The antigen responsible reacts with specific IgE that has been bound to the mast cells and thus initiates the histamine release. Also the bone marrow response appears to require the sensitization of T-lymphocytes.

However, the response to the resultant damage varies in degree; at times the eosinophilia localizes in the affected tissue and is *not* reflected in the blood.

Disorders in which there is a circulating eosinophilia include:

- Staphylococcal hypersensitivity in dogs (and possibly cats).
- *Flea allergy dermatitis (13–20% dogs and cats).
- Other allergic dermatoses, including atopy (although this is not documented in the cat).
- Food allergies.
- Allergies to drugs and vaccines.
- Eosinophilic granuloma complex of the dog.
- Eosinophilic granuloma complex of the cat – a group of related disorders of the skin, lip and oral mucosa.

- Allergic (eosinophilic) tracheobronchitis – both acute (=feline asthma) and chronic.
- Hypersensitivity to exogenous protein.
- *Heartworm disease (= dirofilariasis in the dog, and less commonly, the cat) – not in the UK.
- *Parasitic larval migration, e.g. of ascarids (*Toxocara canis* and *cati*) and also *Ancylostoma caninum* and *Strongyloides stercoralis* (although not in the UK).
- *Parasitic infection of the lower respiratory tract (lungs and airways).
- *Allergic pneumonia (=eosinophilic pneumonia).
- Pneumonia due to chronic infections – the *Mycoplasma* group, fungi (*Aspergillus*, *Histoplasma*), tuberculosis.
- Eosinophilic (gastro)enteritis in the dog and cat, usually associated with malabsorption.
- Steatitis (pansteatitis) in the cat (at times) – associated with neutrophilia.
- Canine panosteitis (eosinophilic panosteitis).
- Pyometra (see below under 'Purulent disorders').
- Eosinophilic myositis, leading to muscle atrophy.

An askerisk * in the above list indicates disorders which almost always result in circulatory eosinophilia.

The parasitic causes of tissue damage are dealt with more fully below.

The term 'hypereosinophilic syndrome' is used in humans to denote diseases of unknown aetiology where there is a persistent circulatory eosinophilia and the infiltration of organs with eosinophils that result in their dysfunction. In the cat it has been applied to include eosinophilic enteritis, disseminated eosinophilic disease and eosinophilic leukaemia.

The most marked eosinophilias arise with respiratory disease having an allergic aetiology. All of these respiratory conditions, and also allergies to drugs and eosinophilic granuloma, *may* be responsible for the syndrome of pulmonary infiltrates with eosinophilia (PIE syndrome in the dog and cat), i.e. the lungs are infiltrated by eosinophils, and this is evident radiographically, and there is a systemic eosinophilia.

DISSEMINATED EOSINOPHILIC DISEASE [RARE] (IN CAT)

This feline disorder has the features of feline eosinophilic enteritis, but eosinophilic infiltration *extends* to other visceral organs (liver, spleen, pancreas, adrenal glands) and the hepatic lymph nodes.

Specific diagnostic features: vomiting and diarrhoea of eosinophilic enteritis *plus* hepatomegaly, splenomegaly etc.

EOSINOPHILIC LEUKAEMIA [RARE]

This very rare feline myeloproliferative disorder (not recorded in the dog) is characterized by significant numbers of developmental stages (eosinophilic meta-myelocytes and myeloblasts) in the circulation, in addition to mature eosinophils. Unlike the majority of hypereosinophilic disorders, it is *unresponsive* to corticosteroid therapy.

PARASITISM

Eosinophilia is most evident with parasites that invade the tissues, and it denotes an *allergic response* to antigens of the parasite (especially helminths). It is least likely to occur with parasites that are free-living in the gut.

In the dog and cat it is most evident with the following.

Larvae migrating through the tissues

Eosinophilia occurs with *Toxocara canis* (dog) and *cati* (cat), and also, although not in the UK, *Ancylostoma caninum* (dog and cat), *Strongyloides stercoralis* (dog and cat), *Spirocerca lupi* (dog) and *Trichinella spiralis* (cat).

Parasites invading the lungs and airways

• *Aleurostrongylus abstrusus* – lungworm of cat.
• *Capillaria aerophilia* (dog).
• *Angiostrongylus vasorum* (dog).

Also (although not in the UK) *Crenosoma vulpis* (dog) and *Paragonimus* spp. of fluke (dog and cat).

Oslerus osleri in the dog (formerly *Filaroides osleri*) is not associated with eosinophilia – presumably because it is well walled off, unlike other respiratory tract parasites.

Parasites initiating cutaneous hypersensitivity reactions

Principally these are fleas in the UK, producing flea allergy dermatitis. (Eosinophilia is *not* a feature of infection with *Demodex* or *Sarcoptes*.)

Dirofilaria immitis, heartworm

This parasite does not occur in the UK. An eosinophilic response to it occurs less often in the cat than in the dog and is often accompanied by an increased basophil count and a variable shift-to-the-left.

Peak eosinophil counts arise when:

• Adult worms first enter the heart.
• Microfilariae are first released into the blood by the female worms.

The presence in the blood of microfilariae of the non-pathogenic filarial worm *Dipetalonema reconditum* does not produce eosinophilia.

Eosinophilia is *not* associated with the presence in the gut of:

• Tapeworms.
• Ascarids and hookworms (although migrating larvae of ascarids and hookworms will initiate eosinophilia).
• Whipworms – occasionally recorded, but the eggs of *Capillaria aerophila* may be mistaken for those of *Trichuris vulpis*.
• Coccidia.

EOSINOPHILIC LEUKAMOID REACTION [VERY RARE]

Very rarely a blood picture resembling eosinophilic leukaemia has been recorded in cats with alimentary lymphosarcoma.

HYPOADRENOCORTICISM (PRIMARY (ADDISON'S DISEASE) AND SECONDARY)

Until recently an absolute eosinophilia was regarded as an invariable feature of hypoadrenocorticism – indeed it formed the basis of the Thorn test for diagnosis. Current opinion is that a minority of cases (possibly the most severely affected) show an eosinophilia, and in many cases the eosinophil counts are within the normal range.

In dogs that are ill this can be regarded as diagnostically significant, because with severe stress an *eosinopenia* might be expected and, indeed, eosinopenia has been recorded in a few cases of hypoadrenocorticism.

DRUG THERAPY

Eosinophilia ($>1.4 \times 10^9/l$) is seen in just over 10% of cats treated for hyperthyroidism with methimazole, and might therefore be expected with the related drug carbimazole used for the same purpose.

OESTRUS

Some bitches demonstrate an eosinophilia only during oestrus, apparently as a response to the release of histamine by mast cells in the uterine wall under the influence of oestrogen.

BREED PREDISPOSITION

Some large breeds, notably German Shepherd Dogs, frequently show evidence of eosinophilia. Indeed the finding is so common that there is a tendency to disregard it as a normal breed characteristic. However, the relatively much higher incidence of eosinophilic enteritis, eosinophilic myositis and panosteitis in the German Shepherd Dog suggests that there is a breed predisposition to hypereosinophilic disorders, and the finding of eosinophilia in apparently normal individuals could denote subclinical disease.

PURULENT DISORDERS

At times, in septic conditions, eosinophilia accompanies neutrophilia, presumably in response to the decomposition of tissue. It seems especially likely to occur in cases of pyometra (in both dog and cat).

REBOUND EOSINOPHILIA

It has been observed that, following the withdrawal of steroid therapy and the disappearance of its eosinopenic effect, there can be a temporary slight increase in the number of circulating eosinophils.

Almost all conditions characterized by eosinophilia can be successfully treated using glucocorticoids, the exception being eosinophilic leukaemia, although obviously where a noticeable underlying cause is present, e.g. parasitism or sepsis, this should be treated specifically.

Causes of eosinopenia

Summary

- Acute stress (adrenaline)
- Chronic stress (glucocorticoids), e.g. pyometra
- Hyperadrenocorticism
- Steroid/ACTH administration
- Acute infection/inflammation

Eosinopenia is a decrease in the number of circulating eosinophils, i.e. in the dog $<0.1 \times 10^9/l$ (<0.1 thousand/µl or mm^3).

In the cat a complete absence of eosinophils can be regarded as normal.

ACUTE STRESS

The release of adrenaline (epinephrine) due to *fear and excitement* (emotional stress, e.g. due to handling or travelling) or *violent muscular activity* (including *convulsions*) causes first a mild eosinophilia followed by a moderate eosinopenia 'peaking' after about 4 hours.

However, this effect is too slow to influence the eosinophil values of blood samples collected under conditions of excitement, e.g. in cats.

The injection of adrenaline will, of course, produce the same effect.

PROLONGED STRESS (e.g. PAIN, SEVERE ILLNESS, INTENSIVE TRAINING)

This provokes the release of endogenous glucocorticoids, principally cortisol, which cause an eosinopenia in addition to neutrophilia, lymphopenia and, in the dog, monocytosis. This is seen, for example, in pyometra and in Greyhounds that are 'trained off' due to the stress of sustained racing.

Glucocorticoids cause eosinopenia by several mechanisms:

• Neutralizing the histamine in the tissues which provokes eosinophil release from the bone marrow.
• Inducing lysis of the eosinophils.
• Increasing phagocytosis of eosinophils by macrophages.
• Stimulating eosinophil migration into the small intestine and lymphoid tissues.
• Reducing bone marrow production of eosinophils.

(The effects of adrenaline (above) *and* corticosteroids will be combined in the stress of surgical procedures and general anaesthesia.)

CUSHING'S SYNDROME (HYPERADRENOCORTICISM)

Eosinopenia (plus neutrophilia, lymphopenia and, in the dog, monocytosis) follows the excessive production and release of cortisol, *either* by an adrenal neoplasm *or* (in 90–95% of canine cases) as a result of adrenal stimulation due to the unregulated output of ACTH by the anterior lobe of the pituitary gland. In cases of Cushing's syndrome in both the dog and the cat, frequently no eosinophils at all are discovered.

The multiplicity of clinical signs, plus the elevated ALP (alkaline phosphatase) activity in dogs (in 95% of cases) and the elevated cholesterol level (in 75% of dogs and cats) greatly aids the diagnosis (see Panel 8.2, p. 401).

ADMINISTRATION OF CORTICOSTEROIDS OR ACTH

The administration of glucocorticoids (or ACTH), e.g. for the control of inflammation or pruritus, will of course produce exactly the same 'steroidal' effects as described above, namely eosinopenia, neutrophilia, lymphopenia and (especially in the dog) monocytosis. Although this 'steroidal blood picture' is usually associated with the injection or oral administration of glucocorticoids, it can also follow their use in eye or ear drops, skin creams or rectal foams. These effects can be termed 'iatrogenic' (= physician-induced) and will be prolonged by long-term therapy, which *may* lead to the creation of iatrogenic Cushing's syndrome, especially where high doses of potent synthetic corticosteroids (betamethasone, dexamethasone, triamcinolone etc.) and long-acting suspensions (e.g. methylprednisolone acetate) are employed.

The dogs that have been on long-term steroid therapy (months/years) that is suddenly stopped may show clinical signs *both* of iatrogenic Cushing's syndrome and of Addison's disease (adrenal insufficiency).

Some drugs which are not regarded as glucocorticoids nevertheless retain some glucocorticoid potency and will also produce an eosinopenia, – principally certain mineralocorticoids (e.g.fludrocortisone) and progestogens (e.g. megestrol acetate in the cat).

However, evidence suggests that *anabolic* steroids do not, in the dog and the cat, have this same effect.

ACUTE INFECTION AND INFLAMMATION

Current opinion is that in these cases there is likely to be another mechanism responsible for the eosinopenia – one that is independent of the release of adrenaline and glucocorticoids due to stress (i.e. as described under 'Acute stress' and 'Prolonged stress' above).

Basophils

Basophils are scarce (indeed they are very rarely reported) in the circulating blood of the dog and cat – particularly the dog, although in part this may be due to a failure to recognize the few which are present. Finding *any* may therefore be regarded as significant.

Basophils, like mast cells in the tissues, have as their major function the promotion of allergic (immediate hypersensitivity) reactions by releasing a number of mediators, including histamine, heparin and serotonin.

Causes of basophilia

Summary

- Allergic (immediate hypersensitivity) disorders
- Localized purulent inflammatory disease
- Heartworm disease (not in the UK)
- Young Basenjis
- Basophilic leukaemia [very rare]
- Hyperlipoproteinaemia (dog)

Basophilia in the dog and cat essentially means the presence of any basophils, which is an unusual occurrence. When it arises it frequently accompanies eosinophilia, particularly in connection with the following.

ALLERGIC DISORDERS

Allergic (immediate hypersensitivity) disorders including in particular those affecting the lung (chronic respiratory disease) or skin (atopy, flea-allergy dermatitis, chronic pyoderma etc.), and also the gastrointestinal tract and reproductive tract.

LOCALIZED PURULENT INFLAMMATORY DISEASE

This would involve the same sites as mentioned above under 'Allergic disorders'.

HEARTWORM DISEASE (DIROFILARIASIS)

Eosinopenia arises particularly when microfilariae are absent. The parasite does not occur in the UK.

YOUNG BASENJIS

In Basenjis around 2 months of age small numbers of basophils are common although by 4 months they are, as usual, rare.

Basophilia may occur *without* eosinophilia, for example, in the following disorders.

BASOPHILIC LEUKAEMIA [VERY RARE]

This does occur extremely rarely and features a high proportion of developmental stages of basophils.

HYPERLIPOPROTEINAEMIA

In humans, and seemingly also in the dog, basophilia, without eosinophilia, occurs where there is an increase in the concentration of lipoproteins in the blood (hyperlipoproteinaemia). This is usually part of a generalized lipaemia, including an increased cholesterol level, e.g. in primary liver disease, diabetes mellitus, hyperadrenocorticism (Cushing's syndrome), nephrosis and, possibly, hypothyroidism.

Mast cells

These cells, which are related to basophils, are also usually absent from the blood but may appear (mastocythaemia) in association with:

- Severe trauma and/or stress.
- Acute inflammation, especially of the gastrointestinal tract.
- Malignant mast cell tumours (mastocytomas).

Mast cell tumours chiefly occur in the skin (especially in the cat), intestine and lymphoreticular tissue (mainly the spleen). Around 50% of those in the skin, and *most* of those found elsewhere, are considered malignant.

The appearance of large numbers of mast cells in the circulation is associated with a disseminated mast cell tumour and has been referred to as mast cell leukaemia. It may involve the bone marrow. The most consistent associated finding is splenomegaly.

Note

Mast cells have been mistaken for basophils and mast cell leukaemia designated basophilic leukaemia.

Causes of basopenia

Basopenia cannot be recognized in dogs and cats since it is usual for there *not* to be any basophils in the blood. However, corticosteroids can decrease the number of basophils in cases of basophilia.

Lymphocytes

NORMAL REFERENCE RANGE

Dog: $1-4.8 \times 10^9/l$ ($1-4.8$ thousand/μl or mm^3).
   In racing Greyhounds the normal range is lower $= 0.8-3.8 \times 10^9/l$.

Cat: $1.5-7 \times 10^9/l$ ($1.5-7$ thousand/μl or mm^3).
   Counts are higher in younger cats.

The vast majority (up to 95%) of lymphocytes are either T-lymphocytes or B-lymphocytes (otherwise known as T-cells or B-cells); the remainder are designated 'null' cells whose functions are not established (they may represent precursors of the other cells).

B-lymphocytes are derived from bone marrow and localize in the lymph nodes (lymphoid follicles and medulla), spleen (red pulp) and the submucosa of the gut and respiratory tract; they are concerned with antibody formation.

T-lymphocytes are derived from the thymus (although originating embryologically in the bone marrow) and localize in the lymph nodes (paracortical areas), spleen (white pulp) and Peyer's patches. They are concerned with cell-mediated immunity and the regulation of immunity (Figure 3.3).

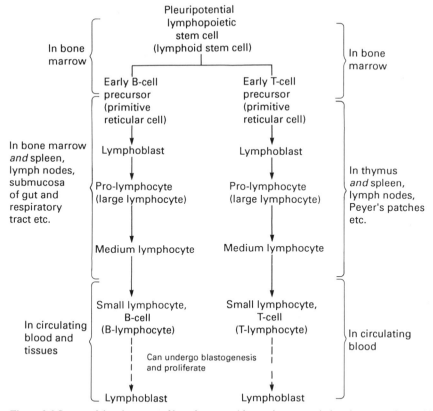

Figure 3.3 Stages of development of lymphocytes. Alternative names in brackets; see also p. 44 for relationship to other cells

The different types of lymphocytes cannot be distinguished by their appearance on a blood smear. However, their age can be determined by size and staining, immature cells being larger and having cytoplasm that appears more basophilic (i.e. blue).

Lymphocytes, especially T-lymphocytes, can recirculate from blood to lymph nodes and then back into the blood again. Given an appropriate stimulus small lymphocytes can transform into *lymphoblasts* and proceed to proliferate. Lymphoblasts, then, are not simply lymphocyte precursors; large numbers of them appear in the acute lymphoproliferative disorders and their presence raises the suspicion of neoplasia (see Panel 3.1, p. 183).

The number of lymphocytes in the blood depends on the number entering and the number leaving; whereas decreased lymphocyte production usually results in lymphopenia, increased production may not result in lymphocytosis – there may be a marked loss into the tissues.

Plasma cells, found in lymphoid tissues, are concerned with the synthesis, storage and release of immunoglobulins, but rarely appear in the circulating blood.

Causes of lymphocytosis

Summary

- Age – young animals
- Physiological – fear/excitement/vigorous activity
- Lymphocytic leukaemia and lymphosarcoma (most common)
- Feline immunodeficiency virus infection
- Prolonged antigenic stimulation – chronic infection/hypersensitivity/ autoimmunity/postvaccination
- Hypoadrenocorticism
- Drug therapy

Lymphocytosis is an increase in the number of circulating lymphocytes.

Dog: $>4.8 \times 10^9$/l (>4.8 thousand/µl or mm^3).
Cat: $>7 \times 10^9$/l (>7 thousand/µl or mm^3).

Lymphocytosis is relatively uncommon and usually does not cause a marked increase in the total WBC count, although total WBC values may be in the upper part of the normal range.

AGE

Lymphocyte counts are higher in puppies and kittens compared with adults.
Dog, rising to a peak of 6.1×10^9/l at 6 weeks old (but within the adult range by 2 months of age).
Cat, rising to a peak of 10.5×10^9/l at 12–13 weeks old (but within the adult range by 4–5 months old).

PHYSIOLOGICAL LYMPHOCYTOSIS

The release of adrenaline due to fear or excitement or violent muscular activity in healthy cats, especially young animals (e.g. when there is difficulty in collecting a blood sample), causes a temporary increase in lymphocyte numbers which is often greater than the modest increase in neutrophils that accompanies it (see p. 152).

The effect is *immediate* and lasts for about 30 minutes. This effect *does not* occur in the dog and is less common in cats that are ill.

An injection of adrenaline will produce the same effect.

LYMPHOCYTIC LEUKAEMIA AND LYMPHOSARCOMA [MOST COMMON]

Lymphocytosis may be a feature of lymphoproliferative disorders in the dog and cat (see Panel 3.1, p. 183).

Usually any increase in lymphocyte numbers is not extensive, with values only slightly above the upper limit of the normal reference range. However, the finding of a normal or very slightly raised lymphocyte count is *diagnostically significant* in cases of obvious systemic illness where lymphopenia would usually be expected.

Occasionally, a very pronounced increase in the number of lymphocytes is seen (e.g. $50–600 \times 10^9/l$) of which a high proportion can be atypical, bizarre forms.

FELINE IMMUNODEFICIENCY VIRUS (FIV) INFECTION

Lymphocytosis occurs in approximately 20% of cases, and in about a third of those it is marked.

PROLONGED ANTIGENIC STIMULATION

This can arise in:

● Chronic infections, e.g. chronic pyoderma, pneumonia and pyometra (very rarely with ehrlichiosis – not in the UK).
● Hypersensitivity diseases.
● Autoimmune diseases.
● Postvaccination: antigenically stimulated lymphocytes (= immunocytes) are commonly seen after vaccination.

In these situations antigens can stimulate lymphocyte production and the resultant lymphoid hyperplasia can result in enlarged lymph nodes. It also causes a slightly elevated lymphocyte count, or at least one in the upper part of the normal range, whereas in most cases of clinically obvious systemic illness, a lymphopenia would be more usual.

The finding of a small number of plasma cells (immunocytes) would support this cause. They may be reported by the laboratory as seemingly larger lymphocytes showing a more basophilic (blue) staining.

HYPOADRENOCORTICISM

An absolute lymphocytosis occurs in some cases of hypoadrenocorticism in the dog (although probably less than 25% overall) but in most of the very few cases reported in the cat.

Most cases of canine hypoadrenocorticism show a lymphocyte count within normal limits. However, in such extremely ill animals as these (under severe stress) a lymphopenia would be a more usual finding, and the fact that they do *not* show lymphopenia is diagnostically *significant*.

DRUG THERAPY

Lymphocytosis ($>6 \times 10^9/l$) is reported in 7% of cats treated for hyperthyroidism with methimazole, and presumably might also arise following carbimazole therapy.

Causes of lymphopenia

Summary

Steroidal effects
- Hyperadrenocorticism
- Administration of steroids/ACTH
- Severe stress

Acute systemic infection – early viral/overwhelming bacterial/uncommon bacterial/acute toxoplasmosis/leishmaniasis
Loss of lymph
Damage to lymph nodes – neoplasia/chronic inflammation
Acquired T-lymphocyte deficiency
Immunosuppressive chemotherapy
Radiation (e.g. therapy)
Hereditary immunodeficiency [rare]
Lymphoid atrophy
Demodicosis – generalized
Chronic renal failure

Lymphopenia is a decreased number of circulating lymphocytes.

Dog: $<1 \times 10^9/l$ (<1 thousand/μl or mm^3).
This value is appropriate to dogs over 2 years of age.
For dogs 3–6 months of age $<2 \times 10^9/l$, and for dogs between 8 and 24 months of age $<1.5 \times 10^9/l$.

Cat: $<1.5 \times 10^9/l$ (<1.5 thousand/μl or mm^3).

Lymphopenia is a relatively common finding in seriously ill animals.

STEROIDAL EFFECTS

These result from:

- Hyperadrenocorticism (Cushing's syndrome).
- Administration of corticosteroids (glucocorticoids) *or* ACTH.
- Severe stress causing release of endogenous steroids, e.g. severe illness (such as chronic pyometra), painful diseases, extremes of body temperature, general anaesthesia etc.

One effect of steroids is to decrease the number of lymphocytes in the circulation, possibly by redistributing them, although, in established Cushing's syndrome, the fall in numbers seems most likely to be due to lympholysis.

A relative fall in lymphocytes (i.e. apparent from the differential WBC count) is a consistent feature of cases of Cushing's syndrome.

In the cat especially, a fall in the *absolute* number of lymphocytes is unusual, although as a *percentage* of all WBC types the lymphocyte count is low.

Lymphopenia is a feature of 'trained-off' Greyhounds due to the stress of sustained racing.

ACUTE SYSTEMIC INFECTION

Lymphopenia is seen in the following infections.

Early viral

Lymphopenia is seen particularly in the early phase of many viral diseases, due to the fact that lymphocytes remain hidden away in lymphoid tissues during the incubation period and viraemic phase, and to changes in their surface properties. It is seen in:

- Infectious canine hepatitis.
- Canine distemper causing lymphoid depletion (this persists in very young dogs with rapidly progressive systemic or neurological signs).
- Enteritis due to canine parvovirus (an inconsistent finding).
- Canine coronavirus infection (without a neutropenia).
- Feline calicivirus disease.
- Feline infectious peritonitis (in *some* cats; usually there is a low–normal lymphocyte count).
- Feline leukaemia virus infection (there is a more marked lymphopenia with *recent* infection than if viraemia has persisted for 4 months or more).
- Feline immunodeficiency virus (FIV) infection (previously termed 'FTLV infection'); lymphopenia occurs in about a third of cases and may be a feature which recurs subsequently.
- Feline infectious enteritis, otherwise known as feline panleucopenia *because* of the characteristic severe reduction in the numbers of all WBC types; *in fact* an absolute lymphopenia is less common in FIE (FPL) than is neutropenia. Where neutropenia and lymphopenia occur together it is more often due to concurrent FeLV infection.

A rebound increase in lymphocyte numbers usually follows recovery from the early stages.

Overwhelming bacterial infections

Lymphopenia is seen in overwhelming bacterial infections (although less often than in viral infections), i.e. septicaemias, and especially endotoxaemias (e.g. salmonellosis).

Uncommon bacterial infections

Lymphopenia is seen in some less common bacterial infections, such as salmon poisoning disease and ehrlichiosis (neither of which occur in the UK).

Acute toxoplasmosis

Lymphopenia is seen along with reductions in the numbers of neutrophils, eosinophils and monocytes.

Leishmaniasis

Lymphopenia is seen, often with thrombocytopenia and anaemia.
  The reduction in lymphocyte numbers may be due to their temporary confinement to the spleen and/or lymph nodes (i.e. for 1–2 days) whilst they are responding to the antigen *or* it may be due to their destruction by the infectious agent.

LOSS OF LYMPH

This can be due to, for example:

- Rupture of the thoracic duct causing chylothorax.
- Feline cardiomyopathy resulting in a chylous thoracic effusion.

- Canine small intestinal disease with a loss of lymph (and protein) into the gut lumen, i.e. a protein-losing enteropathy. The underlying disease may be alimentary neoplasia (especially lymphosarcoma), lymphangiectasia or enteritis with granulomatous lesions and/or ulceration.

In these disorders lymphocytes that are being carried in the lymph are lost and do not return to the circulating blood, reducing their numbers.

DAMAGE TO THE STRUCTURE OF LYMPH NODES

This can occur, for example, by:

- Multicentric (i.e. generalized) lymphosarcoma.
- Diffuse, granulomatous inflammatory diseases.

Generalized lymph node damage interfers with the recirculation of lymphocytes causing lymphopenia, in addition to any disruption of lymphocyte production.

ACQUIRED T-LYMPHOCYTE DEFICIENCY (ACQUIRED CELL-MEDIATED IMMUNODEFICIENCY)

Lymphopenia can result from hypoplasia of the T-lymphocyte system caused by certain *neonatal* infections that result in thymic atrophy, for example FeLV infection in kittens (part of the 'fading kitten' syndrome); it is also seen with canine distemper and feline infectious enteritis (feline panleucopenia).

CHEMOTHERAPY WITH IMMUNOSUPPRESSIVE DRUGS

This occurs with, for example, azathioprine.

RADIATION

Lymphopenia can follow radiotherapy.

In both of the last two causes lymphopenia gradually appears because lymphoid proliferation is suppressed.

HEREDITARY IMMUNODEFICIENCY [RARE]

Lymphopenia may be the result of an *inherited* deficiency of T-lymphocytes (= inherited cell-mediated immunodeficiency) with or without a deficiency of B-lymphocytes, e.g. in Miniature Dachshunds which makes them susceptible to pneumonia caused by *Pneumocystis*.

LYMPHOID ATROPHY

This causes lymphopenia and can arise in old age, malnutrition and vitamin B deficiency.

GENERALIZED DEMODICOSIS

This is probably due *not* to an underlying immunodeficiency but to the effects of the secondary pyoderma (see under 'Acute systemic infection' above).

CHRONIC RENAL FAILURE

In both the dog and cat lymphopenia can develop due to the immunodepressive effect of long-term azotaemia.

Note

- The gradual appearance of lymphopenia (i.e. with repeated blood samples) is an unfavourable sign. If an animal *appears* healthy it can serve as an 'early-warning' sign of illness.
- *Persistent* lymphopenia suggests a continuation of stress; if it persists *despite* therapy the prognosis must be poor.
- The gradual disappearance of lymphopenia, i.e. the restoration of normal lymphocyte numbers, indicates a good prognosis, especially if accompanied by a clinical improvement and other haematological changes (e.g. the disappearance of one or more abnormalities such as eosinopenia, neutrophilia and a shift-to-the-left).

Monocytes

There is normally a small number in the blood.

NORMAL REFERENCE RANGE

Dog: $0.15-1.35 \times 10^9/l$ ($0.15-1.35$ thousand/µl or mm^3).
Cat: $0-0.85 \times 10^9/l$ ($0-0.85$ thousand/µl or mm^3).

Monocytes are formed in the bone marrow and released to circulate for a short time in the blood before entering the tissues and body cavities to become fixed or free macrophages. The blood monocyte:tissue macrophage ratio is approximately 1:400. Taken altogether these cells (bone marrow precursors, blood monocytes and tissue macrophages) comprise the mononuclear phagocyte system (MPS). Previously, the cells in the blood and tissues (but not in the bone marrow) were grouped with reticular and endothelial cells as the reticuloendothelial system.

Cells of the MPS have a large number of functions, including the regulation of immune responses and haemopoiesis, but the prime functions of monocytes are:

- To phagocytose and destroy micro-organisms – bacteria, especially intracellular and/or those producing granulomatous responses, fungi, protozoa and possibly viruses (MPS produces interferon). Usually the disease concerned is chronic.
- To phagocytose foreign material, tissue debris and dead, damaged and non-functional cells.

Monocytes in the blood are, like the neutrophils, divided between a circulating pool and a larger marginal pool, consisting of monocytes adherent to the endothelial wall of blood vessels, and a sudden increase in demand causes the release of cells from the marginal pool into the circulation. Prolonged demand for monocytes may stimulate:

- Their release from the bone marrow reserve pool in the case of the dog, but not in the cat where one does not exist.
- Increased bone marrow production of monocytes.

Tissue macrophages once released *do not* normally re-enter the blood.

Causes of monocytosis

Summary

Steroidal effects:
- Hyperadrenocorticism
- Adminstration of steroids/ACTH
- Severe stress, e.g. pyometra

Acute and chronic infections/inflammation
Immune-mediated disorders
Other disorders causing tissue damage and necrosis
Reduced granulocyte production
Granulopathy in Irish Setters [rare]
Old age
Monocytic leukaemia and myelomonocytic leukaemia
Error: mechanical blood spreaders

Monocytosis is an increased number of circulating monocytes.

$Dog = >1.35 \times 10^9/l$ (>1.35 thousand/μl or mm^3).
$Cat = >0.85 \times 10^9/l$ (>0.85 thousand/μl or mm^3).

STEROIDAL EFFECTS

These are the result of:

- Hyperadrenocorticism (Cushing's syndrome).
- Administration of steroids (glucocorticoids) or ACTH.
- Severe stress causing release of endogenous cortisol, e.g. pyometra.

Monocytosis as a steroidal effect occurs in the dog and sometimes in the cat. It is an inconsistent response in the cat and most often associated with the stress of trauma due to road traffic accidents, less frequently with other accidents, with feline urological syndrome etc.

Monocytosis accompanies the other haematological features of steroid release or administration (neutrophilia, eosinopenia and lymphopenia). It arises because monocytes move from the marginal pool (and in the dog probably also from a bone marrow reserve pool) into the circulation.

Sometimes in the cat the initial response to severe stress may be monocytopenia as monocytes move into the marginal pool, followed *later* by a monocytosis. However, in reality this is impossible to assess (because a total absence of monocytes can be quite normal) unless monocyte counts have been obtained prior to the onset of stress.

Monocytosis due to administration of a single dose of steroids or a single episode of stress is a short-lived effect; it appears within a few hours and lasts less than a day. Persistent steroid administration results in persistence of the monocytosis.

ACUTE AND CHRONIC INFECTIONS AND INFLAMMATION

Monocyte numbers increase whenever phagocytosis is required (in the tissues they transform to macrophages) and monocytosis frequently accompanies or follows neutrophilia, although the increase in monocyte numbers is neither as rapid nor as pronounced as that of the neutrophils.

Monocytosis is not confined to chronic disorders; monocytes will readily phagocytose common pathogenic bacteria, although more slowly than neutrophils. For example they are active in acute bacterial infections, such as septicaemia, bacteraemia and purulent diseases (e.g. pyometra), especially in cats. A monocytosis is also found in about 40% of cases of feline immunodeficiency virus (FIV) infection (previously known as FTLV infection). Monocytosis is also more characteristic of the acute than the chronic phase of ehrlichiosis.

However, the monocytes' particular ability to destroy intracellular pathogens, and organisms that cause granulomatous lesions means that monocytosis is an inevitable feature of chronic infectious diseases; for example, those due to:

- Protozoa (e.g. *Toxoplasma*).
- Bacteria (tuberculosis, actinomycosis, haemobartonellosis).
- Fungi (blastomycosis, nocardiosis, histoplasmosis).

The rate of monocyte production increases in response to the inflammation and to the increased destruction of macrophages.

IMMUNE-MEDIATED DISORDERS

Increased damage to tissues and organs by immune reactions leads to an increased requirement for phagocytosis and therefore to monocytosis (e.g. it is generally marked in autoimmune haemolytic anaemia).

OTHER DISORDERS RESULTING IN TISSUE DAMAGE AND NECROSIS

Phagocytosis is needed in conditions other than those due to infection, inflammation and immune-mediated damage, e.g.

- Intervertebral disc rupture, bone fractures, burns and other forms of trauma.
- Malignant neoplasia, e.g. lymphosarcoma.
- Endotoxaemia.
- Haemolysis and haemorrhage, e.g. anticoagulant poisoning.

It can be a feature of chronic renal failure.

REDUCED PRODUCTION OF GRANULOCYTES (ESSENTIALLY OF NEUTROPHILS AND EOSINOPHILS)

In some cases of feline panleucopenia (feline infectious enteritis) in the cat there may be low numbers of all WBCs *except* monocytes.

GRANULOCYTOPATHY IN IRISH SETTERS

Monocytosis may be a feature when monocytes take over the phagocytic function of neutrophils.

OLD AGE

In old dogs there is a tendency for an absolute monocytosis, lymphopenia and eosinopenia to develop. It is not clear whether this is stress related.

MONOCYTIC LEUKAEMIA AND MYELOMONOCYTIC LEUKAEMIA

Both these myeloproliferative disorders are characterized by pronounced monocytosis and numbers of bone marrow precursors, including monoblasts. Myelomonocytic leukaemia is accompanied by a neutrophilia and developmental granulocytes.
    In both cases affected dogs are usually young. (See Panel 3.2, p. 189.)

ERROR: TECHNIQUE

The use of mechanical blood-spreading devices to produce blood smears, in highly automated laboratories, affects the differential WBC count. More large cells, including monocytes, appear in the smear giving rise to higher differential and absolute monocyte counts.

Causes of monocytopenia

Normal monocyte values are so low that it is difficult to recognize monocytopenia (though experimentally it has been observed to occur in acute toxoplasmosis in cats).

Abnormal white blood cells and white blood cell inclusions

ABNORMAL WHITE BLOOD CELLS (WBCs)

Abnormal WBCs that may be mentioned in reports are as follows.

Neutrophils showing toxic changes

These changes indicate diminished function.

Changes representing defective maturation in the bone marrow
- Diffuse basophilia = bluish cytoplasm.
- Döhle bodies – appear as angular blue granules representing an aggregation of endoplasmic reticulum.
- Giant neutrophils and polyploid neutrophils, band forms and metamyelocytes (large and bizarre).
- Double nuclei – due to a failure of cell division.
- Toxic granulation – blue–black or purple–red (azurophilic) granules in the cytoplasm.

Note

The first three changes listed are common in toxaemic diseases of cats.

Changes due to the effect of toxins in the circulation
The major change is foamy or vacuolated cytoplasm; this is because degenerative changes with the release of lysosomes cause vacuoles to develop at the periphery of the neutrophil.

Neutrophils showing hypersegmentation of the nucleus

In large numbers = a shift-to-the-right. This represents longer intravascular survival due to the effect of steroids, or degeneration in old blood samples.

Small numbers are seen with anaemia due to folate deficiency (and in humans with vitamin B_{12} deficiency).

Lupus erythematosus (LE) cells

Each cell is a mature neutrophil containing a large spherical inclusion of phagocytosed material, probably the nucleus of another neutrophil.

These are seen in many cases of systemic lupus erythematosus, but also in inflammatory conditions and myeloproliferative disorders.

Cells characterizing Pelger–Huët anomaly

In this anomaly neutrophils and eosinophils have unsegmented nuclei, i.e. the nuclei do not form lobules but remain as round or bean-shaped nuclei.

It occurs in dogs and cats and may be confused with a shift-to-the-left.

Cells characterizing Chediak–Higashi syndrome

In this syndrome neutrophils (mainly) and eosinophils contain large, round cytoplasmic granules, that may look like inclusions.

The syndrome is inherited as an autosomal recessive trait in Blue-smoke Persian cats with pale yellow–green irises.

Animals show photophobia but no increased susceptibility to infection, as is the case in humans.

Eosinophils with cytoplasmic vacuoles

This change indicates toxicity. However, *occasional* eosinophils showing the following changes are considered normal:

- Grey-staining granules in Greyhounds.
- Numerous vacuoles (more extensive in Greyhounds).
- A few very large granules.

Mast cells

These occur in 10% of dogs with mast cell tumours and can occur in dogs after severe trauma or with acute inflammation (especially gastroenteritis).

Basophils showing reddish granulation

In the cat this indicates either a toxic effect on basophil cells developing in the bone marrow *or* a response to agents that are stimulating IgE antibody production.

Lymphocytes showing artefacts

These can arise after storage in EDTA for an hour or more, e.g.:

- Lobulation of nuclei.
- Cytoplasmic vacuoles.
- 'Smudging' on staining.

Immunocytes (transformed, reactive or stimulated lymphocytes)

These represent lymphocytes undergoing transformation to lymphoblasts due to antigenic stimulation. They are seen in viral diseases, e.g. infectious canine hepatitis, in autoimmune diseases, following vaccination and (although not in the UK) in salmon disease poisoning.

(Plasma cells appear similar to immunocytes but with an eccentrically placed nucleus. Mott cells are plasma cells with large, clear cytoplasmic pockets.)

Lymphoblasts

These are larger, more basophilic cells, with finer chromatin, compared with lymphocytes. They occur in lymphoproliferative diseases, especially acute lymphoblastic leukaemia (see Table 3.4, p. 184).

Macrophages

These are transformed from monocytes in the circulation. They have abundant, foamy cytoplasm and indicate subacute or chronic bacterial infection, e.g. bacterial endocarditis.

Immature forms

Immature (i.e. developmental) forms of different types of WBCs may occur in the circulation with particular myeloproliferative disorders – see Panel 3.2, p. 189.

WHITE BLOOD CELL (WBC) INCLUSIONS

Granulocytic inclusions in neutrophils

These occur in Birman cats and represent an autosomal recessive disorder.
Despite these fine acidophilic granules the neutrophils appear to function normally.

Inclusions in LE cells

These neutrophils contain phagocytosed material – see under 'Abnormal white blood cells'.

Döhle bodies in neutrophils

These are small basophilic inclusions indicating toxicity – see under 'Abnormal white blood cells'.

Toxic cytoplasmic granules in neutrophils

These are blue–black or purple–red indicating toxicity – see under 'Abnormal white blood cells'.

Distemper inclusions

These are round, eccentrically placed nucleocapsids which occur in lymphocytes (in low numbers) and less frequently in neutrophils and RBCs.

Ehrlichia canis morulae

These are found in lymphocytes and monocytes, and occasionally neutrophils and eosinophils (not in the UK).

Leishmania canis

This *rarely* occurs in monocytes but is not seen in the UK.

Bacteria

These may, although *rarely*, occur in circulating neutrophils, e.g. in septicaemia.

Feline infectious peritonitis inclusions

These represent immune complexes and may occasionally occur in neutrophils.

Granules in lysosomal storage diseases

These may appear in dogs and cats, e.g. in mucopolysaccharidoses and lipidoses which appear to be inherited disorders. The granules accumulate mostly in neutrophils and a few lymphocytes.

Fungi and protozoa

These organisms can appear in the phagocytes (monocytes and neutrophils) in histoplasmosis, toxoplasmosis, trypanosomiasis and hepatozoonosis.

Panel 3.1 Lymphoproliferative disorders (LPDs) or leukaemia complex

Lymphoproliferative disorders are comparatively common disorders (especially in the cat) involving neoplastic proliferation of lymphoid cells. They account for 80–90% of all cases of neoplasia in the cat and about 5–7% of all those in the dog. This incidence is much greater than that of myeloproliferative disorders.

Table 3.3 Classification of lymphoproliferative disorders (LPDs)

Lymphosarcoma (= malignant lymphoma = lymphoma), i.e. solid
tumour
    Lymphoblastic lymphosarcoma
    Lymphocytic lymphosarcoma
    Histiocytic lymphosarcoma (= reticulum cell sarcoma)

Lymphocytic leukaemia
    Acute lymphoblastic leukaemia
    Chronic lymphocytic leukaemia

[*Plasma cell myeloma* (= multiple myeloma)]

Table 3.4 Incidence of the features of lymphoproliferative disorders

Disorder	Percentage (or otherwise) of cases showing each laboratory finding	
	Cat	Dog
1. *Lymphosarcoma (solid tumour)*		
Non-regenerative anaemia	33 of all and 67 of FeLV +ve	50 (mild to moderate anaemia)
Total WBCs ↑	25	40
Total WBCs ↓	12–50	12–15
Lymphocytes ↑	12	20
Lymphocytes ↓	50	25
Neutrophils ↑	25	40
Evidence of lymphocytic leukaemia (lymphoblasts etc.)	25–67	50
Total plasma protein (TPP) ↓	<10 (only seen with histiocytic lymphosarcoma)	45
Plasma Ca^{2+} ↑	Few	Many
2. *Lymphocytic leukaemia (no solid tumour)*		
Acute lymphoblastic leukaemia		
Non-regenerative anaemia	Invariably	Invariably
Lymphocytes ↑	Few	Most (chiefly lymphoblasts)
Lymphoblasts	67–75 show some	Most show ↑ ↑
Total WBCs ↓	Up to 50	–
Platelets ↓	Very few	Most
Chronic lymphocytic leukaemia		
Both the cat and dog show ↑ – ↑ ↑ total WBCs due to ↑ – ↑ ↑ lymphocytes; there *may* be a non-regenerative anaemia		

↑ = increase; ↑ ↑ = marked increase; ↓ = decrease.

Lymphoid proliferation can occur in the lymph nodes, spleen and liver and even the
bone marrow.
    The disorders are of two types:

1. A progressive malignant growth of lymphoid cells into a localized *solid tumour*,
    termed a 'lymphosarcoma', or 'lymphoma' (the latter term being increasingly
    employed). It primarily affects the tissue in which it develops and may or may not
    subsequently involve the peripheral blood.

2. A *diffuse* malignant proliferation of lymphocytes and their precursors in the blood and bone marrow termed 'lymphocytic leukaemia'. It is manifested primarily by changes in the peripheral blood.

Solid tumours and leukaemia represent the two extreme manifestations of lymphoproliferative disorders but all gradations between these two can arise. A number of lymphosarcomas (approximately 50% of those in the dog and 25% in the cat) progress to release cells that invade the bone marrow and blood resulting in leukaemia.

Feline leukaemia virus (FeLV) infection is the major cause of these disorders in the *cat*; only 30% of feline cases are FeLV-negative, i.e. non-viraemic, and this includes cases where FeLV infection is in fact responsible but where replicating virus is absent.

Twenty per cent of persistently viraemic cats will develop a lymphoproliferative disorder.

In the cat virtually all lymphoid malignancies involve T-lymphocytes except alimentary lymphosarcomas in older cats, most of which derive from B-lymphocytes (and which are less likely to be associated with viraemia).

Lymphoproliferative disorders have also arisen in association with feline immunodeficiency virus (FIV) infection.

The cause in the dog is unknown.

Lymphosarcoma (malignant lymphoma = lymphoma)

In the *cat* the most common form is the poorly differentiated lymphoblastic lymphosarcoma; the other two forms frequently found are the mixed lymphoblastic and lymphocytic lymphosarcoma and the histiocytic lymphosarcoma. (The purely lymphocytic lymphosarcoma occurs infrequently.)

In the *dog* three types of lymphosarcomas are found: poorly differentiated lymphoblastic, histiocytic and well-differentiated lymphocytic.

Histiocytic lymphosarcomas are less likely subsequently to invade the blood or bone marrow. They may be misdiagnosed as undifferentiated carcinomas.

The most commonly affected sites vary with the species.

CAT

The following types occur in order of decreasing incidence.

Mediastinal (thymic) [common]

This occurs at all ages, but especially in *young* cats.

It involves the thymus and mediastinal lymph nodes creating a space-occupying mass in the anterior mediastinum.

It results in dyspnoea, incompressible anterior thorax, and sometimes a mass palpable in the thoracic inlet.

CHECK with radiography (mass and fluid line), pleural effusion (examine fluid for lymphocytes, prolymphocytes and lymphoblasts) and possible displaced heart beat etc.

Alimentary [common]

This affects the intestine (especially the anterior ileum) and/or mesenteric lymph nodes – occasionally the stomach.

It is especially seen in older cats, causing anorexia, weight loss, diarrhoea, sometimes constipation, vomiting and a palpable abdominal mass.

CHECK   with radiography, exploratory laparotomy and biopsy.

Multicentric [less common]

This involves a number of lymph nodes, plus the spleen and liver, and possibly the kidneys.

This is a much less common form than in the dog.

Lymph nodes (peripheral, mediastinal, mesenteric etc.) are large (more than three times normal size); very occasionally single nodes are involved.

CHECK   with biopsy: excise the whole node; this is better than lymph node aspiration.

Care

Slight or moderate lymph node enlargement is *more often* due to reactive hyperplasia.

These is also splenomegaly and hepatomegaly and there may be jaundice, and/or abnormal liver function tests, but ALP and ALT activities are often not markedly raised. The liver can be biopsied to confirm the diagnosis.

Rarely the kidneys are involved (enlarged and palpable; biopsy).

Other forms (unclassified)[rare]

These can involve the spinal canal, skin, larynx, nasal passages and/or sinuses, and there may be retrobulbar ocular masses.

DOG

Multicentric (mainly involving B-lymphocytes) [very common]

This type appears as bilateral, painless enlargements of most superficial lymph nodes, especially around the head and neck which may involve the tonsils causing choking and can later cause fluctuating oedema of the head, neck and limbs.

It may also involve the liver, spleen and virtually any other organ.

Specific diagnostic features: there may be weight loss, diarrhoea, vomiting, sudden anorexia, listlessness and/or dehydration; radiography will show thoracic or abdominal masses in 50–75%.

Alimentary [common]

This form affects the gut and the mesenteric lymph nodes, but rarely involves the superficial nodes or spleen.

Specific diagnostic features: there is usually a progressive loss of condition, a palpable abdominal mass and diarrhoea; confirmation is aided by radiography.

Other types [much less common]

These can involve the skin, mediastinum (thymus) and miscellaneous organs.

Breed incidence of these types: Boxers and Scottish Terriers have an increased risk, Dachshunds less risk.

HAEMATOLOGICAL FINDINGS WITH LYMPHOSARCOMA

Cat

At times, especially with solitary tumours, the blood picture is normal.

Total WBC count may be increased, normal or decreased. Lymphopenia occurs in approximately one-half of cases. About one-third of cases show anaemia which is usually persistent and non-regenerative; commonly it arises in mediastinal and multicentric forms, but is uncommon in the alimentary form.

Anaemia and leucopenia may result from myelosuppression due to FeLV infection (FeLV positive cats are seven to eight times more likely to be anaemic) *or* because the bone marrow has been infiltrated by neoplastic cells (infiltration can be moderate or massive).

Rarely anaemia can be due to haemolysis, or haemorrhage which may involve thrombocytopenia.

In between one-quarter and two-thirds of cats some neoplastic lymphocytes from the solid tumour enter the circulating blood and bone marrow. The number is very variable; there may only be a few or sometimes so many as to produce a leukaemic blood picture.

> **Care**
>
> Atypical and immature lymphocytes are not necessarily due to neoplasia; they may appear in response to infection or some other antigenic stimulation and, with recovery, they disappear from the circulation.

Bone marrow aspiration or biopsy clarifies the diagnosis where there is non-regenerative anaemia or some other sign of bone marrow involvement.

Dog

Anaemia is not usually severe but moderate or borderline – usually the anaemia of malignancy (see p. 110). Anaemia may also arise due to haemorrhage, defective production, immune mediation, disseminated intravascular coagulation or bone marrow damage (non-regenerative).

Total WBC count is variable; 40% of cases show leucocytosis (very occasionally extremely high counts; $200-300 \times 10^9/l$) – around 12% show leucopenia. Consequently, almost half have WBC counts in the normal range (usually the upper part): 20% show lymphocytosis, 25% show lymphopenia. Neoplastic lymphocytes appear irregularly in the peripheral blood; just over half of cases show a slight increase in lymphoblasts. Approximately 40% show neutrophilia. Diagnosis therefore cannot be definite on a blood examination.

Lymph node aspiration (rarely bone marrow aspiration) may help diagnosis. Often there is *hypercalcaemia* (especially in St Bernards) because tumour cells produce an osteoclast-activating factor.

Lymphocytic leukaemia

CAT

This accounts for under half of the feline lymphoproliferative disorders (3–40% depending on locality).

The most consistent sign is a non-regenerative anaemia, due to the loss of RBC precursors in the bone marrow.

Usually the total WBC count is normal or low; if low (leucopenia) there *may be* a relative *lymphocytosis* with or without blast cells.

There *may* be a large number of lymphoblasts producing a leucocytosis but this is unusual.

The loss of granulocyte (i.e. neutrophil) precursors in the bone marrow, plus the inability of lymphoblasts to function as lymphocytes in immune responses, facilitates infection.

A loss of platelet precursors (megakaryocytes) produces a tendency towards uncontrolled haemorrhages.

Acute lymphoblastic leukaemia

Most cases are of acute lymphoblastic leukaemia, i.e. primarily involvement of bone marrow and blood with no obvious solid tumours.

Signs are essentially of non-regenerative anaemia (pallor, lethargy, weight loss, anorexia, fever) with or without enlargement of the liver and lymph nodes.

Care

In some infections (e.g. the recovery stage of feline infectious enteritis) there may be a similar picture of transient neutropenia plus atypical lymphocytes. Ideally a diagnosis based on the blood picture needs confirmation with bone marrow aspiration.

Chronic lymphocytic leukaemia

Well-differentiated cases of chronic lymphocytic leukaemia are rare, but usually there is a large number (50–250×10^9/l) of small (mature) lymphocytes, with marked anaemia.

Because the prognosis, i.e. the possibility of chemotherapy proving successful, is so much better in chronic lymphocytic leukaemia than in acute lymphoblastic leukaemia, it is important for laboratory reports to state whether the lymphocytes found are small (mature) or large (lymphoblastic).

DOG

Acute lymphoblastic leukaemia

Over a quarter of dogs affected are German Shepherd Dogs.

The disorder results in non-regenerative anaemia, thrombocytopenia, large numbers of lymphoblasts in the peripheral blood and bone marrow (usually unassociated with solid tumours), plus enlargement of the spleen and liver.

The clinical signs are of lethargy, anorexia, vomiting and diarrhoea and the bone marrow shows reduced RBC and platelet production.

Chronic lymphocytic leukaemia

This shows an excessive number of mature lymphocytes in the peripheral blood and bone marrow (bone marrow infiltration is patchy in early cases, but later becomes more widespread). Signs develop of anaemia, lethargy, inappetance plus ascites, azotaemia and proteinuria.

There may be slight enlargement of the lymph nodes and an enlarged liver and spleen.

This condition is considered to be a disease of the B-lymphocytes and can result in:

- Increased plasma concentrations of IgA, IgM and IgG.
- Bence-Jones protein in the plasma in 50% of cases.
- Monoclonal antibody peaks in more than 50% of cases (see p. 296).
- Very occasionally, development of the hyperviscosity syndrome.

Three per cent of affected dogs have very high white blood cell counts, i.e. $>100 \times 10^9/l$ (85–97% of these WBCs are lymphocytes); half of these cases are in Boxers.

Most canine cases show anaemia, thrombocytopenia, enlarged lymph nodes and an enlarged spleen.

CHECK   for long-standing depression, periodic vomiting, attacks of diarrhoea, inappetance, weight loss, polydipsia (sometimes) and pyrexia.

Panel 3.2 Myeloproliferative disorders (MPDs)

Myeloproliferative disorders are rare, neoplastic disorders of bone marrow cells. There is uncontrolled proliferation of cells belonging to one or more of the different cell lines in the bone marrow, i.e. those which give rise to the RBCs, the platelets and the various types of WBC, with the exception of the lymphocytes (see Figure 2.1, p. 44). (On very rare occasions the rapidly multiplying cells are the primitive stem cells (pleuripotential haemopoietic stem cells) from which *all* the other cells derive.) These proliferating neoplastic cells replace a variable proportion of the normal bone marrow tissue.

The large number of immature cells resulting from this uncontrolled multiplication may:

- Either develop more or less normally into mature cells of that particular cell line (e.g. mature RBCs, mature neutrophils etc.).
- Or fail to mature further and remain as immature cells.

Large numbers of these proliferating cells pass from the bone marrow into the circulating blood.

Examination of the blood

This will show the following.

INCREASED NUMBER OF CELLS OF THE CELL LINE(S) AFFECTED

These may be either predominantly mature or immature (developmental, precursor or 'blast') cells. Diagnosis therefore requires expert examination of stained blood smears.

MPDs are described as *chronic* if these cells are mainly mature forms, and *acute* if they are predominantly immature.

Acute leukaemia is diagnosed on finding neoplastic immature cells predominating in the blood and bone marrow.

NON-REGENERATIVE ANAEMIA

This is often severe. The exception is primary polycythaemia (see Panel 2.6, p. 123) where there is a great increase in mature RBC numbers.

On the basis of the MCV and MCHC the anaemia may be classified as either normocytic/normochromic *or* macrocytic/normochromic (i.e. the MCHC is normal and the MCV is either normal or raised).

A raised MCV is seen principally in erythraemic myelosis and erythroleukaemia in cats, and at times with monocytic leukaemia and myelofibrosis, whenever there are *enough* large cells (macrocytes) present, i.e. nucleated RBCs.

NUCLEATED RED BLOOD CELLS [FREQUENTLY]

When these are present, they occur *without* increased numbers of reticulocytes, whatever the type of MPD. In large numbers, the nucleated RBCs (which are larger than normal RBCs) will result in anisocytosis (i.e. disparity in size of the RBCs), and even an increase in the MCV; they will also produce a red tinge in the lower part of the buffy coat on performing the haematocrit and in the lower part of the plasma column when measuring the ESR (see p. 122).

DEFICIENCY OF PLATELETS [USUALLY]

There is usually a deficiency of platelets and those present are abnormally large and of bizarre appearance. (However, in primary polycythaemia, megakaryocytic leukaemia in the cat and a case of basophilic leukaemia in the dog, thrombo*cytosis* has been reported.)

A VARIABLE NUMBER OF WBCs (LOW, NORMAL OR HIGH)

In developing disorders counts are frequently low, but in chronic disorders leucocytosis is often a feature.

Examination of a sample of bone marrow obtained by biopsy helps in diagnosing equivocal cases.

Other features

1. Myeloproliferative disorders are *much more common in the cat* than in the dog, although in both species they are less common than lymphoproliferative disorders.

2. In the cat the vast majority of cases of myeloproliferative disorders have been linked with FeLV infection. More recently, their association with some cases of FIV (feline immunodeficiency virus) infection has been recorded. Therefore testing for FeLV and FIV infections can provide a check on the diagnosis.
3. Enlargement of the spleen, liver and lymph nodes (splenomegaly, hepatomegaly and lymphadenopathy) commonly occurs in acute MPDs as the immature haemopoietic cells proliferate in the vascular spaces of these organs, a phenomenon termed 'extramedullary haemopoiesis'.
4. Hyperbilirubinaemia (and consequently jaundice) may arise due to:
   (a) atrophy of liver parenchymal cells, as the liver becomes packed with the haemopoietic cells,
   (b) increased phagocytosis of RBCs giving an extravascular haemolytic anaemia.

Recognized MPDs

The following MPDs are recognized (Table 3.5).

Table 3.5 Classification of myeloproliferative disorders (MPDs)

Disorder	Predominant abnormal cells in circulation
Acute MPDs	
Acute granulocytic (myelogenous) leukaemia*	Early neutrophil precursors (chiefly myeloblasts)
Erythraemic myelosis*	Rubriblasts
Erythroleukaemia*	Rubriblasts and myeloblasts
(Acute) monocytic leukaemia	Monoblasts
(Acute) myelomonocytic leukaemia	Myeloblasts and monoblasts
Eosinophilic leukaemia	Eosinophils and precursors
Basophilic leukaemia	Basophils and precursors
(Acute) megakaryocytic leukaemia	Megakaryoblasts
Reticuloendotheliosis (= undifferentiated leukaemia)	Haemopoietic stem cells
Chronic MPDs	
Chronic granulocytic (myelogenous) leukaemia	Neutrophils and late precursors
Primary polycythaemia	Mature RBCs
Myelofibrosis (with myeloid metaplasia)	Megakaryocytes, fibroblasts (confined to bone marrow)
Related disorders	
Multiple myeloma	Plasma cells
Mast cell leukaemia	Mast cells

* These are the most common MPDs in dogs and cats.

GRANULOCYTIC LEUKAEMIA (MYELOGENOUS LEUKAEMIA = MYELOID LEUKAEMIA)

The blood shows neutrophil precursors – myeloblasts, progranulocytes, myelocytes and metamyelocytes.

Acute granulocytic leukaemia

This is the type of granulocytic leukaemia *most commonly seen* in dogs and cats. The total WBC count may be increased, normal or decreased and up to 90% of the WBCs are *early* neutrophil precursors (myeloblasts, progranulocytes and myelocytes) and there may be mature neutrophils without nuclear lobulation (Pelger–Huët cells). (With rough handling or prolonged storage in EDTA these immature WBCs show vacuolation or 'smudging'.)

Chronic granulocytic leukaemia

This features a leucocytosis and a neutrophilia with a shift-to-the-left, but in general with only a small number of early neutrophil precursors that are often *unevenly* arranged (i.e. the most immature are not necessarily the least numerous). Some neutrophils may be hypersegmented.

Preleukaemic (or subleukaemic) granulocytic leukaemia (haemopoietic dysplasia)

This may occur in the cat; the blood shows a persistent *leucopenia* and *neutropenia* and small numbers of neutrophil precursors, with or without nucleated RBCs.

Granulocytic leukaemia having a blood picture that strongly *resembles* that of leukaemia but which is, in fact, due to some other cause is termed a 'leukaemoid reaction'.

The most common type of leukaemoid reaction resembles chronic granulocytic leukaemia – there is neutrophilia and a shift-to-the-left that includes some developmental forms of neutrophils. It develops principally in cases of severe bacterial infection, i.e. purulent inflammation, in immune-mediated disorders (e.g. autoimmune haemolytic anaemic) and in association with malignant neoplasia. (Leukaemoid reactions involving other cells, such as lymphocytes and eosinophils, occasionally arise.)

Distinguishing features of a *leukaemoid reaction* are:

● Evidence of an infectious or inflammatory cause, an immune-mediated disorder or malignant neoplasia at a site other than the bone marrow.
● Repeated (i.e. serial) samples show this blood picture to be only temporary.
● Toxic changes in the neutrophils (see p. 180).

Distinguishing features indicating *leukaemia* are:

● Very severe anaemia, thrombocytopenia and splenomegaly.
● An uneven shift-to-the-left, i.e. in the blood the more immature the neutrophil precursors the more numerous they are.
● Neutrophils showing hypersegmentation and considerable variation in size and shape.

ERYTHRAEMIC MYELOSIS (ERYTHROBLASTIC LEUKAEMIA)

In association with a severe non-regenerative anaemia there are large numbers of nucleated red blood cells, i.e. without a corresponding increase in reticulocytes. Anisocytosis is prominent.

ERYTHROLEUKAEMIA

The blood shows features of both erythraemic myelosis and granulocytic leukaemia, i.e. there is neoplastic proliferation of both erythroid and granulocytic cells. It is considered to be an intermediate stage in the progression of erythraemic myelosis to granulocytic leukaemia, and is an example of a leucoerythroblastic reaction.

Note

The presence of many nucleated RBCs *and* immature neutrophils in the blood can be referred to as a leucoerythroblastic reaction. Usually it arises without any, or with a disproportionately small, increase in reticulocyte numbers. WBC numbers are variable, and may be below or slightly above the normal range. If anaemia is present it can be termed 'a leucoerythroblastic anaemia'.

A leucoerythroblastic reaction may be a feature of:

- Myeloproliferative diseases, especially erythroleukaemia.
- Disseminated haemangiosarcomas.
- An intense response to acute haemorrhage or acute haemolysis.

MONOCYTIC LEUKAEMIA

There is marked monocytosis with developmental monocytes (monoblasts), and a mild non-regenerative anaemia. Affected dogs are young.

MYELOMONOCYTIC LEUKAEMIA

The blood shows marked monocytosis and neutrophilia with primitive cells of both the granulocyte and monocyte series. Affected dogs are young.

EOSINOPHILIC LEUKAEMIA

There is marked eosinophilia plus a large number of developmental eosinophils. It is not recorded in the dog, only the cat (particularly in association with haemorrhagic ulcerative colitis). Until recently no case positive for FeLV infection had been recorded.

The blood picture may be confused with that due to allergy (including parasitism), eosinophilic enteritis or disseminated eosinophilic disease (see 'Causes of eosinophilia', p. 164), although in those conditions the majority of cells are mature. Very rarely a similar picture (*eosinophilic leukaemoid reaction*) develops in feline cases of alimentary lymphosarcoma.

BASOPHILIC LEUKAEMIA

The blood shows a high proportion of developmental basophils. One canine case was associated with *thrombocytosis*.

MEGAKARYOCYTIC LEUKAEMIA

This is characterized by the presence of megakaryoblasts (early stages in platelet formation) with *thrombocytopenia* in the dog and *thrombocytosis* in the cat.

RETICULOENDOTHELIOSIS (UNDIFFERENTIATED MPD = UNDIFFERENTIATED LEUKAEMIA = POORLY DIFFERENTIATED MPD = ACUTE ERYTHROLEUKAEMIA)

The primitive pleuripotential haemopoietic cell proliferates and numbers of these large primitive cells appear in the blood.

PRIMARY POLYCYTHAEMIA (POLYCYTHAEMIA VERA)

This is a chronic MPD that has little in common with other MPDs (see Panel 2.6, p. 123). In particular there is the reverse of anaemia – a massive increase in RBC numbers, usually with leucocytosis and thrombocytosis.

MYELOFIBROSIS (WITH MYELOID METAPLASIA)

Primary myelofibrosis

This is characterized by the proliferation of fibroblasts and the deposition of collagen in the bone marrow cavity, so that the normal haemopoietic (blood-forming) tissue is replaced by fibrous tissue and collagen. It may result from an excessive accumulation of megakaryocytes. Often this disorder develops as the end-stage of an MPD in dogs and cats (e.g. of erythroleukaemia in cats).

Usually there is proliferation of haemopoietic cells in other organs (spleen, liver and lymph nodes) – termed 'myeloid metaplasia' and this often produces enlargement, especially splenomegaly but also hepatomegaly and lymphadenopathy. The large numbers of RBC precursors (reticulocytes and nucleated RBCs) appearing in the blood due to this proliferation have been misinterpreted as indicating a regenerative response to the anaemia. Mis-shapen RBCs (poikilocytes) may appear, especially oval and tear-shaped RBCs (ovalocytes and dacrocytes).

Secondary myelofibrosis

This can be a non-specific reactive change, the result of bone marrow damage by drugs (particularly oestrogens), radiation or metastatic neoplasms, or the end-stage of pyruvate kinase deficiency in the Basenji and Beagle.

Related disorders

Two other neoplastic disorders produce very similar signs – multiple myeloma and mast cell leukaemia.

MULTIPLE MYELOMA (see panel 5.1, p. 295)

A myeloma is a plasma cell tumour of the bone marrow. Typically it affects bone marrow at more than one site (i.e. is multicentric) and the condition is then termed 'multiple myeloma'. (Plasma cell tumours other than in bone marrow are termed 'plasmacytomas'.)

Myelomas can:

- Release large numbers of plasma cells into the blood.
- Decrease the production of RBCs, granular WBCs and platelets (i.e. can result in anaemia, granulocytopenia and thrombocytopenia).

• Secrete a large amount of a monoclonal immunoglobulin, which is usually non-functional IgM. The large amount of identical immunoglobulin coming from a single clone of cells produces a typical high 'spike' or 'church spire' in the globulin region when electrophoresis of plasma or serum is performed, i.e. this is a monoclonal gammopathy. (Monoclonal gammopathy is also a feature of some lymphomas.)

In the urine the following may appear:

• Light chains of immunoglobulin (Bence-Jones protein). Urine testing dipsticks are not sensitive to it and it is best detected by urinary electrophoresis.
• Excess albumin, as a result of glomerular damage.

MAST CELL LEUKAEMIA (MAST CELL NEOPLASIA)

Mast cells are tissue cells, not blood cells, but they have functions in *common* with basophils with which they may be confused. In cases of disseminated malignant mast cell neoplasia, particularly in cats, large numbers of mast cells may appear in the blood (termed 'mast cell leukaemia') and infiltrate the bone marrow, lymph nodes, liver and spleen (which often enlarges). They can phagocytose RBCs to produce anaemia, and a further complication may be ulceration of the stomach or duodenum.

Chapter 4

Platelets (thrombocytes)

Platelet count (thrombocyte count)

The platelet count represents the number of platelets in a stated volume of blood, which in SI units is one litre.

The recommended SI units are 10^9/litre (e.g. 320×10^9/l). Previously the platelet count was reported in terms of 10^3/μl, 10^3/mm^3, thousand/μl or thousand/mm^3, which are all numerically equivalent to 10^9/l and to each other (e.g. 320×10^9/l = 320×10^3/μl). Alternatively, the number of platelets can be expressed in terms of 10^5/μl; in this case the number preceding the units has to be divided by 10^2, i.e. 320×10^9/l = 3.2×10^5/μl.

NORMAL REFERENCE RANGE

Dog: 200–500 $\times 10^9$/l.
Cat: 300–700 $\times 10^9$/l.

Platelet counts are generally only made in cases that have a bleeding disorder. An abnormally low number of platelets (thrombocytopenia) could account for frequent, multiple haemorrhages and impaired blood clotting. However, *spontaneous* haemorrhage would not be expected until platelets had fallen below 50×10^9/l and usually not until they were below 20×10^9/l.

But other factors besides thrombocytopenia could be responsible for a bleeding defect (see Panel 4.1, p. 212).

Platelet production (megakaryocytopoiesis) is controlled by the number of circulating platelets via thrombocytosis stimulating factor (TSF) or thrombopoietin, manufactured, at least in part, in the kidney.

PLATELET FUNCTION

The main function of the blood platelet is the prevention of blood loss (haemostasis) by:

- Routinely maintaining the normal continuity or integrity of the lining of the blood vessels (i.e. endothelium), especially the capillaries. The platelets act to prevent any weakening of the endothelium and plug any gaps that might appear. If this routine repair is left undone, RBCs can escape, resulting in petechial haemorrhages.
- Repairing minor damage to the endothelium by adhering to the exposed underlying collagen and then forming a plug of platelets (primary haemostatic plug) to seal the hole and stop blood loss. Later this plug is strengthened by a fibrin clot.
- Activating and accelerating the process of blood clotting.

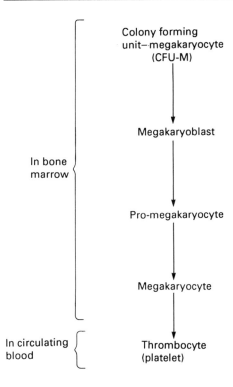

In bone marrow

In circulating blood

Colony forming
unit–megakaryocyte
(CFU-M)

Megakaryoblast

Pro-megakaryocyte

Megakaryocyte

Thrombocyte
(platelet)

Figure 4.1 Stages of development of blood platelets. (See also p. 44 for relationship to blood cells)

METHOD OF PLATELET COUNTING

Platelets are counted *either* with an automated blood counter (which is regarded as reliable with canine platelets, but not always with feline, because of their tendency to aggregate, particularly where there has been some difficulty withdrawing the blood sample) *or* using a haemocytometer.

The *accuracy* may be no more than ± 25%.

Blood must be collected into EDTA and counts made as soon as possible, ideally within half an hour and certainly within 2 hours. Otherwise the platelets aggregate producing falsely low values, because a clump of platelets is either counted as a single platelet *or* exceeds the threshold for counting and does not register at all.

Other ways of assessing the number of platelets (if counts cannot be speedily made by the above methods) involve either examining a Romanowsky or supravitally stained blood smear or using the QBC-V system. A *smear* should be made at the time of blood collection, fixed and then despatched to the laboratory (see Appendix I, p. 468).

Counting platelets on a stained smear

Counting the number of platelets per oil immersion field
Six to seven platelets per oil immersion field are roughly equivalent to a count of 100×10^9/l.

Counting the numbers of platelets and RBCs over the same area of smear
This requires the RBC count in $10^{12}/l$ to be known.

$$\text{Platelet count (in } 10^9/l) = \frac{\text{No. platelets counted} \times \text{RBC count (in } 10^{12}/l) \times 10^3}{\text{No. of RBCs counted}}$$

One platelet per 70 RBCs is roughly equivalent to a count of $100 \times 10^9/l$.

Counting the numbers of platelets and WBCs over the same area of smear
This is the most accurate method and can be combined with performance of the differential WBC count.

$$\text{Platelet count (in } 10^9/l) = \frac{\text{No. of platelets counted} \times \text{WBC count (in } 10^9/l)}{\text{No. of WBCs counted}}$$

All three methods of estimation can have considerable errors due to the clumping of platelets and uneven platelet distribution within the smear.

The QBC-V system (see Appendix I, p. 470)

This sytem allows the simple measurement of platelet numbers in the practice immediately after blood collection. It appears sufficiently accurate for most clinical purposes, but in the cat the platelet counts can be lower than they should because platelets tend to stick to the float.

Causes of increased platelet count (thrombocytosis)

In the *dog* = $>500 \times 10^9/l$ and in the *cat* = $> 700 \times 10^9/l$.
Increases are generally short lived and relatively modest.

Summary
Summary
• Excitement
• Exercise
• Pregnancy
• Posthaemorrhage
• After trauma, fractures and surgery
• Postsplenectomy – dog
• Acute or chronic infection/inflammation
• Iron deficiency – dog
• Drug-induced
• Myeloproliferative disorders
• Malignant neoplasia

EXCITEMENT

In the cat this can be for as little as 3 minutes and can increase the platelet count due to the influence of adrenaline mobilizing platelets from the splenic pool.

EXERCISE

When mild, platelets come from the non-splenic pool (mainly pulmonary); when strenuous, from the splenic pool as well.

PREGNANCY

In the bitch, counts rise from the third week of pregnancy and are almost always above $500 \times 10^9/l$ just before parturition.

All the following causes are termed 'reactive'.

POSTHAEMORRHAGE

This arises especially after chronic haemorrhage, e.g. associated with blood-sucking parasites and ulcerating neoplasms.

After severe, acute haemorrhage, the platelet count rises 36 hours later, this thrombocytosis following a thrombocytopenia.

Continuing thrombocytosis (more than 3 weeks) suggests persistent haemorrhage and possible causes should be checked (see Panel 2.1, p. 75).

AFTER TRAUMA, FRACTURES AND SURGERY

This occurs 3–10 days after major surgery and platelet numbers return to normal in approximately 2 weeks. This is associated with posthaemorrhage thrombocytosis (see above).

FOLLOWING SPLENECTOMY (IN THE DOG)

Platelets that would normally be sequestered (hidden) in the spleen are now obliged to return to the circulation.

ACUTE OR CHRONIC INFECTIONS AND INFLAMMATORY DISORDERS

Examples of these include bronchitis and enteritis.

IRON DEFICIENCY (IN THE DOG)

Thrombocytosis is often associated with chronic haemorrhage.

DRUG-INDUCED

Thrombocytosis can be induced by glucocorticoids, adrenaline and especially vincristine, which increases platelet production and can lead to a considerable rise in numbers. In the early stages of oestrogen therapy, platelet numbers increase (although long term they fall).

SOME MYELOPROLIFERATIVE DISORDERS

These are essentially primary polycythaemia, megakaryocytic leukaemia in the cat and basophilic leukaemia in the dog. (Most myeloproliferative disorders give rise to the opposite effect – thrombocytopenia.)

MALIGNANT NEOPLASIA

Causes of decreased platelet count (thrombocytopenia)

Summary

Decreased platelet production
- Toxic drugs and chemicals
- Other toxins – uraemic/bacterial/mycotic
- Infection
- Radiation [rare]
- Stem cell replacement in bone marrow
- Severe iron deficiency [unusual]
- Defective thromopoietin production [very, very rare]
- Rebound thrombocytopenia – after transfusion
- Hypoadrenocorticism

Increased platelet destruction or usage
- Infection
- Disseminated intravascular coagulation
- Anaphylaxis
- Immune-mediated disorders
- Functional platelet defects

Excessive platelet loss
- Massive external haemorrhage [very rare]

Abnormal platelet distribution
- Spenomegaly

Error:
- Platelet clumping
- Clotted sample

Thrombocytopenia is due mainly to decreased platelet production by the bone marrow and/or increased destruction or usage of platelets.

However *always* **CHECK** that *clotting* in the sample is not the cause; it can result in very low platelet counts.

Strictly thrombocytopenia exists when the number of platelets falls below $200 \times 10^9/l$ in the dog or $300 \times 10^9/l$ in the cat, but generally only counts below $100 \times 10^9/l$ are considered clinically significant.

DECREASED PRODUCTION OF PLATELETS BY THE BONE MARROW

Many of the causes below can also result in decreased production of RBCs and WBCs, i.e. they produce aplastic anaemia (see 'Causes of hypoproliferative anaemia', p. 111).

Drug and chemical toxicity

- Oestrogens, both administered (natural and synthetic) and endogenous (e.g. from Sertoli cell tumours and granulosa cell tumours).

  CHECK for anaemia, plus, in the early stage, thrombocytosis and leucocytosis due to neutrophillia – later thrombocytopenia and leucopenia.

- Chloramphenicol in the cat.
- Ribavirin (antiviral drug) in the cat.
- Levamisole.
- Dapsone.
- Phenylbutazone.
- Aspirin.
- Paracetamol (acetaminophen).
- Phenobarbitone.
- Chlorpromazine and promazine.
- Penicillin.
- Streptomycin.
- Thiazide diuretics.
- Sulphonamides.
- Tetracycline.
- Acetazolamide.
- Frusemide (furosemide).
- Propylthiouracil.
- Methimazole (and ?carbimazole).
- Gold compounds.
- Anticancer drugs.

Most commonly oestrogens, phenylbutazone and thiazide diuretics are involved.

Drugs suppressing the bone marrow usually result in a decrease in WBC count *before* they cause a reduced platelet count, because the platelets have a longer lifespan.

Effect of other toxins on bone marrow

- Uraemia (depresses platelet manufacture).
- Bacterial toxins.
- Mycotoxins.

Infection

Reduced platelet production can be due to FeLV infection and (although not in the UK) chronic canine ehrlichiosis.

It may occur in other viral, bacterial and protozoal infections, although it is believed that the thrombocytopenia is primarily due to *increased platelet destruction* (see below) in these conditions.

Radiation [rare]

Replacement of platelet stem cells in bone marrow

Replacement by non-functional cells occurs in:

- Lymphoproliferative disorders and the majority of myeloproliferative disorders.
- Other myelophthistic diseases, e.g. due to infiltration by metastatic tumours from elsewhere, myelofibrosis and osteopetrosis.

In association with severe iron deficiency [unusual]

CHECK   for low levels of serum iron *and* total iron-binding capacity.

Some defect in the production of thrombopoietin [very, very rare]

'Rebound' thrombocytopenia

This can follow thrombocytosis due to the transfusion of blood containing large numbers of platelets.

Addison's disease (hypoadrenocorticism)

Thrombocytopenia is due to the low cortisol level.

INCREASED PLATELET DESTRUCTION OR USAGE

Infection

Many viral, bacterial and protozoal diseases are associated with thrombocytopenia which can arise in a number of ways: direct damage to the platelets, disseminated intravascular coagulation (DIC), platelets binding to the blood vessel endothelium and immune-mediated platelet destruction.

Important examples are:

- Feline infectious peritonitis.
- Feline infectious enteritis (= feline panleucopenia).
- Canine parvovirus infection.
- Infectious canine hepatitis.
- Neonatal canine herpes virus infection.
- Leptospirosis.
- Salmonellosis.
- Histoplasmosis.
- Disseminated candidiasis.
- Bacteraemia.

Also, although not in the UK, Rocky Mountain spotted fever, babesiosis and haemobartonellosis (in the dog) and ehrlichiosis (Breitschwerdt, 1988).

Disseminated intravascular coagulation

This is discussed in Panel 4.2 (p. 216).

Anaphylaxis

Immune-mediated disorders

Thrombocytopenia is especially a feature of autoimmune thrombocytopenia and systemic lupus erythematosus (see Panel 2.7, p. 125).

Functional defects of platelets

These can contribute to an increased rate of platelet destruction.

EXCESSIVE LOSS OF PLATELETS

Massive external haemorrhage

This may (although very rarely) result in a massive loss of platelets.

ABNORMAL DISTRIBUTION OF PLATELETS

Splenomegaly

In conditions where there is a large increase in the size of the spleen more platelets can be hidden away in this organ and this may lead to thrombocytopenia.

ERROR

Clumping of platelets

This can result in a *falsely low* count because an aggregation of platelets may be counted as if they were a single one. This is more likely to happen with:

- Electronic counting, especially of feline blood samples in which clumping commonly occurs, because the clumps are not seen and therefore not allowed for.
- Delayed counting, i.e. samples collected more than 2 hours previously.
- Difficulty in venepuncture (especially in cats), because the blood sample can become contaminated with tissue thromboplastin which initiates clumping.

Clotted sample

The liquid part of a blood sample which has clotted may contain very few platelets, e.g. $<10 \times 10^9/l$.

Changes in platelet appearance (morphology)

This includes changes in size, shape and granularity.

SIZE

Young platelets are large; as they grow older, they lose membrane fragments and become smaller. Therefore a high proportion of large platelets (megathrombocytes) suggests a rapid turnover.

Size is more variable in the cat and some platelets are as large as RBCs.

Very small platelets (microthrombocytes) can occur in autoimmune thrombocytopenia.

SHAPE

Normal platelets are irregular discs, without nuclei, appearing more rounded in blood containing EDTA.

Numbers of large, bizarre-shaped platelets and reduced total numbers (thrombocytopenia) suggest increased destruction or consumption, and are especially seen in myeloproliferative disorders.

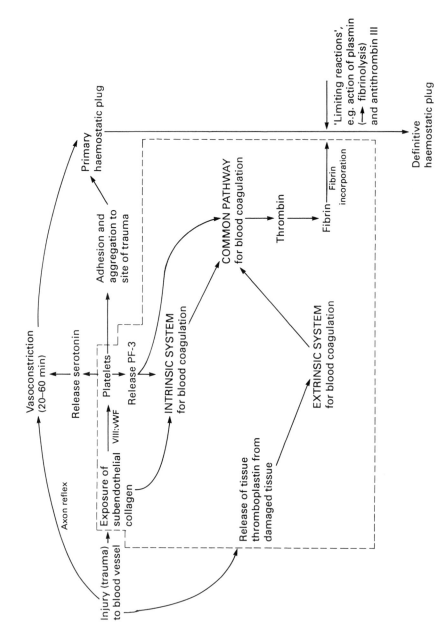

Figure 4.2 Normal haemostatic mechanisms. PF-3 = platelet factor 3; VIII:vWF = von Willebrand's factor. For details of blood coagulation (intrinsic system, extrinsic system and common pathway), i.e. the area within the dotted lines, see Figure 4.3

GRANULARITY

Normally feline platelets show marked granularity; it is less obvious in the dog.
An absence of granules, or the presence of vacuoles is abnormal and is seen, for example, with:

- Disseminated intravascular coagulation.
- Disorders associated with FeLV infection.
- Chediak–Higashi syndrome in Persian cats.

Panel 4.1 Haemostasis (including defects and tests)

Normal haemostasis

Normal haemostasis (i.e. prevention of blood loss) depends upon three interrelated processes (Figure 4.2):

1. Temporary vasoconstriction to reduce the flow of blood from the damaged blood vessel, and thereby make it easier to plug the leak.
2. The formation of a plug of platelets to seal the damaged blood vessel (referred to as the primary haemostatic plug).
3. Strengthening this initial platelet plug with an insoluble fibrin clot that is formed as the result of blood coagulation.

Relevant features of each of these steps are as follows.

TEMPORARY VASOCONSTRICTION

Vasoconstriction starts as a reflex axonal response and continues as a response to substances (e.g. serotonin) released by the platelets.

FORMATION OF THE PRIMARY HAEMOSTATIC PLUG

The platelets must *first* adhere to the exposed subendothelial collagen (outside the body it will be to some other abnormal surface, such as glass or plastic in the case of a blood collecting tube) and *then* aggregate (i.e. clump together) forming further layers of platelets over the first layer. Adhesion and aggregation can be induced by adrenaline (epinephrine), bacterial endotoxins, viruses and particulate matter. In addition to adhering and aggregating, the platelets release factors required for vasoconstriction and blood clotting (coagulation).

BLOOD CLOTTING

Formation of the fibrin clot requires a series of 'clotting factors' to act upon each other in a fixed sequence of steps. These factors are conventionally numbered in Roman numerals and, with the exception of factor III, tissue thromboplastin, are already present in the blood plasma. (The numbering of the clotting factors is related *not* to the order in which they act in blood coagulation *but* to the order in which they were

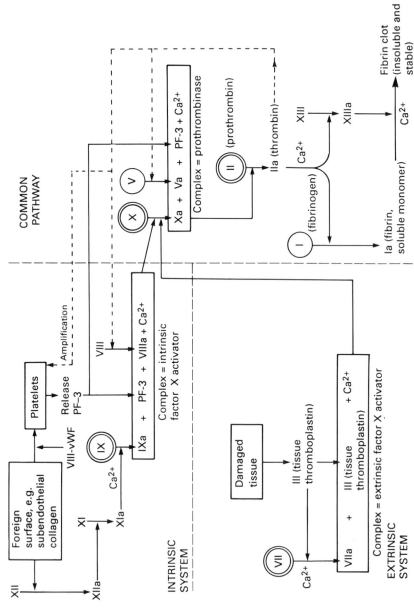

Figure 4.3 Pathways for blood coagulation. PF-3 = platelet factor 3; VIII:vWF = von Willebrand's factor; circles around those clotting factors produced by the liver; double circles around those clotting factors also requiring vitamin K. Factor XII activation is enhanced by prekallikrein and high-molecular-weight kininogen. The foreign surface initiating the intrinsic system may also be glass or polystyrene etc. Prothrombinase is also known as thrombokinase or thromboplastin. (Note: calcium ions are factor IV; there is *no* factor VI)

discovered.) Many of them are produced by the liver, some requiring vitamin K for their synthesis. They are generally considered to interact as shown in Figure 4.3, with each factor in turn being converted to an 'activated' factor, represented by the same Roman numeral plus an a. This activated factor, or in some cases *complex of activated factors*, functions as an enzyme to catalyse the activation of the next factor in the chain, and so on. (Factors may therefore also be referred to as pro-enzymes.) Calcium ions (otherwise known as factor IV) must be present for some of these conversions to take place. Each step *magnifies* the initial stimulus so that ultimately a comparatively large amount of fibrin is formed. In reality the process is even more complex with some factors influencing the formation of those *earlier* in the sequence, such as the effect of thrombin (IIa) both on the platelets and in the activation of factors V and VIII.

The first part of the clotting process can proceed along one of two pathways, the intrinsic and extrinsic systems, both of which result in the formation of a complex to activate factor X, after which a single (*common*) pathway is followed that results in the formation of the insoluble fibrin clot.

The intrinsic system is initiated by the activation of factor XII in plasma following its contact with an abnormal surface, which in the blood vessel is usually subendothelial collagen. The extrinsic system begins with the release by the damaged tissue of factor III, a phospholipid–protein complex called tissue thromboplastin. Usually following an injury *both* systems will operate but the intrinsic system appears to be more necessary than the extrinsic in triggering the steps of the common pathway. For example, a deficiency of factor VIII produces a severe haemorrhagic disorder whereas a deficiency of factor VII causes a comparatively mild bleeding defect.

Effective haemostasis depends upon all three processes. In particular it can be impaired by:

- Deficiency of platelets (thrombocytopenia).
- Reduced ability of the platelets to adhere and/or aggregate, referred to as functional platelet defects.
- A lack of one or more clotting factors, including prothrombin or fibrinogen.

Defects in haemostasis

THROMBOCYTOPENIA

The causes are listed in the section 'Causes of decreased platelet count', p. 200).

FUNCTIONAL PLATELET DEFECTS

These may be acquired or, very rarely, inherited.

Inherited platelet defects

Those recognized in small animals are:

- Glanzmann's thrombasthenia, due to an autosomal recessive gene. Reduced adhesion of platelets (caused by a lack of glycoprotein) prolongs the bleeding time, and clot retraction is also defective.
- Hereditary thrombopathia in the Basset hound and Otterhound (autosomal inheritance). Abnormal platelet function results in a variable bleeding time, but clot retraction is normal.

- Chediak–Higashi syndrome in Blue-smoke Persian cats. There is abnormal platelet aggregation in this autosomal recessive syndrome, causing a prolonged bleeding time.

Acquired platelet defects

These are far more common and may be the result of:

- Uraemia (primarily in chronic renal failure).
- Severe liver disease (e.g. cirrhosis).
- Amyloidosis.
- Myeloproliferative disorders.
- Lymphoproliferative disorders.
- Myelomas and macroglobulinaemia.
- Autoimmune diseases, e.g. systemic lupus erythematosus.
- Autoimmune thrombocytopenia and autoimmune haemolytic anaemia.
- The administration of a number of drugs, most of which inhibit platelet adhesion, including aspirin, phenylbutazone and other non-steroidal anti-inflammatory drugs, corticosteroids, dextran, local analgesics, antihistamines, ampicillin, frusemide (furosemide), promazine tranquillizers, inhalational anaesthetics, nitrofurantoin, sulphonamides and live (viral) vaccines.

DEFICIENCIES OF CLOTTING FACTORS

These may also be either inherited or acquired.

Hereditary clotting factor deficiences (congenital coagulopathies)

These are inherited deficiences of a single coagulation factor, and affected animals often have a history of bleeding problems beginning early in life.

So far deficiences have been recognized of factors I (fibrinogen), II (prothrombin), VII, VIII (including the component known as von Willebrand's factor or VIII:vWF), IX, X, XI and XII.

Factor VIII deficiency is the most common in dogs, followed by a deficiency of factor IX and von Willebrand's factor. Deficiences of factors I, II and V are very rare.

Deficiencies of factors VIII and IX are sex linked, due to X-chromosome defects. Consequently, they appear only in males and in homozygously affected females, that arise only very rarely. Mild forms of the disease are occasionally discovered in heterozygous females.

Factor I (fibrinogen) deficiency
Hypofibrinogenaemia in St Bernards (autosomal incomplete dominant) and dysfibrinogenaemia in Borzois (autosomal dominant) cause severe bleeding.

Factor II (prothrombin) deficiency
Dysprothrombinaemia in Boxers causes a mild bleeding defect. It has also been recorded in a Miniature Pinscher and American Cocker Spaniel.

Factor VII deficiency
This autosomal recessive disorder causes mild bleeding in Beagles and Alaskan Malamutes.

Factor VIII deficiency
This is now known to comprise two interrelated factors: VIII:C and VIII:vWF or von Willebrand's factor. A *portion* of the latter factor, known as VIII:RAg or, in full, factor VIII-related antigen, induces antibodies which can be tested for.

A deficiency of factor VIII:C causes haemophilia A, a sex-linked, recessive bleeding disorder, often severe (although variable), affecting many dog and cat breeds. It is the *most common* inherited clotting factor deficiency.

Factor VIII:vWF deficiency causes von Willebrand's disease. This factor is required to ensure adhesion of platelets to an abnormal surface, and a deficiency results in a (usually) mild bleeding disorder (although it varies in severity). It affects many breeds and is believed to be an autosomal recessive condition in the Scottish Terrier and an autosomal incomplete dominant in other breeds such as Golden Retrievers, Miniature Schnauzers, German Shepherd Dogs and Dobermann Pinschers.

The activity of factor VIII is low in both of these disorders (haemophilia A and von Willebrand's disease) but the activity of factor VIII-related antigen is normal in haemophilia A and low in von Willebrand's disease.

Factor IX deficiency (haemophilia B, Christmas factor deficiency)
This sex-linked, recessive deficiency produces a moderate disorder in many canine breeds (Cairn Terrier, Alaskan Malamute, St Bernard, Cocker Spaniel, French Bulldog, English Sheepdog, Shetland Sheepdog, Scottish Terrier etc.) and in British Shorthaired cats.

Factor X deficiency (Prower factor deficiency)
This autosomal recessive condition in American Cocker Spaniels causes a severe problem in puppies but is a comparatively mild disorder in adults.

Factor XI deficiency (haemophilia C)
This autosomal recessive deficiency causes a mild disorder in English Springer Spaniels, Kerry Blue Terriers and Pyrenean Mountain Dogs (Great Pyreneans).

Factor XII deficiency (Hageman factor deficiency)
This deficiency, seen primarily in the domestic cat but occasionally in dogs (Standard Poodle and German Shorthaired Pointer), is *asymptomatic* and haemostasis appears normal.

The severity of these disorders can vary and bleeding can become severe following marked trauma or surgical procedures.

Acquired deficiencies of clotting factors

These are chiefly the result of liver damage or a deficiency of vitamin K.

Vitamin K deficiency may be due to poor nutrition but is usually the result of ingesting anticoagulant rodenticides (e.g. warfarin) which are vitamin K antagonists. (As little as 5 mg/kg body weight of warfarin *can* result in impaired clotting in the dog.) Some drugs, e.g. aspirin, chloramphenicol and phenylbutazone, potentiate the anticoagulant effects of warfarin and related drugs. Other drugs, such as barbiturates, griseofulvin, phenytoin and corticosteroids, will antagonize these anticoagulant effects.

Diagnosis of haemostasis: Tests

Essentially, it is necessary to decide whether there is a genuine *defect* in haemostasis (i.e. a haemorrhagic diathesis), as distinct from bleeding due to other causes (trauma, neoplasm, ulcer) and, if so, the type of defect and whether it is likely to be acquired (and potentially 'curable') or inherited (and therefore permanent).

All defects of haemostasis present similarly, i.e. with an increased tendency to haemorrhage, often at multiple sites, although the severity can range from mere bruising to acute blood loss. A major handicap to diagnosis is that most of the relevant tests cannot be performed on samples despatched to a laboratory through the post in the usual way. This is because the normal haemostatic mechanisms begin to operate the instant the blood is withdrawn from the body, and so measurements need to be made either immediately or very soon afterwards.

However, four comparatively simple tests – bleeding time, clotting time (or activated clotting time), clot retraction and the platelet count (or, often more convenient, an estimation of platelet numbers from a stained blood smear or measurement using the QBC-V system (see Appendix I, p. 470)) – can together indicate the general nature of the disorder. The first three of these tests have to be started with the animal present but can easily be performed within a veterinary practice. Most other tests involve collecting blood into special tubes and separating the plasma and need to be started after no more than half an hour's delay, unless, in some cases, the plasma can be deep frozen. In general, the options are either to perform these initial screening tests within the practice and have other tests to refine the diagnosis performed at centres close by (e.g. human hospital laboratories) or, if that is not feasible, to have all or most of the tests performed at a specialized centre to which the animal must be referred.

Table 4.1 lists the findings of the major tests for each condition, and indicates other appropriate procedures. A brief description of these tests follows and, although this is essentially not a book of techniques, in order that they can be performed in the practice details of how to carry out the bleeding test, clotting time (or activated clotting time) and clot retraction are given in Appendix I (p. 466). Also there are details of fixing a blood smear, so that it can be stained later and the number of platelets estimated (estimation of platelets from a blood smear is described on p. 197), and a description of the QBC-V system.

BLEEDING TIME

This can only be determined in the patient, i.e. it is *not* a 'laboratory' test. It measures the ability of the platelets to adhere, aggregate and form the primary haemostatic plug, and hence to halt bleeding. A prolonged bleeding time therefore indicates:

● A deficiency of platelets (thrombocytopenia).

CHECK   platelet count.

● A functional platelet defect, usually acquired.

CHECK   values for urea, creatinine, ALT and ALP, albumin and globulin, and for evidence of myeloproliferative or lymphoproliferative disorders etc.

● Von Willebrand's disease, i.e. a deficiency of factor VIII:vWF.

Deficiencies of other clotting factors are not associated with a prolonged bleeding time, apart from I and II (fibrinogen and prothrombin) which rarely occur.

Bleeding time in the dog and cat <5 minutes.

CLOTTING TIME AND ACTIVATED CLOTTING TIME (ACT)

These tests measure the efficiency of the entire blood coagulation mechanism from start to finish. Because of the greater importance of the intrinsic system compared to the extrinsic, a deficiency of factor VII has no appreciable effect, whereas deficiences of factors VIII (both VIII:C and, often, von Willebrand's factor, VIII:vWF), IX, X, XI and XII (and also I, fibrinogen, and II, prothrombin) result in these times being prolonged. The clotting time and ACT are not dependent on platelet numbers or platelet function, other than a lack of platelet factor 3.

- The clotting time is performed with blood contained in fine capillary tubes.
  Clotting time in the dog <13 minutes.
  Clotting time in the cat <9 minutes.
- The activated clotting time (ACT) is preferred because it is a less variable and more sensitive test than clotting time, and the time is shorter because of the improved contact of the platelets with an abnormal surface. It uses a special Vacutainer tube that will allow the clot retraction time to be measured later *on the same sample*. It is an acceptable alternative to the activated partial thromboplastin time (APTT) where it is not possible for that test to be performed.
  In the dog ACT <95 seconds at 37°C (at room temperature <130 seconds).
  In the cat the ACT <90 seconds at 37°C.

To increase these clotting times the amount of one or more relevant clotting factors must be less than 5% of normal. They may also be slightly prolonged if the platelet count is <10 × 10⁹/l, due to a lack of platelet factor 3 (PF-3).

In addition the clotting times can be prolonged by prior administration of anticoagulants, barbiturates and salicylates (e.g. clotting takes longer in samples collected during barbiturate anaesthesia), and they can also be falsely prolonged by:

- Failure to recognize the appearance of the clot.
- When being performed at 37°C, failure to pre-warm the tube to that temperature.
- Inadequate mixing in the ACT tube.

They can be falsely shortened by excessive tissue damage during blood collection (i.e. difficult venepuncture) which adds a large amount of tissue thromboplastin to the sample.

CLOT RETRACTION

Clot retraction can be assessed as normal or otherwise by observing the amount of serum appearing around the blood clot. The test can be performed in a clean glass tube or using the same specialized Vacutainer tube used for the ACT. *After 1 hour* the clot is inspected, and normally the presence of clear serum around a firm clot is obvious. When separated, the volume of serum normally measures at least 25% of the original blood volume (since 2 ml of blood is used the volume of serum should be at least 0.5 ml). If retraction is poor after 1 hour the clot can be re-inspected after 2 and 4 hours, and finally after 24 hours.

Table 4.1 Diagnosis of bleeding defects

Test[a]	Bleeding time	Clotting time (or ACT)	Clot retraction time	Platelet count	Activated partial thromboplastin time (APTT)	Prothrombin time (PT) (or OSPT)	Thrombin time (TT)	Level of fibrinogen	Level of FDPs	Other diagnostic tests
Blood sample needed	None collected	Fill capillary tube or 3 × 1 ml in glass tubes or 2 ml in special Vacutainer	2 ml into glass tube	EDTA sample or make blood smear immediately	(2.5–)5 ml blood into liquid sodium citrate tube. Separate plasma[b]			EDTA sample	2 ml blood into 'Thrombo-Wellcotest' tube. Separate serum	
'Normal' values Dog:	<5 min	<13 min (for ACT see[c])	1–2 hours	>200 × 10^9/l	<11 seconds	7–10 seconds	<11 seconds	1–5 g/l	<10 µg/ml	
Cat:	<5 min	< 9 min	1–2 hours	>300 × 10^9/l	<15 seconds	7–12 seconds	<20 seconds	0.5–3 g/l	<10 µg/ml	
Deficiency of intrinsic factors, VIII (= VIII:C), IX, XI or XII	N	↑	N	N	↑	N	N	N	N	N VIII:RAg[d] Repeat APTTs[e]
Deficiency of extrinsic factor, VII	N	N	N	N	N	↑	N	N	N	
Deficiency of common factors: X	N or ↑[s]	↑	N[f]	N	↑	↑	N←N	N	N	
I (fibrinogen)	N or ↑[r]	↑ variable	↑[f]	N	N or ↑[r]	↑	N←N	N→N	N	
II (prothrombin)		↑ variable	N	N	N	↑	N	N	N	
Vitamin K deficiency or antagonism (i.e. anticoagulant poisons)	N	↑[h]	N	N	↑[g,h]	↑[h]	N	N	N	
von Willebrand's disease	↑	Variable, often ↑	↑[i]	N	Variable, often ↑	N	N	N	N	↓ VIII:RAg[d]
Platelet defects, acquired and inherited	↑	N or ↑	N or ↑[i,j]	N	N	N	N	N	N	CHECK for ↑ urea, ↑ creatinine, ↑ ALT, ↑ ALP, ↓ albumin, ↑ globulin, evidence of myeloproliferative and lymphoproliferative disorders

										Notes
Thrombocytopenia										
Bone marrow suppression	↑	N[k]	↑	↓	↑			N	N	Bone marrow biopsy[l]
Immune mediated	↑	N[k]	↑	↓	↑			N	N	+ve ANA, +ve LE cell, +ve PF-3
Disseminated intravascular coagulation (DIC)	↑	Often ↑[m]	↑	↓	↑			↑	↑	↑
Severe liver disease	↑ variable	↑ variable	↑ variable	N or ↓	↑	↑ variable[o]	↑ variable[p]	↓ late stage[q]	↑ variable	CHECK for ↑ ALT, ↑ ALP, ↓ TP, ↓ albumin, ↓ urea, ↑ ammonia, ↑ bile acids, ↑ BSP etc.

Acquired defects (i.e. liver disease, DIC, vitamin K antagonism, acquired platelet defects and factors causing thrombocytopenia) are variable in their effects, and the finding of abnormal results depends on the severity of the defect.

Clotting factor activities need to be <30% of normal before they will affect APTT or PT (OSPT) and <5% of normal before affecting clotting time or ACT.

Haemorrhages occurring with *no abnormal results* on these tests, or with increased platelet numbers are due to some other cause. (See 'Causes of haemorrhagic anaemia', p. 91, and 'Causes of increased platelet count', p. 198.)

N = normal value, ↑ = increased value, ↓ = decreased value, variable = variable result.

a The first six tests are the most generally useful; the first four tests can be performed, or estimated, in a veterinary practice.

b Nine parts blood to one part liquid sodium citrate (0.38% soln). Ideally separate plasma within half an hour of blood collection and perform test, *or* deep freeze (−20°C) and transport deep frozen. APTT and PT need 0.1 ml plasma each, thrombin time 0.2 ml plasma, but allow for repeat estimations.

c ACT (activated clotting time) values are (at 37°C) dog <95 seconds, cat <90 seconds, and at room temperature, dog <130 seconds.

d Activity of factor VIII is reduced in both haemophilia A (deficiency of VIII:C) and von Willebrand's disease (deficiency of VIII:vWF), but in haemophilia A the activity of factor VIII:RAg (factor VIII-related antigen) is normal and in von Willebrand's disease it is low. Von Willebrand's factor can be measured in citrated samples up to 3 days after collection by specialist centres (Littlewood and Bevan, 1989).

e Deficiencies of intrinsic factors can be distinguished by repeating the APTT successively, on each occasion adding a plasma which is known to be deficient in just one of the factors and observing whether the result becomes normal or not.

f Small clots produced. Can be confused with fibrinolysis.

g Modest rise appearing later in severe cases.

h In early cases or, if only mild, the PT (OSPT) alone may increase, with clotting time (or ACT) and APTT *both remaining normal*.

i Reduced platelet adhesiveness can be checked with glass bead columns or other tests.

j Inherited defects; clot retraction is *slow* in thrombasthenia but *normal* in thrombocytopathia (in Basset Hounds).

k Slightly prolonged clotting time (or ACT) when platelet counts are below 10×10^9/l.

l With bone marrow aplasia, biopsy will show few or no megakaryocytes, whereas with increased platelet destruction the number of megakaryocytes is normal or increased plus fewer granulocyte WBCs and a non-regenerative anaemia.

m Clotting time (or ACT) is prolonged where clotting factors are markedly depleted.

o PT (= OSPT) is only *increased* in acute liver damage, it is *normal* in chronic cases.

p Thrombin time is prolonged where the level of fibrinogen is reduced and that of FDPs increased.

q Fibrinogen level is decreased in the *terminal* stage of liver disease; indicates a poor prognosis. Although a normal bleeding time and prolonged APTT would be anticipated, rare cases of dysprothrombinaemia are reported so show the opposite.

r Bleeding time may be prolonged due to a deficiency of platelet-associated fibrinogen.

Poor clot retraction will occur due to:

- Thrombocytopenia ($<100 \times 10^9$/l).
- A functional platelet defect (in association with normal platelet numbers), including von Willebrand's disease.
- A deficiency of fibrinogen.

A crumbly, soft clot which liquefies after ½–1 hour denotes a lack of fibrinogen or excessive fibrinolysis (clot breakdown).

PLATELET COUNT (THROMBOCYTE COUNT)

The platelet count loses accuracy after half an hour and is hardly worth performing after 2 hours.

An alternative is to make and stain a blood smear (or make and fix a blood smear for later staining) at the time the blood is withdrawn, and use it later to estimate platelet numbers (see p. 192).

Alternatively the number of platelets can be quickly assessed after blood collection using the QBC-V system.

Strictly thrombocytopenia exists when the number of platelets falls below 200×10^9/l in the dog or 300×10^9/l in the cat, but generally only counts below 100×10^9/l are considered clinically significant. Spontaneous haemorrhage, due to thrombocytopenia alone, does not arise above levels of 50×10^9/l and generally not above 20–25×10^9/l.

Thrombocytopenia can have many causes including bone marrow suppression, immune-mediated disease, splenic sequestration, DIC and severe liver disease (see 'Causes of decreased platelet count', p. 200).

ACTIVATED PARTIAL THROMBOPLASTIN TIME (APTT)

This is otherwise known as the kaolin–cephalin clotting time.

This test evaluates the efficiency of the clotting factors in the intrinsic system plus the common pathway. Citrated plasma is incubated with kaolin, or celite, which activates factor XII, plus cephaloplastins as a substitute for platelet factor 3. The time between adding calcium ions (to overcome the effect of the citrate) and the formation of fibrin is then measured.

In the dog APTT <11 seconds.
In the cat APTT <15 seconds.

These times vary with the reagents but should not exceed 20 seconds.
APTT is prolonged with:

- Deficiences (<30%) of any one of factors VIII (including von Willebrand's factor), IX, X, XI or XII; in this respect it gives a similar result to the clotting time or ACT (although for *those* times to be prolonged the activity of clotting factors must be *reduced further, i.e. below 5% of normal*).
- A deficiency of fibrinogen, factor I (<0.5 g/l).
- Inhibition by an anticoagulant, e.g. heparin.

(To distinguish between them the test is repeated after adding an equal amount of normal plasma to the sample; the APTT will return to normal with a factor deficiency but stay low if due to heparin inhibition.)

See the Note below (p. 215).

PROTHROMBIN TIME (PT)

This is otherwise known as the one-stage prothrombin time (OSPT).

This test evaluates the efficiency of the extrinsic system plus the common pathway. Citrated plasma is added to thromboplastin (with platelet factor 3) and calcium ions, and the time taken to form fibrin is measured.

In the dog prothrombin time = 7–10 seconds.
In the cat prothrombin time = 7–12 seconds.

The prothrombin time (OSPT) is prolonged if there is a deficiency of factors VII or X (<30% of normal activity) or of factors II (prothrombin) or I (fibrinogen, <0.5 g/l).

It is prolonged with severe liver disease, DIC or vitamin K deficiency, including vitamin K antagonism by coumarin-like anticoagulants (e.g. warfarin). Because of the short half-life of factor VII, it is very sensitive to vitamin K deficiency or vitamin K antagonism.

See the Note below.

THROMBIN TIME (TT)

This is otherwise known as thrombin clotting time (TCT).

This is the time taken for fibrin to be formed after the addition of thrombin to a citrated plasma sample. It is a measure of the amount of fibrinogen present and the ability to convert it to fibrin.

A prolonged thrombin time is found with a deficiency of fibrinogen or with difficulty in the production of fibrinogen (<1 g/l in the dog) *or* the presence of inhibitors such as heparin or fibrinogen degradation products (FDPs), associated with severe liver disease or disseminated intravascular coagulation.

See the Note below.

In the dog, thrombin time = <11 seconds.
In the cat, thrombin time = <20 seconds.

Note

The activated partial thromboplastin time (APTT), prothrombin time (PT or OSPT) and thrombin time (TT), are probably best performed at a specialist centre to which the animal is taken. If performed on a sample sent to a laboratory, blood should be taken into citrate (nine volumes of blood added to one volume of 0.38% sodium citrate solution). Ideally the plasma should be separated within half an hour of blood collection. The test is best performed within 2 hours (certainly no more than 4 hours) of blood collection; alternatively the sample can be deep frozen before, and during, transport to the laboratory. However, unfrozen postal samples *usually* give clinically useful results. Von Willebrand's factor (vWF) can also be measured in citrated samples up to 3 days after collection, by specialist centres (Littlewood and Bevan, 1989).

FIBRINOGEN ESTIMATION

This is performed on a sample of blood taken into *EDTA* (*not* into heparin).

Low levels of fibrinogen can be due to:

- Reduced fibrinogen production, usually acquired (e.g. the terminal stage of liver failure), or rarely an inherited disorder.
- Increased fibrinogen consumption, as in DIC.

High levels can indicate generalized disease.

Normal reference range

Dog = 1–5 g/l.
Cat = 0.5–3 g/l.

FIBRINOGEN DEGRADATION PRODUCTS (FDPs)

Blood is collected into special Thrombo-Wellcotest tubes containing thrombin, to cause clotting, plus a plasmin inhibitor. The serum is collected, diluted and mixed with antibodies to FDPs absorbed onto latex particules. A sufficient concentration of FDP results in microagglutination on a microscope slide. By using different dilutions of serum the approximate concentration of FDPs can be determined.

Normal level of FDPs in the dog and cat = <10 µg/ml.

Increased levels of FDPs are usually the result of disseminated intravascular coagulation, but in severe liver disease the liver may have reduced ability to remove them, resulting in their accumulation.

High concentrations may also result from profuse internal haemorrhage.

Panel 4.2 Disseminated intravascular coagulation (DIC) (= consumption coagulopathy)

This complex haematological disorder is characterized by intravascular clotting, haemolysis and multiple haemorrhages. It is recognized relatively infrequently in dogs and cats.

Causes

Tissue damage results in the release of tissue thromboplastin which initiates the coagulation of blood (see Figure 4.2). If thromboplastin release is excessive, or if the normal simultaneous enzyme breakdown of the blood clots (fibrinolysis) designed to limit their deposition is inadequate, massive *intravascular* clotting occurs. This uses up so many platelets and clotting factors that any subsequent haemorrhage cannot be efficiently controlled.

The *major causes* of tissue damage that trigger DIC in dogs are:

- Malignant neoplasia (especially metastasizing carcinomas, haemangiosarcomas and lymphosarcomas).
- Acute pancreatitis.
- Chronic active hepatitis.
- Heat stroke.

Less information is available concerning cats but malignant neoplasia is certainly important.

Other causes include:

- Septicaemia, especially in cats (liposaccharides of Gram-negative bacteria, e.g. *Salmonella*, initiate coagulation).
- Other infective organisms, including the viruses causing feline infectious peritonitis, feline panleucopenia, canine parvoviral enteritis and infectious canine hepatitis, plus leptospirae and *Histoplasma*. (Other causal organisms which do *not* occur in the UK are *Rickettsia rickettsii* causing Rocky Mountain spotted fever, *Babesia* spp. in the dog, and *Ehrlichia canis*).
- Other toxins (e.g. aflatoxin).
- Severe intravascular haemolysis, e.g. following snake bite or incompatible blood transfusion (adenosine diphosphate (ADP) liberated from the RBCs activates the platelets and hence coagulation).
- Massive trauma.
- Aortic thromboembolism in cats.

It is also reported with vasculitis, acidosis, endocarditis and a variety of obstetric complications.

Mechanism (pathophysiology)

IN COAGULATION

- The enzyme thrombin splits fibrinogen into fibrin monomers which then join together (polymerize) to form a solid clot.
- Platelets and clotting factors are consumed in forming the clot, often in large quantities. If they cannot be replaced quickly enough, the amounts in the blood become seriously depleted.

IN FIBRINOLYSIS

- The enzyme plasmin can degrade (i.e. break down) clotting factors, thereby reducing their amounts.
- But particularly plasmin degrades fibrinogen and fibrin to fibrinogen degradation products (FDPs) which interfere with clot formation by preventing polymerization of the fibrin monomers, i.e. they have an anticoagulant effect.

FDPs are normally removed by the mononuclear phagocyte system (=reticuloendothelial system), for instance in the liver, but in disease this system may not function efficiently.

Consequences

The outcome of any case depends upon the balance between coagulation and fibrinolysis.

EXCESSIVE COAGULATION

Without adequate fibrinolysis, this leads to fibrin clots (thrombi) forming in, and blocking, small blood vessels (microthrombosis). The fibrin deposited in these vessels damages the circulating RBCs and this produces haemolysis (microangiopathic haemolysis). Haemolysis is both intravascular (due to the fibrin strands shearing the RBC's membranes) and extravascular (with phagocytosis of mis-shapen and fragmented RBCs, i.e. poikilocytes and schistocytes).

EXCESSIVE FIBRINOLYSIS

Activation of fibrinolysis limits coagulation and haemostasis. If there is also inadequate replacement of clotting factors and platelets, and/or inadequate removal of FDPs, it increases the tendency for haemorrhages to be uncontrolled.

In most cases there is extreme intravascular coagulation which depletes the supply of platelets and clotting factors leading to multiple secondary haemorrhages.

Diagnosis

CLINICAL SIGNS

The principal clinical signs of DIC are:

* Shock, varying in degree.
* Generalized or localized bleeding, often severe and especially obvious in the skin and mucous membranes (petechial haemorrhages and ecchymoses).
* Signs of intravascular haemolysis (e.g. haemoglobinaemia and haemoglobinuria).
* Specific signs that indicate damage to particular organs (e.g. kidney, liver, pancreas etc.).

Any resultant anaemia may be haemorrhagic and/or haemolytic.

LABORATORY FINDINGS

There is no single laboratory test that will confirm the disorder and no test can be relied upon to give abnormal results in *every* case.

Laboratory diagnosis (see Table 4.1) is usually based upon:

* A decreased number of platelets – less than $200 \times 10^9/l$ (dog) or $300 \times 10^9/l$ (cat), and often less than $20 \times 10^9/l$.
* An increased prothrombin time (PT), otherwise called the one-stage prothrombin time (OSPT) – more than 10 seconds (dog) or 12 seconds (cat).
* A low plasma level of fibrinogen – less than 1 g/l (dog) or 0.5 g/l (cat).
* An increased level of fibrinogen degradation products – more than 10 µg/ml.

Additional laboratory findings that may be present include:

* RBC fragments (schistocytes) and 'burr cells' (markedly crenated echinocytes) accounting for more than 5% of the RBCs (this would require blood smears to be reported upon).
* An increased activated partial thromboplastin time (APTT); more than 11 seconds in the dog or more than 15 seconds in the cat.

- An increased blood urea level – more than 7 mmol/l in the dog or 11 mmol/l in the cat.
- A prolonged clotting time (more than 13 minutes in the dog or 9 minutes in the cat) *and/or* a prolonged activated clotting time (ACT) (in the dog, more than 103 seconds at room temperature, or more than 95 seconds at 37°C; in the cat, more than 90 seconds at 37°C).
- An increased thrombin time (TT) – more than 11 seconds in the dog, more than 20 seconds in the cat.
- Decreased activity of antithrombin III – less than 90% of normal.
- Decreased activities of factors V and VIII:C – less than 80% of normal and less than 75% of normal respectively.

Part 2 Plasma biochemistry

Introduction

Biochemical estimations on blood may include measurement of any of the wide variety of substances found in blood plasma – substrates, metabolites, enzymes, electrolytes, metals and hormones. Guidance has already been given on the choice of biochemical tests in certain common diagnostic situations (see 'Appropriate tests for various clinical signs', p. 9); suffice it to say that unless it is simply a matter of confirming a diagnosis the initial use of a general profile has much to recommend it. To the profile can be added such other tests as appear necessary from the history and clinical features of the case.

Collection and preparation of blood samples

Generally it is advisable to collect fasting samples, i.e. ideally after 12 hours fasting. This avoids temporary increases in the levels of some substrates and metabolites and decreases the risk of lipaemia which can lead to haemolysis. The exception, however, is bile acids where samples collected 2 hours post-feeding can be more informative. Some fasted animals with liver or biliary disorders may produce normal or only slightly elevated bile acid values whereas after feeding much higher values occur which allow them to be distinguished from normal individuals. Often samples for bile acid estimations are collected after fasting *and* 2 hours after feeding for comparison.

As with the collection of samples for haematological tests, the jugular vein is most appropriate but the cephalic vein is most often used, and the saphenous vein is a good alternative especially in animals that prove difficult to handle. In exceptional circumstances, the marginal ear vein may be incised to allow a few drops of blood to be applied directly to a strip, e.g. Glucostix or Azostix or any of those used with the Reflotron. Again appropriate needle sizes would be 20–21 gauge in cats or small dogs and 19–20 gauge in other dogs.

The correct sample container should be used for the purpose: usually those containing EDTA are reserved for haematological tests, those containing (lithium) heparin are used for obtaining plasma samples, those with *no* anticoagulant serve for obtaining serum samples (most biochemical estimations can be performed on either plasma or serum) *and* containers with fluoride–oxalate are used for glucose estimations to inhibit the glycolytic enzymes in the RBCs. However, samples containing fluoride must not be used with any of the strip tests for glucose, e.g. Glucostix or those used with the Seralyzer or Reflotron, because this enzyme inhibitor will also inhibit the enzymes used in the reagent strips. Sample containers with anticoagulants should be filled to the level indicated and the blood and anticoagulant mixed (by repeated gentle inversion of the container) immediately after replacing the cap.

Haemolysis of the sample is undesirable, for all the reasons mentioned in the section 'Effects of haemolysis on laboratory tests' (p. 19) but partial clotting, whilst an inconvenience, does not render a sample totally unsuitable for biochemical tests as it does with haematological examination.

The same methods of collection may be used as described for haematological tests, i.e. direct collection through a needle, into a syringe, into an evacuated tube (although if paediatric size (2 ml) tubes are used to avoid haemolysis two or more tubes may need to be filled to obtain sufficient plasma), into a Monovette or S-Monovette.

Serum and plasma

Nowadays plasma is widely preferred to serum because there is no delay in separation and a greater volume of sample material can be obtained. Samples for serum containing no anticoagulant should be left for at least 2 hours at room temperature to ensure complete clotting and clot separation (or 2 hours in an incubator at 37°C and half an hour in a refrigerator at 4°C). Prior to centrifuging clotted samples it is necessary to detach the clots from the side of the container with a swab stick or mounted needle; if done carelessly this can cause haemolysis.

Calcium levels should not be estimated on samples collected into fluoride, oxalate or citrate since these anticoagulants bind the calcium and will result in falsely low values.

The addition of a silicone material (e.g. Serasieve) to plasma samples prior to centrifuging (or with Sure-Sep *during* centrifuging) allows the separated plasma to be poured off. Alternatively, plastic beads can be added (these are already contained in Monovettes) and, by forming a barrier between the cells and the plasma, greatly facilitate drawing off the plasma cleanly using a pipette. If neither material is used care must be taken in removing the plasma because, if the tip of the pipette is placed next to the RBC layer, it is easy to draw up RBCs as well.

Serum and plasma samples which are not being tested immediately should be refrigerated (or frozen/deep frozen if there is to be a considerable delay). This preserves especially the activity of enzymes. However, all samples must be allowed to return to room temperature before testing.

Amount of sample

The increasing use of micromethods means that a lot of routine tests require comparatively little sample material and, in general, if 5 ml of heparinized blood is obtained this will be adequate for almost all tests. Nevertheless, it is advisable to check a particular laboratory's requirements, especially if an unusual test is required.

Chapter 5

Nutrients and metabolites

Plasma urea

SI units of measurements are millimoles per litre (mmol/l).
The previous units used were mg/dl (=mg/100 ml).

Conversion factors

- To convert mg/dl to mmol/l multiply by 0.17.
- To convert mmol/l to mg/dl multiply by 6.0.

IMPORTANT NOTE – UREA AND BUN

It is important to appreciate that in the past urea concentrations have been expressed as *either* the concentration of *urea* itself *or* the concentration of the *nitrogen* component of that urea.

The latter is widely referred to as the *blood urea nitrogen* (BUN) even though it is generally measured in plasma or serum; sometimes it is termed 'serum urea nitrogen' (SUN).

Because nitrogen is only *part* of the urea molecule the level of BUN will necessarily be lower than that of urea (molecular weights: BUN=28, urea=60), and factors for conversion are:

- To convert BUN (mg/dl) to urea (mg/dl) multiply by 2.14.
- To convert urea (mg/dl) to BUN (mg/dl) multiply by 0.47.
- To convert BUN (mg/dl) to urea (mmol/l) multiply by 0.36.
- To convert urea (mmol/l) to BUN (mg/dl) multiply by 2.8.

Both urea and BUN can be expressed in mg/dl but only urea can properly be expressed in mmol/l – obviously it is not possible to record the number of molecules of BUN when nitrogen forms only a *part* of each molecule of urea.

Unfortunately, in the UK some commercial laboratories confuse urea and BUN, and use the terms as if they were interchangeable, i.e. they state that they are reporting the BUN concentration whereas in fact they actually report the urea concentration (in mmol/l).

If the unsuspecting clinician 'converts' this 'BUN' into urea he or she will obtain a urea value which is *twice* the true value and this might lead to errors in diagnosis.

The best CHECK on whether urea or BUN is being reported is to compare the laboratory's normal reference range with the reference range given below.

NORMAL REFERENCE RANGE FOR UREA

Dog: 2.5–7 mmol/l (= 15–40 mg/dl).
Cat: 5–11 mmol/l (= 30–65 mg/dl).

In terms of *true BUN* (see Note above):

Dog: BUN=7–20 mg/dl.
Cat: BUN=14–32 mg/dl.

SOURCE

Urea is synthesized in the liver from ammonia, most of which comes from the breakdown (catabolism) of amino acids derived from tissue proteins or dietary proteins. Also some ammonia is absorbed from the bowel, where it is formed by the action of bacteria on dietary amino acids and re-circulated endogenous urea, and carried to the liver.

Urea is largely excreted by the kidney, although about a quarter is excreted by the gut, converted to ammonia as previously described, absorbed and re-converted to urea.

In the kidney, urea is freely filtered through the glomeruli and then passively reabsorbed in the tubules; normally about half is reabsorbed but this depends on the animal's hydration and the rate of urine formation.

In essence then urea is formed in the liver and excreted via the kidney. Therefore *higher levels of urea* in the plasma result from:

- Either increased breakdown of tissue proteins or dietary proteins (with high protein diets).
- Or impaired excretion.

A slightly raised urea level is not necessarily the result of renal failure.
Urea levels of 17–20 mmol/l and above (>100–120 mg/dl = BUN >50–60 mg/dl) are significant.

- Values >16 mmol/l (>96 mg/dl = BUN>45 mg/dl) are unlikely to be be due solely to increased protein breakdown.
- Urea levels above 35 mmol/l (>210 mg/dl = BUN>100 mg/dl) are unlikely to be due solely to impaired renal perfusion (even if severe), i.e. they are due to chronic renal failure, primary acute renal failure, or obstruction or rupture of the urinary tract.
- Urea levels above 67–70 mmol/l (>400 mg/dl = BUN>190–200 mg/dl) carry a poor prognosis.

Lower levels of urea in the plasma (<2.5 mmol/l = <15 mg/dl = BUN<7 mg/dl) result from reduced synthesis because of defective liver function or the reduced intake or breakdown of protein.

Urea is in fact only one of a number of non-protein nitrogenous substances that accumulate in the plasma when renal excretion is reduced. The others include creatinine, creatine, guanidine, cyanate, aliphatic amines and organic acids – among them guanidinoacetic acid and phenolic acids etc., many of which are far more toxic than urea. Technically, urea is the simplest of these substances to measure and it is therefore conveniently used to indicate an increase in all their levels.

Conventionally the presence of elevated concentrations of nitrogenous protein-breakdown products in the blood is termed 'azotaemia'.

The specific clinical syndrome that develops due to the presence of high levels of these toxic substances in the blood, e.g. in renal failure, is termed 'uraemia'.

Purely as an indicator of *renal function*, creatinine is preferable to urea, because it is *less* affected by the variety of non-renal factors which influence urea levels.

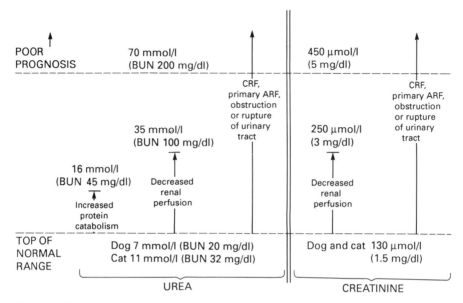

Figure 5.1 Urea and creatinine levels in urinary disorders

However, compared with creatinine, urea will:

• Provide information about disorders other than those of the kidney.
• Be less affected by delays in analysis and the presence of interfering substances (see p. 235).

Overall it would be preferable to:

• Either measure urea and creatinine levels together routinely.
• Or measure the urea level first and, if found to be raised, then to check it by measuring the creatinine level.

ACCURACY

Blood strip tests do not give precise values but *can* indicate whether or not urea levels are *significantly* raised.

The presence of ammonium salts (e.g. ammonium oxalate as anticoagulant) will falsely elevate readings and ammonium vapour (or tobacco smoke) will falsely affect test strips (e.g. Azostix or Urastrat).

Causes of increased plasma urea levels

Summary

Prerenal azotaemia
Increased rate of protein breakdown
- High protein diet
- Carbohydrate deficiency
- Intestinal haemorrhage
- Fever and necrosis
- Hyperthyroidism
- Prolonged exercise
- Catabolic drugs
- Reduced anabolism
Decreased renal perfusion
- Dehydration [most common cause]
- Severe haemorrhage
- Shock
- Hypoadrenocorticism
- Reduced cardiac output
- Hypoalbuminaemia

Renal azotaemia
Primary (renal) acute renal failure
- Acute interstitial nephritis – infection
- Acute tubular necrosis – nephrotoxins/ischaemia/diffuse nephrocalcinosis/acute glomerulonephritis
- Chronic renal failure
- Chronic interstitial nephritis
- Chronic glomerulonephritis
- Chronic amyloidosis
- Chronic pyelonephritis
- Diffuse nephrocalcinosis
- Neoplasia
- Familial renal diseases [relatively rare]
- Other disorders [rare]

Postrenal azotaemia
Obstruction to urinary flow
- Congenital disorders
- Calculi
- Neoplasms
- Blood clots
- Feline urological syndrome
- Surgical ligation
- Herniation
- Prostatic disorders
Bladder rupture
Error: Ammonia contamination

The term 'uraemia' would *seem* to be appropriate for this state but is in fact used to denote the specific toxic syndrome that can develop from the accumulation of protein-derived nitrogenous substances, i.e. in cases of renal failure.

The causes of elevated plasma urea levels, and azotaemia, generally can be divided into prerenal, renal and postrenal.

PRERENAL AZOTAEMIA

This is the most usual cause and the increase in urea is usually mild/modest.

An increased rate of protein breakdown (increased protein catabolism)

A higher urea level is *unaccompanied* by an increase in the plasma creatinine level. (Indeed, if the muscle mass is seriously depleted, as in starvation, the creatinine level may fall slightly.)

Increased dietary intake of protein

- Surplus amino acids are catabolized. (If a large amount of poor quality (low biological value) protein is eaten the non-essential amino acids are broken down.)
- Urea levels usually rise only *slightly*, e.g. up to 10–12 mmol/l (60–72 mg/dl; BUN = 30–35 mg/dl) in the dog. Exceptionally, levels may reach 16 mmol/l (= 95 mg/dl; BUN = 48 mg/dl).
- Urea levels higher than this, which are triggered by giving a high protein diet, suggest that there is an underlying loss of renal function making it difficult to eliminate the urea.
- Temporary rises can follow feeding and for this reason urea estimations should be made on samples from *fasted animals*.

Deficiency of carbohydrate or complete starvation
This is therefore caused by a lack of calories.

The body's protein stores (e.g. in the liver) and ultimately its tissue proteins (e.g. muscles) are catabolized to provide energy. In severe cases urea levels can rise to 15–20 mmol/l (90–120 mg/dl; BUN = 45–60 mg/dl).

Intestinal haemorrhage
Blood is digested in the small intestine and its protein components are absorbed and catabolized.

CHECK   PCV, total protein and albumin levels and the reticulocyte count. After 4 days' avoidance of meats and offals (and all blood-containing foods), test faeces for occult blood.

Fever and necrosis
These occur, for example, in infectious diseases and in neoplasia. Both are causes of increased tissue protein breakdown.

Hyperthyroidism
An elevated urea level is a feature in over 40% of cats, but in less than 20% of dogs with hyperthyroidism.

It is due to increased protein catabolism and reduced renal perfusion following from decreased cardiac output.

Prolonged exercise
This causes increased protein catabolism.

Drugs causing increased tissue catabolism
Examples of such drugs are glucocorticoids and thyroid hormone.

Decreased anabolism
This may be due to:

- A lack of growth hormone and somatomedin in pituitary dwarfism.
- Tetracyclines.

By reducing anabolism more protein is directed into catabolism.

Decreased renal perfusion (prerenal acute renal failure)

The reduction in blood flow through the kidneys reduces the overall glomerular filtration rate and so the plasma urea level rises (although up to 6% dehydration causes little change).

Values are often above 15 mmol/l (>90 mg/dl; BUN = >40 mg/dl) and exceptionally rise to 35 mmol/l (210 mg/dl; BUN = 100 mg/dl).

This may be due to the following causes.

Dehydration
This is the most common cause of raised urea levels, e.g. with vomiting, diarrhoea and polyuric disorders (such as diabetes mellitus, especially in cats, and particularly non-ketotic hyperosmolar diabetes mellitus).

CHECK   for increases in PCV and total protein level.

Severe haemorrhage

CHECK   decreases in PCV after 2–3 hours.

Shock

Hypoadrenocorticism
In dogs urea is increased in almost all primary cases (Addison's disease) and two out of three secondary cases; in cats all recorded cases show increased urea levels.

Reduced cardiac output
This is caused by congestive heart failure or cardiac arrhythmias.

Hypoalbuminaemia
This reduces the plasma osmotic pressure.

Care

Polyuria plus a slightly raised urea level does not necessarily denote renal failure. In any polyuric disorder (see 'Causes of polyuria', p. 415) failure to replace body water fast enough can cause dehydration, reduced renal perfusion and a *modest* rise in the plasma urea level. Clinically, cases showing decreased renal perfusion, especially cardiac disorders and Addison's disease, *may* be mistaken for renal failure cases because of the associated vomiting, weakness and depression.

Whatever the cause two characteristic features should distinguish decreased renal perfusion from renal failure due to a loss of nephrons.

1. A urinary specific gravity >(1.025–)1.030 in the dog, or >1.035 (–1.040) in the cat, reflecting renal concentrating ability; with nephron loss the specific gravity is *lower*.
2. Failure of the creatinine level to increase to the same extent. In prerenal acute renal failure (ARF), the reabsorption of urea from the renal tubules back into the blood is increased but creatinine, a larger, less diffusible molecule, stays in the tubules. Therefore the usual urea:creatinine ratio is increased. (Arguments that the urea:creatinine ratio is not helpful in diagnosis (Finco and Duncan, 1976) have since been countered (Michell, 1988).)

Consequently the ratio urea (in mmol/l)/creatinine (in μmol/l) is more than 0.08. (If both metabolites are measured in mg/dl the ratio is >43 – and if in addition BUN is substituted for urea (both in mg/dl) the ratio is >20.)

Note

The prolonged absence of any appreciable renal perfusion will result in ischaemia and, if this persists for around 2 hours (0.75–4 hours), it will cause irreversible damage, i.e. acute tubular necrosis (ATN). At this stage the blood urea level rises further and all the signs of ATN appear, including an elevated creatinine level.

RENAL AZOTAEMIA (PRIMARY RENAL AZOTAEMIA)

When around three-quarters of the nephrons are lost or non-functional, as in chronic renal failure (CRF) and primary (renal) acute renal failure (ARF) those that remain cannot maintain an adequate glomerular filtration rate (GFR); therefore urea, and likewise creatinine, are not filtered from the blood plasma at the same rate as usual. But at any GFR the amount of urea removed from the plasma will increase as the level of urea in the plasma increases, i.e. plasma urea level × GFR = a constant.

Consequently urea accumulates in the plasma until it reaches a level at which its rate of removal equals the rate at which it is being formed, i.e. if the GFR is halved the rate at which urea is removed will be the same when the plasma urea level has doubled.

Consequently, the rise in urea level reflects the degree of nephron loss, although this assumes a constant rate of urea formation, i.e. the same intake of the same diet.

Note

When the intake of protein is restricted the plasma urea level will inevitably be reduced and therefore will not provide a true indication of renal function; in this situation the level of creatinine will provide a truer guide.

In primary renal ARF and CRF (in comparison with decreased renal perfusion):

- The urinary specific gravity is lower, with a loss of two-thirds of nephrons <1.029 in the dog and <1.034 in the cat, and with a loss of three-quarters of nephrons <1.012 in the dog and <1.025 in the cat.

  However, a very dilute urine (specific gravity <1.007) cannot be formed. Ultimately, in both species, isosthenuria exists (i.e. urinary specific gravity lies between 1.008 and 1.012).

Note

There is a rare disorder characterized by a reduced GFR but the retention of tubular function; consequently, the urine is well concentrated although distinguished by proteinuria.

- The ratio urea (in mmol/l)/creatinine (in μmol/l) is maintained at or below 0.08, i.e. plasma urea and creatinine concentrations rise *together* as the GFR falls.

(If both metabolites are measured in mg/dl the ratio is at or below 43 and if, in addition, BUN is substituted for urea (both in mg/dl) the ratio is at or below 20.)

Primary (renal) ARF

Glomerular filtration rate falls dramatically without there being time for compensation. As well as rises in urea and creatinine levels there is also:

- An increased plasma phosphate level, usually with a slightly low or low/normal calcium level (found also in CRF).
- An increased plasma potassium level.
- Initially minimal urinary output (oliguria), until the later (polyuric) phase.

These last two features are chiefly confined to ARF, although oliguria can be found in the terminal stage of CRF.

The major causes of primary renal ARF are toxic substances (nephrotoxins) and prolonged deprivation of an adequate blood supply (ischaemia). Details are given in Panel 5.2 (p. 299).

Acute interstitial nephritis (AIN)
This is due to infectious agents, i.e. in the dog, canine adenovirus-1, canine herpes virus, *Leptospira canicola* (causing acute leptospirosis) and *Klebsiella*, and in both dog and cat infection with *E. coli*, *Proteus* spp., staphylococci and streptococci.

Acute tubular necrosis (ATN)
This is due to:

- Nephrotoxins including compounds of lead, arsenic, gold, mercury and bismuth, the rodenticide thallium, amphotericin B, 5-fluorocytosine and the antibiotics of the polymyxin/bacitracin and aminoglycoside (streptomycin, neomycin, gentamicin etc.) groups, plus the less soluble sulphonamides, organic compounds such as carbon tetrachloride, chloroform, methyl alcohol, phenol and ethylene glycol (in anti-freeze – incidentally radio-opaque), the analgesics phenacetin and phenylbutazone, cyclophosphamide, methoxyflurane, chlorinated hydrocarbons and radio-opaque contrast media.

  Also large amounts of myoglobin following muscle breakdown (rhabdomyolysis) or crush injuries, or haemoglobin, following massive haemolysis, contribute by obstructing the tubules.

  These effects are enhanced by dehydration and, in the case of drugs excreted via the kidney, pre-existing renal damage.
- Ischaemia due to severe, irreversible hypoperfusion of the kidney (i.e. with hypotension and/or hypovolaemia), e.g. following prolonged surgery or anaesthesia, severe acute haemorrhage, disseminated intravascular coagulation (DIC), burns, heart failure, shock, trauma, incompatible blood transfusion, obstruction of the renal blood vessels by infarcts or thrombi and prolonged prerenal ARF, i.e. decreased renal perfusion.

  Also high blood calcium levels, by producing hypercalcaemic nephropathy (diffuse nephrocalcinosis) can result in ischaemia.

  Acute glomerulonephritis can also be the cause of considerable renal damage, resulting in oliguria.

CHECK – in ATN there may be large amounts of protein, RBCs, casts and renal tubular cells in the urine, plus oxalate crystals in ethylene glycol poisoning.

Chronic renal failure (CRF)

The progressive loss of nephrons, and therefore of renal function, occurs slowly. This allows time for each surviving nephron to increase its individual GFR to compensate for the overall reduction in GFR and to re-adjust its tubular absorptive and secretory mechanisms.

The renal disorders that result in chronic renal failure are listed in Panel 5.2 (p. 299) but they include chronic interstitial nephritis, chronic glomerulonephritis, neoplasia, and many other progressively damaging disorders.

Apart from increased levels of urea and creatinine, findings include:

- A high plasma phosphate level, usually accompanied by a slightly low or low to normal calcium level (seen also in ARF).
- Often a mild depression (non-regenerative) anaemia, showing slightly low or low–normal PCV and an absence of reticulocytes.
- Thrombocytopenia due to defective platelet production.
- Lymphopenia.
- Polyuria (until the terminal oliguric stage) due to the increased GFR of each individual surviving nephron exceeding its tubular reabsorptive capacity.

In hypercalcaemia, urea levels rise less than creatinine, probably because of reduced permeability of the collecting ducts to both water and urea.

When raised plasma levels of urea (and creatinine) appear renal failure is *already present*.

Methods of detecting diminished renal function *before* the onset of renal failure have been investigated (see Panel 5.2, p. 299) including a decrease in the ratio of urea in the urine to that in the plasma. A ratio of less than 10:1 is common in CRF, and 30:1 or less should raise suspicion of reduced function.

The addition of renal perfusion problems, or other types of ARF, in cases of CRF quickly causes decompensation and further increases in the blood urea level, referred to as 'acute-on-chronic' renal failure.

POSTRENAL AZOTAEMIA

This is due to abnormalities in the lower urinary tract.

Obstruction to the flow of urine

This can be caused, for example, by calculi, neoplasms or blood clots anywhere along the urinary tract (most commonly the urethra; above the bladder these blockages need to be bilateral), feline urological syndrome (FUS), congenital urinary tract abnormalities, surgical ligation of both ureters (e.g. at spaying), herniation (perineal or inguinal) of the bladder or severe prostate gland enlargement. It may follow prostatectomy or drainage of an abscessed prostate gland.

At times there may be complete anuria. Urine accumulates and the pressure in the urinary tract builds up until it equals the filtration pressure in the kidney; then urine formation stops.

Increases in the plasma urea level are related to the duration and completeness of the obstruction.

High plasma urea levels (60 mmol/l or more = 360 mg/dl or more; BUN = 170 mg/dl or more) appear within 24 hours of complete urinary tract obstruction.

Bladder rupture

This is usually due to trauma (especially road traffic accidents).

A raised plasma urea level occurs within hours and can reach >100 mmol/l (>600 mg/dl; BUN >280 mg/dl). It is *not* attributable to renal failure, because this does not develop, but to the inability to eliminate urea and other waste products from the body. They continue to be reabsorbed from the urine in the peritoneal cavity.

ERROR: AMMONIA CONTAMINATION

Since many urea determinations require urea to be converted to ammonia for measurement, existing high levels of ammonia will cause false results, e.g. ammonium oxalate should be avoided as an anticoagulant. With strip tests (e.g. Urastrat) ammonia vapour or even tobacco smoke can cause false positive reactions.

Causes of decreased plasma urea levels

Summary
- Low protein diet
- Anabolic steroids
- Liver failure
- Portosystemic shunt
- Diabetes insipidus and psychogenic polydipsia
- Primary hyperammonaemia [very rare]

LOW PROTEIN DIET

A low (though good quality) protein diet which is providing adequate energy can be a cause.

Decreased protein catabolism reduces plasma urea levels to the lower part of the normal range or just below it, although generally not less than 2 mmol/l (i.e. not <12 mg/dl; BUN not <6 mg/dl).

Almost all the ingested protein is used for protein synthesis.

ANABOLIC STEROIDS

These divert proteins from catabolism to tissue formation.

LOSS OF LIVER FUNCTION

This means severe loss of liver function; the liver is unable to convert ammonia to urea in the usual way. Consequently the level of plasma urea is often low, i.e. <2.5 mmol/l (<15 mg/dl; BUN <7 mg/dl), whilst that of ammonia is raised. A significantly high level of ammonia impairs the brain, producing a variety of CNS signs (hepatic encephalopathy – see p. 291); whether or not they appear depends on the severity of the defect.

Hepatic failure (a loss of more than three-quarters of the functional hepatocytes) may be due to:

1. Replacement of functional liver cells by
   (a) fibrous tissue, i.e. cirrhosis, e.g. in chronic active hepatitis (following damage to the cells, see below), so that on radiography the liver appears small;
   (b) neoplastic tissue, e.g. carcinomas, hepatomas etc. (on radiography the liver often appears large);
   (c) amyloid (rarely) giving a large liver.
2. Damage of liver cells by toxins (e.g. drugs and aflatoxin), infectious agents or the abnormal storage of copper.

CHECK – toxins and infection can produce haematological signs of acute inflammation plus biochemical changes indicative of liver damage and loss of liver function, see Panel 6.1 (p. 333).

In general with liver dysfunction, levels of albumin and urea are low and that of bile acids is high, and with obstruction to the outflow of bile, ALP activity and the level of bilirubin are high. Also BSP clearance is prolonged and ALT activity may be raised depending upon the degree of damage.

Urea values which are within the normal range do not rule out this condition, although in general in the dog, they would be less than 4 mmol/l (<24 mg/dl; BUN <12 g/dl).

PORTOSYSTEMIC SHUNT

This includes portacaval shunt and acquired hepatocellular insufficiency. One of a number of possible congenital defects in the vasculature results in blood in the portal vein, carrying absorbed nutrients from the gut, effectively by-passing the liver cells. The portal vein may empty directly into the posterior vena cava or the azygos vein, or empty into a patent ductus venosus which opens into the posterior vena cava. The liver atrophies and often levels of albumin, urea, cholesterol and prothrombin are low (although in the *cat* urea and albumin values are often normal). However, urea values within the normal range *do not* rule out this condition, although they would generally be less than 4 mmol/l in the dog (<24 mg/dl; BUN <12 mg/dl). The level of bile acids is increased and BSP clearance is prolonged. ALT and ALP activities and the bilirubin level are usually barely affected because there is no liver damage or obstruction.

The vascular abnormalities are demonstrable by portal angiography.

DIABETES INSIPIDUS AND PSYCHOGENIC POLYDIPSIA

Excessive loss of urea through the kidneys decreases plasma urea levels to around the bottom of the normal range, i.e. in the dog 1.8–3.6 mmol/l (11–22 mg/dl; BUN = 5–10 mg/dl).

PRIMARY HYPERAMMONAEMIA [VERY RARE]

This is a very rare *congenital* defect in the urea cycle – lack of an enzyme prevents ammonia from being converted into urea. The blood supply to the liver is normal (as demonstrated by portal angiography) and no other functions of the liver are affected (i.e. levels of albumin, cholesterol and clotting factors are normal, as is the BSP clearance). The condition is recognized in dogs but not yet in cats.

Plasma creatinine

This is often referred to in North America as *serum* creatinine and abbreviated to SC.

SI units of measurement are micromoles per litre (μmol/l). Previous units used were mg/dl (= mg/100 ml).

CONVERSION FACTORS

- To convert mg/dl to μmol/l multiply by 88.4.
- To convert μmol/l to mg/dl multiply by 0.0113.

NORMAL REFERENCE RANGE

Dog and cat: 40–130 μmol/l (0.5–1.5 mg/dl).

Probably animals with 100% renal function have creatinine levels below 110 μmol/l (1.2 mg/dl) and any higher level could indicate reduced renal function.

SOURCE

Plasma creatinine is derived almost solely from the catabolism of creatine found in the body's muscle tissues. Creatine is used to store energy in muscle (as phosphocreatine) and its breakdown to creatinine occurs at a steady rate (around 2% per day).

The pool of creatine from which creatinine is liberated depends on the total muscle mass, so wasting or other muscular disease results in lowered creatinine production and, conversely, severe prolonged exercise can increase creatinine levels. In practice production is fairly constant and is barely affected by increased catabolism of dietary or tissue proteins (factors which *do* affect urea synthesis), even though a small amount of creatinine is obtained from muscle tissue in the diet.

Excretion of creatinine is solely via the kidneys; it is freely filtered and not reabsorbed. In the dog a small amount is actively secreted in the proximal tubules. Essentially plasma creatinine levels reflect excretion, high levels indicating deficient renal function.

Note

GFR and creatinine levels are not linearly related. Consequently, the loss of half the functional nephrons produces only a marginal increase in creatinine (to 180 μmol/l = 2 mg/dl) but following the loss of three-quarters of the nephrons any further losses produce substantial increases in the creatinine concentration.

Abnormally *low* creatinine levels are not genuinely encountered but see 'Accuracy' below.

IMPORTANT NOTE

The enzyme creatine kinase (CK), otherwise known as creatine phosphokinase (CPK), present in muscle tissue, is used as an indicator of muscle injury and is *not* directly concerned with renal function (see p. 327).

Although reflecting renal function more accurately than urea (since there is no reabsorption), creatinine does not provide information about other types of disorders and it is also more subject to interference when measured (see below). Therefore it is best performed in conjunction with urea estimations, or following the finding of a raised urea level. An elevated level of creatine with a normal urea value may arise in animals with decreased renal function receiving a low protein diet.

ACCURACY

Falsely low values

These can be due to:

- Progressive, although slow, disappearance from samples with time.
- High levels of bilirubin (using kinetic Jaffé reactions).

Falsely high values

These can be due to:

- High levels of ketones (specifically acetoacetate) in cases of ketotic diabetes mellitus.
- Drugs – chiefly the presence of certain cephalosporins which interfere with the analytical method (although with some methods for creatinine measurement, cephalosporins can decrease the values); less so by those drugs which inhibit tubular secretion, i.e. salicylates, trimethoprim (e.g. in co-trimoxazole) and cimetidine.

Causes of increased plasma creatinine levels

Summary

Prerenal azotaemia
- Decreased renal perfusion, e.g. dehydration etc.

Renal azotaemia
- Primary (renal) acute renal failure
- Chronic renal failure

Postrenal azotaemia
- Obstruction to urinary flow
- Bladder rupture

Severe exercise

Error: presence of ketones/drugs – especially cephalosporins

As with plasma urea, the renal causes can be classified as prerenal, renal and postrenal.

PRERENAL AZOTAEMIA

Decreased renal perfusion (prerenal acute renal failure)

This can be due to dehydration (although compared with urea, creatinine is much less affected), severe haemorrhage, shock, hypoadrenocorticism, reduced cardiac output and hypoalbuminaemia.

Values may reach $250\,\mu mol/l$ (3 mg/dl).

This cause can be distinguished from renal and postrenal causes, i.e. primary renal failure and urinary tract obstruction, by two features:

1. The level of creatinine increases much less than that of urea, because the reabsorption of urea from the tubules is increased but creatinine remains in the tubules.

   Consequently the ratio urea (in mmol/l)/creatinine (in $\mu mol/l$) is more than 0.08.

   (If both metabolites are measured in mg/dl the ratio is more than 43, and if in addition BUN is substituted for urea (both BUN and creatinine being in mg/dl) the ratio is >20.)

2. The urinary specific gravity is higher – >(1.025–)1.030 in the dog, >1.035(–1.040) in the cat, mirroring renal concentrating ability.

RENAL AZOTAEMIA (PRIMARY RENAL AZOTAEMIA)

The functional loss of three-quarters of the total nephrons, i.e. in chronic renal failure and primary (renal) acute renal failure, results in a reduction in GFR and an accumulation of creatinine, as with urea. But because there is no reabsorption of creatinine this rise is apparent earlier than with urea, allowing the abnormality to be detected sooner. (Likewise any reduction in levels affects creatinine first.)

Levels above 250 μmol/l (>3 mg/dl) are clinically significant, i.e. unlikely to be due just to poor renal perfusion, but probably due to primary renal azotaemia (primary ARF or CRF) or postrenal azotaemia (urinary tract obstruction or rupture).

Above 450 μmol/l (>5 mg/dl) the prognosis is poor.

Distinguishing features from prerenal ARF (i.e. decreased renal perfusion) are:

1. A lower urinary specific gravity;
   (a) with a loss of two-thirds of nephrons: <1.029 in the dog and <1.034 in the cat;
   (b) with a loss of three-quarters of the nephrons a specific gravity of less than 1.012 in the dog and less than 1.025 in the cat, although a very dilute urine (specific gravity <1.007) cannot be formed.
       Ultimately in both species isosthenuria develops (i.e. a urinary specific gravity lying between 1.008 and 1.012).
2. The urea:creatinine ratio in plasma is higher, i.e. urea (in mmol/l)/creatinine (in μmol/l) is at or below 0.08.
   (If urea and creatinine are measured in mg/dl the ratio is at or below 43, and if in addition BUN is substituted for urea (both BUN and creatinine being in mg/dl) the ratio is at or below 20.)

Primary (renal) acute renal failure

With a dramatic drop in glomerular filtration rate the creatinine level can rise rapidly, at times to >1000 μmol/l (>12 mg/dl).

In addition to rises in creatinine and urea there is also:

- An increased plasma phosphate level, usually with a slightly low or low–normal calcium level (in both ARF and CRF).
- An increased plasma potassium level.
- Initially minimal urinary output (oliguria) until the later (polyuric) phase.

The last two features are chiefly confined to ARF, although oliguria can be found in the terminal stage of CRF.

Major causes of this condition are:

- Acute interstitial nephritis (AIN), due to infectious agents.
- Acute tubular necrosis (ATN) which can be due to either nephrotoxins or ischaemia.

Further details are given in Panel 5.2 (p. 299).

Chronic renal failure (CRF)

As with urea, the progressive loss of nephrons results in an overall reduction in glomerular filtration rate (despite the increased GFR of each individual remaining nephron) resulting in an accumulation of creatinine in the blood.

As well as elevated levels of urea and creatinine there is:

- A high plasma phosphate level, usually accompanied by a slightly low or low–normal calcium level.
- Often a mild (non-regenerative) anaemia.

- Defective platelet production.
- Lymphopenia.
- Polyuria, until the terminal oliguric stage.

The causes of chronic renal failure are detailed in Panel 5.2 (p. 299), and include the end-stage of many progressive renal disorders.

Unfortunately by the time levels of creatinine are high the animal is already in renal failure.

POSTRENAL AZOTAEMIA

The causes are

- Obstruction to the outflow of urine.
- Bladder rupture.

Individual conditions are detailed in Panel 5.2 (p. 299).

SEVERE EXERCISE

A marginal increase in plasma creatinine is present immediately after severe exercise in Greyhounds (Snow et al., 1988).

ERROR: FALSELY ELEVATED VALUES

These can arise from:

- High levels of ketones (especially acetoacetate) in cases of ketotic diabetes mellitus.
- Drugs, particularly certain cephalosporins which interfere with the analytical method.

Drugs which inhibit tubular secretion, i.e. salicylate, trimethoprim and cimetidine, are less likely to cause elevated values.

Total plasma protein

- SI units of measurements are grams per litre (g/l).
- Total protein cannot be measured in millimoles per litre (mmol/l) because it contains a variety of proteins having *different* molecular weights.
- Previous units were g/dl (= g/100 ml).

CONVERSION FACTORS

- To convert g/dl to g/l multiply by 10.
- To convert g/l to g/dl multiply by 0.1.

NORMAL REFERENCE RANGE (ADULTS)

Dog: 57–77 g/l (= 5.7–7.7 g/dl).
Cat: 58–80 g/l (= 5.8–8.0 g/dl).

In the past total protein has most frequently been measured in *serum* in veterinary laboratories.

Values obtained from serum will be slightly lower, by approximately 5% (i.e. by 2 g/l (1–4 g/l) = by 0.2 g/dl), because of the loss of fibrinogen (a globulin fraction) in clotting.

Total serum protein = albumin + globulins without fibrinogen.

Total plasma protein = albumin + globulins including fibrinogen.

AGE

With age total protein levels increase (in fact globulins increase and albumin decreases) and therefore in animals under 6 months old values at the lower end of the adult ranges would be expected.

SOURCE

Albumin and all other proteins except the immunoglobulins are synthesized by the liver – this includes fibrinogen and the α-globulins. These proteins are catabolized in all active tissues.

The immunoglobulins (IgG, IgM, IgA and IgE) are produced by the plasma cells and B-lymphocytes in lymphoid tissue in response to antigenic stimulation. They are included in the β- and γ-globulin fractions, principally the latter, as shown in Figure 5.2.

The globulin fraction comprises the following.

α-Globulins

These include haptoglobin (which binds free haemoglobin), transcortin (which binds cortisol), α_1-lipoprotein (which transports lipids) etc.

α-Globulin concentrations increase in acute inflammatory disorders.

β-Globulins

These include transferrin (which binds iron), complement (conferring cell-mediated immunity), β-lipoprotein (which transports lipids), some immunoglobulins (conferring humoral immunity), fibrinogen (clotting factor I) etc.

The concentration of β-globulins increases when there is severe antigenic stimulation and with neoplasia.

γ-Globulins

These include most immunoglobulins. The concentration of γ-globulins increases with antigenic stimulation, especially with chronic infections and autoimmune disorders.

OTHER PROTEIN CONCENTRATIONS

Albumin

This is dealt with on p. 250 and the following pages.

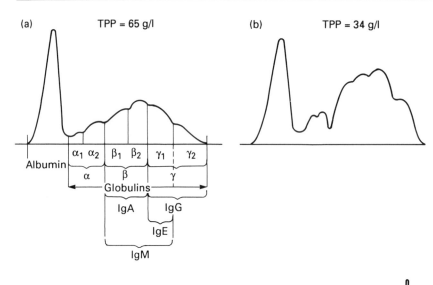

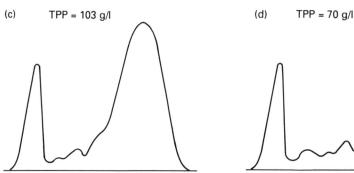

Figure 5.2 Protein electrophoretic patterns. (a) Normal electrophoretic trace (dog) showing the globulin fractions and how the immunoglobulins are disposed. Note that they are not confined to the γ-globulin fraction, although that *is* the site of IgG, which represents 85% of the immunoglobulins. (b) Trace of a dog with hypoalbuminaemia due to the nephrotic syndrome. There is a *relative* increase in the globulin fractions. (c) Trace of a cat with feline infectious peritonitis. There is an enormous increase in γ-globulins – an example of a polyclonal gammopathy. (d) Trace from a dog with a plasma cell myeloma showing the characteristic 'church spire' peak of a monoclonal gammopathy. TPP = total plasma protein

Globulin

This equals the difference between the values obtained for total plasma protein and for albumin.

Dog: 25–45 g/l (2.5–4.5 g/dl).
Cat: 28–55 g/l (2.8–5.5 g/dl).

Albumin:globulin ratio (A:G ratio)

Dog: 0.5–1.3.
Cat: 0.4–1.3.

Fibrinogen

Dog: 1–5 g/l (0.1–0.5 g/dl).
Cat: 0.5–3 g/l (0.05–0.3 g/dl).

METHOD OF MEASUREMENT

It is usual to measure the total protein concentration and the albumin concentration (see p. 250) and to assume that the difference between them represents the concentration of the globulins. From these figures the albumin:globulin ratio (A:G) can be calculated, a ratio which may assist diagnosis by accentuating the relative changes in the two major protein components. However, much more valuable is a careful comparison of albumin and globulin fractions derived from electrophoresis.

Total protein concentration

This is usually measured by the Biuret method.
Accuracy is good except at low levels (<10 g/l = <1 g/dl).
Bilirubin (>85 μmol/l = >5 mg/dl) will elevate the readings if a sample blank is not used.

A quick alternative is to use a previously calibrated refractometer to assess the total protein level.
Accuracy is generally sufficient for clinical purposes but:

- This method assumes that other solutes remain in normal concentrations. Very high levels of other solutes (e.g. urea, glucose, cholesterol and sodium, or substances such as dextran which may be infused in large amounts in hypoproteinaemic disorders) will falsely increase the protein readings.
- Samples showing haemolysis or lipaemia will be falsely elevated (because of the turbidity).

Note

If the albumin value is subtracted from a *falsely elevated* total protein value the globulin fraction will appear (erroneously) to be elevated and similarly the A:G ratio will be falsely decreased.

Changes in total protein levels are due primarily to increases or decreases in the albumin level; changes in globulin concentrations generally have less effect.
Abnormalities of protein levels are termed 'dysproteinaemias'.

Protein electrophoresis and globulin fractions

Zone electrophoresis is a technique whereby the different types of plasma proteins are separated, making it possible to determine their relative proportions in a particular sample. At an alkaline pH, serum or plasma, supported on a polyacrylamide gel or other medium, is placed in an electrical field, causing the different protein fractions to migrate at varying speeds towards the anode. Following staining, these fractions appear as bands of varying intensity of colour which can be scanned by a densitometer to produce an electrophoretic trace (Figure 5.2).

Table 5.1 Normal albumin and globulin reference ranges (adults)

Protein	Dog		Cat	
	g/l	(g/dl)	g/l	(g/dl)
Albumin	25–40	(2.5–4)	25–40	(2.5–4)
Globulin fractions				
α_1	2–5	(0.2–0.5)	2–11	(0.2–1.1)
α_2	3–11	(0.3–1.1)	4–9	(0.4–0.9)
Total α	5–13	(0.5–1.3)	6–16	(0.6–1.6)
β_1	6–13	(0.6–1.3)	3–9	(0.3–0.9)
β_2	6–14	(0.6–1.4)	4–10	(0.4–1)
Total β	12–22	(1.2–2.2)	7–16	(0.7–1.6)
γ_1	4–13	(0.4–1.3)	3–24	(0.3–2.4)
γ_2	4–9	(0.4–0.9)	12–19	(1.2–1.9)
Total γ	8–18	(0.8–1.8)	15–35	(1.5–3.5)
Total globulin	25–45	(2.5–4.5)	28–55	(2.8–5.5)

The length and height of each section of the trace indicates the relative amount of a particular protein or group of proteins. This can be translated into percentage readings and, by combining this information with the total protein concentration, absolute values for the concentration of each protein, or protein group, can be calculated. This can serve as a check on the value obtained for albumin concentration by chemical means, and provide quantitative information about the globulin fractions. Normal reference values are shown in Table 5.1.

Albumin (the fastest-migrating protein) appears as a distinct high peak at one end of the trace – in most cases this is placed on the extreme left hand side, although in North American publications it generally appears on the right. Behind it are arranged the globulins, in the order α, β and γ and, in many instances, each of these can be clearly subdivided into two bands (i.e. α_1, α_2, β_1, β_2, γ_1 and γ_2) although at times, especially with the β bands, this separation cannot be made.

The appearance of the electrophoretic trace can be distinctive in particular disorders, e.g. hypoalbuminaemia and polyclonal and monoclonal gammopathies (see Figure 5.2).

PLASMA AND SERUM

Plasma contains fibrinogen, which serum does not, and if plasma is subjected to electrophoresis the fibrinogen appears as a prominent peak between the β- and γ-globulin peaks, seemingly in the γ_1 position. It is especially evident in acute inflammatory diseases.

HAEMOLYSIS

Haemolysed serum or plasma results in an increase in the β- and α_2-globulin fractions and some blurring of the β peaks.

Causes of increased total protein levels (hyperproteinaemia)

Summary

Dehydration [common]
Increased globulin level
* Acute inflammation
* Subacute inflammation
* Chronic inflammation
* Liver disease
* Neoplasia
* Viral and rickettsial diseases [unusual]
* Fungal and protozoal infections
* Autoimmune disorders
* Newborn animals [transient]
* Pyodermas
* Primary glomerular diseases
* Haemolysis
Anabolic steroids
Increased fibrinogen level
Error: haemolysis and lipaemia (with refractometer)

Increases may be relative (i.e. due to dehydration) or absolute (due to an increase in the globulin fraction); *true hyperalbuminaemia* is unknown. Raised globulin levels are a common non-specific finding in sick cats.

DEHYDRATION [RELATIVELY COMMON]

For example following prolonged non-availability of drinking water, severe vomiting and polyuric disorders such as pyometra and diabetes mellitus. The increase in protein is only relative, i.e. its total quantity is unchanged.

CHECK – dehydration is also indicated by finding:
* An increased PCV (although PCV can be falsely elevated by splenic contraction is animals that are stressed, i.e. afraid or excited; in such cases the total plasma protein remains normal) – hyperproteinaemia is often a surer guide to the degree of dehydration than the PCV, unless the fluid loss is small.
* An elevated albumin level, because a *true* absolute increase does not occur.
* A normal A:G ratio – loss of water elevates the albumin and globulin concentrations to the same degree.

AN INCREASED LEVEL OF GLOBULINS

This is associated with an increase in the globulin fraction:
* The albumin level remains normal, or even declines (particularly in cases of liver disease).
* The A:G ratio is reduced.

Information about the possible cause may be obtained from an electrophoretic trace (see p. 241), allowing changes in the globulin fractions to be detected.

Acute inflammation and tissue injury

Acute inflammation (e.g. acute hepatitis), tissue injury (e.g. due to cold, heat or fractures) and fever produce an increase in α-globulins (acute phase reactants), sometimes accompanied by an increase in β-globulins, e.g. fibrinogen (estimations of fibrinogen and haptoglobin may be used as indicators of acute inflammation).

Subacute inflammation

Subacute inflammation, especially when due to bacteria, produces an increase in α- and γ-globulins.

Chronic inflammation

For example chronic hepatitis leading to cirrhosis, abscess formation, pyometra and other chronic infections e.g. tuberculosis, produce an increase in γ-globulins.

Liver disease

- Acute hepatitis produces an increase in α-globulins.
- Chronic active hepatitis produces an increase in β_2- and γ_1- globulins with 'bridging' on the electrophoretic trace, i.e. no clear separation of these two fractions.
- Cirrhosis is characterized by increases in γ-globulins.
- β_2-Globulins are increased in jaundice.
- β_1-Globulins increase in liver neoplasia (although they are decreased in other liver diseases).
- Non-specific increases in α_2 -globulins may also be seen.

Neoplasia

In many cases this is associated with increases in α_2- and β-globulins, although with lymphosarcomas and hepatic carcinomas an increase in β- and γ-globulins is common.

Viral and rickettsial diseases

In general, these do not significantly increase the absolute (or relative) amounts of proteins – the major exception being *feline infectious peritonitis* where there is usually an increase in total protein despite a fall in albumin, due to a massive increase in γ-globulins; the height of the γ-globulin peak often exceeds that of albumin. In feline infectious peritonitis there is also a less pronounced increase in α_2- and β-globulins. Not unusually the albumin level is less than 20 g/l and the globulin level more than 100 g/l. The diagnosis of FIP can be CHECKED by finding a positive serological titre.

Raised γ-globulin levels are a feature in a third of cats infected with feline immunodeficiency virus (FIV), due to increases in IgG (γ- globulin).

An increase in α_2- and γ-globulins is a feature of canine distemper.

Increases in α_2-, β- and γ-globulins also occur in ehrlichiosis.

Fungal and protozoal infections

Leishmaniasis produces an increase in IgG (γ-globulin) which can increase the total protein level to more than 100 g/l (>10 g/dl) despite a decrease in the albumin component.

Blastomycosis results in increases in α_2-, β- and γ-globulins, and globulin increases are also seen in histoplasmosis and coccidioidomycosis, although in all these conditions there may be a balancing decrease in albumin.

Autoimmune disorders

These show an increase in γ-globulins (e.g. with glomerulonephritis caused by pyometra, and systemic lupus erythematosus).

In rheumatoid arthritis there is often mild hypoalbuminaemia with increases in α- and γ-globulins, including fibrinogen.

Lymphocytic cholangitis in cats probably has an autoimmune cause, and it resembles feline infectious peritonitis by showing a similar massive increase in the level of globulins (together with increases in conjugated bilirubin, ALP and GGT, plus lymphopenia, neutrophilia and a non-regenerative anaemia).

In newborn animals

Immediately after suckling colostrum, but for only a short while, the electrophoretic trace may appear similar to that shown in feline infectious peritonitis (see above) with a high γ-globulin level.

Pyodermas

These produce an increase in β-globulins.

Primary glomerular disease

Primary glomerular disease (glomerulonephritis and amyloidosis) frequently produce increases in α-, β and γ-globulin concentrations. Amyloidosis, in particular, is associated with an increased α-globulin level, e.g. some cases of spontaneous amyloidosis, a familial disease of young Abyssinian cats, show a marked hyperglobulinaemia with elevation of the α_2-globulins.

ERROR: HAEMOLYSIS

Haemolysis will cause increases in the α_2- and β-globulin fractions with blurring of the β peaks.

Note

If *plasma* is employed instead of serum for electrophoresis, a peak will appear between the β- and γ-globulins, seeming to be in the γ_1 position, due to the presence of fibrinogen.

The increases in γ- and β-globulins (occasionally also α_2-globulins) that are especially evident in chronic infectious inflammatory diseases (particularly of the liver), immune-mediated disorders and (occasionally) lymphosarcomas (as described previously) produce a broad peak in those regions on electrophoretic traces. This is because more than one immunoglobulin is involved. Consequently they are termed 'polyclonal gammopathies'.

But, in addition, 'monoclonal gammopathies' can arise, i.e. where there is proliferation of a single 'clone' of plasma cells that produce a large quantity of just one immunoglobulin (termed a 'paraprotein') causing a narrow globulin peak ('church spire') on electrophoresis. Monoclonal gammopathies are associated with plasma cell myelomas, macroglobulinaemia, lymphoproliferative disorders and (rarely) other tumours, and sometimes chronic inflammatory or immune-mediated diseases (see Panel 5.1, p. 295).

ANABOLIC STEROIDS

These are reported to increase levels of total protein and albumin.

AN INCREASED LEVEL OF FIBRINOGEN [RARE]

This, when associated with inflammation (e.g. moderate liver damage), neoplasia or fractures can in *extreme cases* elevate the total protein level.

ERROR: A FALSE INCREASE IN TOTAL PROTEIN LEVEL

When estimated using a refractometer, or using the Biuret method but without employing a sample blank, a false increase will occur with samples that are:

• Either haemolysed.
• Or lipaemic.

If an accurate albumin concentration is subtracted from the falsely elevated total protein concentration the globulin fraction will appear to be increased. This erroneous value will result in a falsely decreased A:G ratio.

Causes of decreased plasma total protein levels (hypoproteinaemia)

Summary

Relative decrease – overhydration and errors
Age – young animals
Decreased protein synthesis
• Protein starvation
• Small intestinal malabsorption
• Liver disorders
• Congestive heart failure
Increased protein loss
• In urine
• From the gut
• From burns
• Haemorrhage
• Sepsis and bacteraemia

RELATIVE DECREASE (INCLUDING ERROR)

There can be relatively more water present in the plasma due to:

• Overhydration with intravenous fluids.
• Collecting the blood sample from a vein into which fluid was administered either simultaneously or shortly beforehand.
• Collecting a blood sample from the same needle or cannula used to administer intravenous fluid.

The total quantity of protein is not decreased but is diluted by the additional fluid. Provided there are no complicating factors (i.e. other conditions present concurrently) confirmatory features would be:

• A PCV which is equally low.
• An A:G ratio which remains unaltered.

AGE

Young animals (<6 months old) have lower total protein levels than adults.

DECREASED PROTEIN SYNTHESIS

Liable to be responsible for poor wound healing.

Protein starvation

Diets *very* low in protein fed over a long period, or alternatively complete starvation, will result in low total protein and albumin levels, but lesser deficiencies of protein usually cause no change in the plasma protein values.

Small intestinal malabsorption

Failure to absorb an adequate amount of amino acids from the small intestine (e.g. due to a bacterial overgrowth problem or exocrine pancreatic insufficiency) will result in a low total protein level and particularly in a low albumin level.

Malabsorption usually accompanies a *protein-losing* enteropathy, and is often of greater significance in producing hypoproteinaemia, especially where there is marked villous atrophy (atrophy of the absorptive villi) as in canine 'sprue'.

Liver disorders

These include sepsis and acute toxoplasmosis.

Failure of the liver to synthesize proteins (chiefly albumin) will reduce the total protein level and especially the albumin level. Consequently the A:G ratio may be decreased.

CHECK   whether there is an elevated bile acid level, and reduced urea level and BSP clearance. These are some of the changes indicating reduced liver function (see Panel 6.1, p. 333).

> **Note**
>
> There will not necessarily be concurrent liver *damage* or *cholestasis* and therefore liver enzyme levels (ALT, ALP, GT etc.) will not necessarily be raised.

Congestive heart failure

In general total plasma protein concentrations are decreased, due not only to reduced synthesis (mainly of albumin) in the liver but also to:

- Dilution of proteins by retained water.
- Protein losses into ascitic fluid.
- Diminished intake of food.
- Protein malabsorption, and possibly protein losses into the gut.

INCREASED PROTEIN LOSS

Liable to be responsible for poor wound healing.

Protein loss in the urine

This is most marked in primary glomerular diseases (glomerulonephritis and renal amyloidosis) and may lead to development of the nephrotic syndrome (see p. 300).

Mainly *albumin is lost* because it has the smallest molecule, and consequently the A:G ratio is reduced, although as glomerular damage increases, and with it the loss of protein, an increasing *proportion* of globulin is lost.

(Alongside the loss of albumin, which causes the fall in total plasma protein, there may be (smaller) increases in α_2-globulins (in acute glomerulonephritis) and γ-globulins (in chronic glomerulonephritis, for example that associated with pyometra).)

CHECK   for proteinuria (commercial test strips are most sensitive to albumin) and an increase in the cholesterol level which accompanies the fall in albumin.

Other causes of proteinuria (see p. 431), such as chronic renal failure, are of lesser degree and usually do not result in hypoproteinaemia. Indeed the accompanying dehydration may be responsible for a relative *hyper*proteinaemia.

Protein loss from the gut

In certain inflammatory, ulcerative and neoplastic disorders protein can leak from the wall of the gastrointestinal tract into the lumen and be lost in the faeces.

Chiefly this occurs in the small intestine, particularly in cases of lymphosarcoma but also with other neoplasms, enteric parvovirus infection, inflammation (e.g. eosinophilic enteritis), lymphangiectasia and histoplasmosis. These disorders are referred to as protein-losing enteropathies. They are closely bound up with malabsorption (see under 'Decreased protein synthesis' above).

There may at times be significant protein losses from ulcers in the stomach and/or proximal duodenum (peptic ulcers) and from ulcers in the colon and rectum (ulcerative colitis). Such protein losses involve both albumin and globulin affecting most severely proteins with a longer half-life, i.e. albumin and the γ-globulins.

Because albumin and globulin are generally lost equally there is usually no change in the A:G ratio.

Gastrointestinal parasites may accentuate these losses, although alone they usually produce no detectable change in protein levels.

Protein loss from burns or severe exudative inflammatory lesions

Usually the animal's history simplifies the diagnosis. Losses from skin abrasions and other lesions are *usually not sufficient* to disturb the total protein level.

Haemorrhage

A severe loss of blood will reduce the albumin and globulin pools equally, and will become obvious in estimations performed 2–3 hours after the incident when sufficient fluid has been transferred into the circulation to dilute the proteins.

These changes will be accompanied by a lower PCV.

After haemorrhage it is probable that at least half of the albumin will be replaced within 24 hours and this *might* lead to a relative increase in the A:G ratio.

Sepsis and bacteraemia

Increased capillary permeability (and possibly vasculitis, which is immune mediated or due to an embolus) allows albumin to leak into the extravascular compartment. Reduced albumin production by the liver may accentuate the loss.

(This is probably the reason for changes in protein levels in the rickettsial disease Rocky Mountain Spotted Fever in the USA.)

Causes of normal total plasma protein levels with changes in the protein fractions

These are detected by the altered albumin:globulin ratio.

Summary

Decreased A:G ratio
- Increased globulin
- Decreased albumin

Increased A:G ratio [rare]
- Hypogammaglobulinaemia
- Congenital immunodeficiency
- Acquired immunodeficiency

DECREASED A:G RATIO

Increased globulin content

Increases in the level of the various globulin fractions, which can raise the total plasma protein level (due to those causes given in the section 'Causes of increased total plasma proteins', p. 243), may be of *lesser* magnitude and simply decrease the A:G ratio leaving the total plasma protein level within the normal range. For example, an increase in α_2-globulin with mast cell tumours (mastocytomas).

These increases may be accompanied by a decrease in the albumin level, e.g. in severe trauma where an increase in α_2-globulin level occurs with a fall in albumin concentration.

Reduction in the albumin content of plasma

This can reduce the A:G ratio without being of such severity as to decrease the total plasma protein level. They may be due to decreased albumin synthesis or increased losses through the kidney or gut or (rarely) skin burns, or they may be due to increased albumin catabolism (as in Cushing's syndrome, hyperthyroidism, uncontrolled diabetes mellitus, infection with fever, trauma, pregnancy, lactation and malignant neoplasia).

INCREASED A:G RATIO [RARE]

Since an absolute increase in albumin is unknown, the increased ratio arises due to decreased levels of globulins, which may indicate severe immunodeficiency.

Hypogammaglobulinaemia

This is normal in newborn animals and, if they are not allowed to take colostrum, the condition will persist, i.e. maternal antibodies will not be transferred.

Congenital immunodeficiency

- Combined (humoral and cell-mediated) immunodeficiency in Long-haired Dachshunds and Bassett Hounds.
- Selective IgA deficiency in Beagles, German Shepherd Dogs and Shar Peis.
- Deficiency of growth hormone resulting in severe thymic deficiency in Weimeraners.

Acquired immunodeficiency

Viral and bacterial diseases

A number of viral and bacterial diseases result in deficiencies in specific immune defences, e.g.

- Canine distemper (in neonates).
- Canine parvovirus infection.
- Staphylococcal infection secondary to demodicosis.
- Feline leukaemia virus infection.
- Feline immunodeficiency virus (FIV) infection.
- Feline infectious peritonitis (exceptionally).

In general though, it would *not* be expected that these would result in significant reductions in plasma globulin content.

Uraemia

This can reduce immunoglobulin levels. There is also a possibility of reduced immunoglobulin levels arising in association with lymphosarcoma and with the use of immunosuppressive drugs.

Plasma albumin

SI units of measurement are grams per litre (g/l). Although albumin could be measured in mmol/l, for the sake of consistency, the same units are used as for the estimation of total protein (which is measured in g/l because it consists of many proteins which have *differing* molecular weights).
Previous units used were g/dl (=g/100 ml).

CONVERSION FACTORS

- To convert g/dl to g/l multiply by 10.
- To convert g/l to g/dl multiply by 0.1.

NORMAL REFERENCE RANGE (ADULTS)

Dog and cat: 25–40 g/l (2.5–4 g/dl).

Normal reference ranges may vary considerably between laboratories; therefore checking is advisable.

AGE

With advancing age the level of albumin tends to fall *slightly*.
The difference between the total plasma protein level and the albumin level represents the amount of globulins present and, from the albumin and globulin levels, the albumin:globulin ratio (A:G ratio) can be calculated.

ALBUMIN:GLOBULIN RATIO (A:G RATIO)

Dog: 0.5–1.3.
Cat: 0.4–1.3.

SOURCE AND FUNCTION

Albumin is synthesized in the liver from amino acids (approximately 0.15–0.2 g/kg body weight per day) and it usually accounts for 35–50% of the total plasma proteins. It is the main storage form of protein and source of amino acids to the tissues and is chiefly responsible for the colloid osmotic pressure of the blood. It binds and transports many substances (including unconjugated bilirubin, free fatty acids and thyroxine (in part), and many drugs). Calcium is also transported bound to albumin and hypoalbuminaemia results in hypocalcaemia (but not in hypocalcaemic tetany as only the bound fraction is reduced, not the ionized).

Albumin has a lower molecular weight than other plasma proteins and there is frequent interchange of albumin between the plasma and interstitial fluid, some of it being returned to the blood via the lymphatic circulation.

METHOD OF MEASUREMENT

The albumin concentration is usually determined by binding it to the dye bromocresol green (BCG).

ACCURACY

Inaccurate results arise at times, especially because:

- Low albumin levels can give *falsely high* readings because the dye attaches to other protein fractions.
- *Falsely low* readings can arise when certain drugs (aspirin, carbenicillin) or bilirubin are present, because they compete with albumin for the binding of BCG.

CHECK – absolute albumin levels, derived from a combination of the total protein estimation and the relative proportions obtained from an electrophoretic trace, can serve as a check on the result obtained by the BCG method.

Causes of increased plasma albumin levels (hyperalbuminaemia)

Absolute increases in albumin levels are generally thought not to arise, although there have been reports of increases following anabolic steroid therapy (in Greyhounds). Increases are almost always due to one of the following.

DEHYDRATION

This may follow severe vomiting, diarrhoea and polyuric disorders as well as prolonged deprivation of drinking water which will aggravate increased losses.

In association with the elevated albumin level there will be an increased PCV but a normal A:G ratio (because albumin and globulin are affected to the same extent by plasma water losses).

ERROR: DRUG INTERFERENCES

- Penicillins interfere with the BCG method. Ampicillin therapy has produced *slight* increases in albumin values although, in practice, the effect is probably insignificant.
- The addition of heparin in very large amounts to blood samples can produce considerable variations (increases and decreases) in the albumin value.

Causes of decreased plasma albumin levels (hypoalbuminaemia)

Summary

Relative decrease – overhydration and error
Decreased protein synthesis
- Protein starvation
- Small intestinal malabsorption
- Liver disorders
- Severe trauma
- Congestive heart failure
- Pituitary dwarfism
- Primidone therapy
Increased protein loss
- In urine
- From the gut
- From burns
- Haemorrhage
- Sepsis and bacteraemia
Diet (s/d)
Error: interference with measurement (BCG method)

RELATIVE DECREASES (INCLUDING THOSE ARISING FROM ERROR)

These are due to increased plasma water content.
Relatively more water will be present in the plasma if:

- The patient is overhydrated with intravenous fluids.
- The blood sample is collected from a vein into which fluid has been administered.
- The sample is collected from the same needle or cannula used for intravenous fluid administration.

Note

Dextran 70 given for a number of days can cause a considerable fall in plasma albumin concentration (e.g. 30–40%) due to haemodilution.

DECREASED PROTEIN SYNTHESIS

Protein starvation

This refers to starvation due to diets extremely low in protein fed for prolonged periods, or to complete starvation.

Small intestinal malabsorption

This may accompany a protein-losing enteropathy, and may be the more important feature.

Liver disorders

These include disorders in which the liver fails to synthesize adequate amounts of protein, e.g. in severe hepatic dysfunction (hepatic failure) and with portosystemic shunts.

In the *cat* this effect of these disorders is less common, hypoalbuminaemia occurring only rarely with chronic hepatic disease and usually not being a feature of portosystemic shunts.

Severe trauma

Decreased synthesis with unchanged catabolism can cause a rapid fall reaching a minimum after 3–6 days. (In humans a 25–30% reduction is a feature of moderate injury.)

Congestive heart failure

Dilution of albumin by retained water, protein losses into ascitic fluid, diminished food intake, protein malabsorption and gastrointestinal protein losses combine to reduce the albumin level.

Pituitary dwarfism

Reduced albumin concentration is due to the lack of the anabolic effect of growth hormone.

Primidone therapy

Primidone therapy in the long term decreases albumin levels in approximately 70% of dogs due to reduced hepatic function.

INCREASED PROTEIN LOSS

Protein loss in the urine

This is particularly a feature of primary glomerular diseases (glomerulonephritis and renal amyloidosis) and may lead to development of the *nephrotic syndrome* (see p. 300). Chiefly it is albumin which is lost (being a smaller molecule), which therefore leads to a decreased A:G ratio.

CHECK – other features would be proteinuria and an increase in cholesterol related to the fall in albumin.

In other proteinuric conditions, hypoalbuminaemia is not usually a feature although it does occur in extreme cases, e.g. familial nephropathy in Soft-coated Wheaten Terriers.

Protein loss from the gut

Usually both albumin and globulin are lost equally from the intestines in protein-losing enteropathies, e.g. lymphosarcoma and other neoplasms, enteric parvovirus infection, inflammation (e.g. eosinophilic enteritis), lymphangiectasia and histoplasmosis. Losses may be significant from ulceration affecting the stomach and/or proximal duodenum (peptic ulcers) or in the large bowel (colon and rectum) with ulcerative colitis. Ulceration is probably the cause of the increased gastrointestinal losses of albumin seen in uraemia.

Protein loss from burns

Albumin is lost from burns and from severe inflammatory lesions with exudation.

Haemorrhage

Two to three hours after severe haemorrhage the reduction in albumin (and globulin) levels will be obvious, accompanied by a lower PCV (see 'Causes of haemorrhagic anaemia', p. 91).

Sepsis and bacteraemia

Increasing capillary permeability allows albumin to leak into the extracellular fluid. This effect may be enhanced by reduced hepatic albumin production.

DIET

The long-term use of Hill's s/d diet for the dissolution of struvite calculi in dogs may lead to some degree of hypoalbuminaemia.

ERROR: INTERFERENCE WITH MEASUREMENT BY THE BCG METHOD

Interference, producing falsely low values can be due to the presence of bilirubin in large amounts, or some drugs, including:

- Carbenicillin.
- Aspirin.
- Anticonvulsants – these are reported to produce low albumin values but this is not supported by the human literature (Seist and Galteau, 1988).

Note

Also associated with low albumin levels are:

- A low urea level, due to reduced protein catabolism.
- A low calcium level due to a reduction in the protein-bound fraction.

Almost all of the causes of low total protein levels (hypoproteinaemia) will also result in a low albumin level. Further detail is provided in the section 'Causes of decreased total plasma proteins' (p. 246).

Plasma bilirubin

The SI units of measurement are micromoles per litre (μmol/l). Previously the units used were mg/dl (= mg/100 ml).

CONVERSION FACTORS

- To convert mg/dl to μmol/l multiple by 17.1.
- To convert μmol/l to mg/dl multiple by 0.059.

NORMAL REFERENCE RANGE (ADULTS)

Dog: 1.7–10 μmol/l (= 0.1–0.6 mg/dl).
Cat: 2–5 μmol/l (= 0.12–0.3 mg/dl).

Total bilirubin = unconjugated bilirubin + conjugated bilirubin. The two forms of bilirubin can be distinguished by the van den Bergh reaction. Normally almost all the bilirubin is unconjugated in both dog and cat.

Both forms of bilirubin are yellow/orange pigments that give a yellow colour to the plasma and, in sufficient quantity, to the mucous membranes and sclera – referred to as *jaundice* or *icterus*. Jaundice is evident clinically with total levels of 35–50 μmol/l (2–3 mg/dl), although bilirubin levels are significant above 10 μmol/l in the dog (>0.6 mg/dl) and above 5 μmol/l in the cat (= 0.3 mg/dl) even though jaundice is absent.

If a plasma (or serum) sample does not *appear* abnormally yellow (jaundiced), it is unlikely that the bilirubin level will be elevated.

ACCURACY

Falsely elevated values can be the result of haemolysis in the sample interfering with measurement of the bilirubin.

SOURCE

Most of the bilirubin in the plasma derives from the breakdown (i.e. phagocytosis) of aged RBCs by the mononuclear phagocyte system (essentially the same as the reticuloendothelial system), especially the spleen. The remaining bilirubin comes from the breakdown of myoglobin, cytochromes and immature RBCs in the bone marrow.

The haemoglobin released from the RBCs is split into globin (which is conserved in the body's protein pool) and haem. After removal of the iron molecule (which is stored and/or reutilized) the haem is converted into bilirubin. In the event of *intravascular* haemolysis the haemoglobin in the plasma is cleared mainly by the mononuclear phagocyte system (MPS), apart from small amounts removed by hepatic cells and renal tubular cells.

The bilirubin formed is unconjugated bilirubin which is transported to the liver bound to plasma albumin. It is alternatively known as free, prehepatic or indirect-reacting bilirubin. It is not water soluble (but *is* fat soluble), and therefore is not filtered by the renal glomerulus and is not normally excreted in the urine.

Rarely unconjugated bilirubin is found which is not bound to albumin, when:

- Albumin levels are extremely low.
- There is competition for albumin binding sites, e.g. with thyroxine, salicylates, sulphonamides, digoxin, cortisol or diazepam.
- When unconjugated bilirubin levels are extremely high – >340 μmol/l (>20 mg/dl).

In the liver the attachment to albumin is broken and, within its cells (hepatocytes), bilirubin is conjugated with glucuronic acid to form conjugated bilirubin (otherwise known as posthepatic or direct-reacting bilirubin). This *is* water soluble, and is actively secreted into the small bile canaliculi and subsequently excreted in the bile (Figure 5.3).

Very little conjugated bilirubin is normally present in the plasma; in healthy animals most of the bilirubin in the plasma is unconjugated.

Conjugated bilirubin in the intestine cannot be reabsorbed but, in the ileum and colon, bacterial enzymes convert it to (colourless) urobilinogen (faecal urobilinogen or stercobilinogen) some of which (10–15%) is reabsorbed and passes in the portal circulation to the liver. Most of this urobilinogen is re-excreted in the bile but a little is excreted in the urine (see 'Urinary urobilinogen', p. 444).

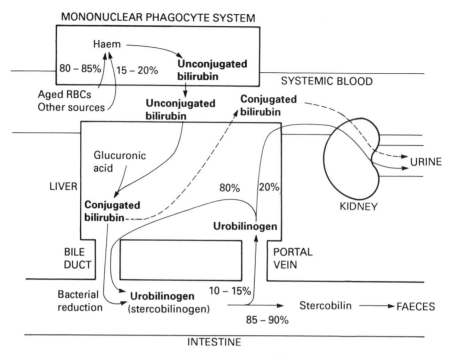

Figure 5.3 Formation, circulation and excretion of bile pigments. Usually only a minimal amount of conjugated bilirubin (if any) is excreted in the urine

The urobilinogen remaining is oxidized to stercobilin, which gives the faeces the characteristic brown colour.

Increased levels of bilirubin in the *plasma* (=hyperbilirubinaemia) can result from the following six major defects.

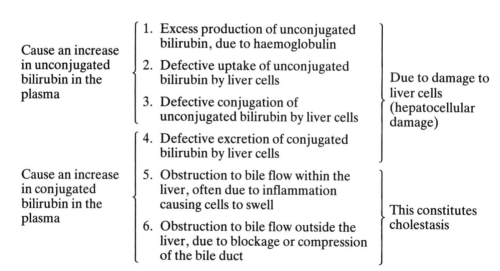

Cause an increase in unconjugated bilirubin in the plasma

1. Excess production of unconjugated bilirubin, due to haemoglobulin

2. Defective uptake of unconjugated bilirubin by liver cells

3. Defective conjugation of unconjugated bilirubin by liver cells

Due to damage to liver cells (hepatocellular damage)

Cause an increase in conjugated bilirubin in the plasma

4. Defective excretion of conjugated bilirubin by liver cells

5. Obstruction to bile flow within the liver, often due to inflammation causing cells to swell

6. Obstruction to bile flow outside the liver, due to blockage or compression of the bile duct

This constitutes cholestasis

Jaundice is essentially classified as being haemolytic, hepatocellular or obstructive (= cholestatic), although there is some overlap especially between the last two types. In inflammatory liver diseases (toxic and infectious hepatitis) causes (2) to (5) above are present and, therefore, both forms of bilirubin accumulate in the plasma.

The test often used to measure bilirubin is the van den Bergh reaction. Using an alcoholic solution in the test *all* the bilirubin (i.e. both unconjugated and conjugated) is measured, using an aqueous solution only the conjugated (direct-reacting) is measured. The difference between them is the level of unconjugated (indirect-reacting) bilirubin.

Causes of increased plasma bilirubin levels (hyperbilirubinaemia)

Summary

Mainly unconjugated bilirubin
Severe acute haemolysis
Absorption of large haematoma or massive internal haemorrhage
Transfusion of stored RBCs
Almost equally unconjugated and conjugated bilirubin
Loss of hepatocellular function (see below)
Obstruction to bile flow (see below)
Following severe acute intravascular haemolysis (or large haematoma, or massive internal haemorrhage)
Largely conjugated bilirubin
Loss of hepatocellular function [common]
- Toxic damage (poisons, drugs)
- Infectious diseases
- Parasites – flukes (not in the UK)
- Severe trauma
- Feline liver disorders
- Chronic active hepatitis
- Myeloproliferative disorders
- Secondary liver damage (dog – rare/cat – possible)
Obstruction to bile flow [common]
- Pressure of inflamed liver cells
- Space-occupying lesions (tumours, abscesses)
- Abnormal tissue deposition in liver
- Pyogranulomatous hepatitis
- Bile duct blockage
- Inflammation of biliary tract
- Right-sided heart failure
- Congenital cystic disease (dog – rare)
Rupture of the biliary tree [unusual]

If the total bilirubin level is raised it may assist diagnosis to know whether the increase is mainly in one type or in both. Generally, of course, there will be other diagnostic indicators.

DUE MAINLY TO UNCONJUGATED (INDIRECT-REACTING) BILIRUBIN (75% OR MORE)

Severe acute haemolysis (haemolytic crisis) [uncommon]

See Panel 2.3 (p. 95).

The rapid release of a large amount of haemoglobin into the plasma is generally only a feature of *intravascular* haemolysis, primarily:

- Certain cases of autoimmune haemolytic anaemia (see Panel 2.7, p. 125),
- Dissociated intravascular coagulation (DIC), and splenic torsion.
- Certain types of *toxicity*, e.g. oxidant drugs (causing Heinz body anaemia) or snake venom.
- Physical lysis – the intravenous injection of hypotonic solutions (especially water), heat, i.e. severe burns, and radiation.
- Incompatible blood transfusion.
- Haemolytic disease of the newborn.
- Feline haemobartonellosis – bilirubinaemia is not generally expected but may sometimes occur with an acute haemolytic crisis.
- Babesiosis (but not in the UK).

The large amount of (unconjugated) bilirubin formed greatly exceeds the liver's capacity to conjugate it.

After haemolysis hyperbilirubinaemia will not be apparent for 8–10 hours – it takes that long for an appreciable quantity of bilirubin to form. Consequently a plasma sample collected too soon afterwards will *not* show this change.

Other anticipated features include:

- A low PCV (i.e. anaemia).
- Free haemoglobin in the plasma giving it a pink/red colour (haemoglobinaemia).
- Free haemoglobin in the urine (haemoglobinuria) probably sufficient to cause a pink/red colour.
- Reticulocytosis in the blood *after 3 (2–4) days* (i.e. an increased number of reticulocytes and possibly, if very severe, of nucleated RBCs also).

Note

- In the early stages *bilirubinuria is not a feature*, since unconjugated bilirubin (tightly bound to albumin) is not filtered by the kidney. This inability of unconjugated bilirubin to escape can result in a high plasma level of bilirubin.

    However, *slightly* more bilirubin than usual *may* be present in the urine because the renal tubular cells are able to clear a small amount of haemoglobin, to convert it to unconjugated bilirubin, to conjugate it and to excrete the conjugated bilirubin.

- One to two days *after* severe intravascular haemolysis there is *also* an increased amount of conjugated bilirubin in the plasma, although usually less than 50% of the total. This is because conjugation has been taking place but the capacity of the liver cells to excrete the conjugated bilirubin has been exceeded and/or there is liver cell damage due to hypoxia caused by the lack of RBCs.

    At this stage the plasma levels of unconjugated and conjugated bilirubin are almost equal and significant bilirubinuria occurs, because the conjugated bilirubin can be excreted.

- Haemoglobinaemia and bilirubinaemia are not generally associated with *extravascular haemolysis* (i.e. due to increased tissue phagocytosis of RBCs) because the rate of haemolysis is less and a large amount of haemoglobin is not usually liberated all at once. This slower release of haemoglobin enables the formation and excretion of conjugated bilirubin to proceed normally without accumulation at any stage. However, slight increases in plasma bilirubin levels have been recorded in aspirin poisoning in the cat and in pyruvate kinase deficiency in Basenjis.

Absorption of a large haematoma or following massive internal haemorrhage

A cause of such internal haemorrhage would be with poisoning by an anticoagulant rodenticide.

Tissue macrophages phagocytose the RBCs and degrade their haemoglobin to unconjugated bilirubin which is then conveyed to the liver. The sequence of events is then the same as for intravascular haemolysis. Jaundice is improbable except in very young animals.

Note

Both severe haemolysis and massive haemorrhage will result in a regenerative anaemia, i.e. a fall in packed cell volume and reticulocytosis, but regeneration is *more* marked with haemolysis (i.e. reticulocyte production index (RPI) >3).

Transfusion of stored RBCs

Hyperbilirubinaemia results if the blood was collected more than 3 weeks beforehand. These old RBCs are rapidly broken down and a large amount of unconjugated bilirubin is formed.

DUE TO ALMOST EQUAL AMOUNTS OF UNCONJUGATED AND CONJUGATED BILIRUBIN

Loss of hepatocellular function following liver damage (see below)

Generally, this is due to a more chronic liver disorder or to moderate damage (e.g. chronic active hepatitis). Between 20% and 60% of the bilirubin is conjugated, the lower level being more common in cats.

Obstruction to the flow of bile

This is usually intrahepatic (=regurgitation hyperbilirubinaemia) – see below under 'Obstruction of the biliary tract' (p. 262) for more detail.

With extrahepatic obstruction the bilirubin is, generally, predominantly conjugated.

A few days after severe acute intravascular haemolysis

Hyperbilirubinaemia of this type can also occur (rarely) after a massive haematoma or internal haemorrhage – when the level of conjugated bilirubin has risen. The causes of such haemolysis are described above under 'Severe acute haemolysis'. Usually conjugated bilirubin is less than 50% of the total. The usual features of haemolytic anaemia would be expected (see Panel 2.3, p. 95).

DUE LARGELY TO CONJUGATED BILIRUBIN (i.e. >50%)

Loss of hepatocellular function [common]

This is consequent upon damage to the liver cells. Their ability to excrete bile is more affected than their ability to conjugate bilirubin, with the result that there is an accumulation of conjugated bilirubin. The cell walls of the hepatocytes become more permeable and conjugated bilirubin diffuses out.

In addition some degree of intrahepatic obstruction appears inevitable where there is hepatocellular damage, because:

- Swollen, inflamed liver cells compress the bile canaliculi slowing the flow of bile.
- In chronic inflammation fibrosis interferes with the bile flow.
- Also, where there is necrosis, the bile canaliculi may rupture releasing bile.

In hepatocellular disorders the plasma levels of both conjugated and unconjugated bilirubin are raised, but generally conjugated predominates. Most cases have a toxic or infectious cause, although trauma may be more important than previously suspected.

Toxic damage [common]
This occurs by poisons or drugs.
Those substances most consistently associated with bilirubinaemia and icterus are:

- Phosphorus – yellow phosphorus is still used as a rodenticide.
- Phenolic compounds – tar, creosote and phenolic disinfectants.
- Aflatoxins – aflatoxin B_1 poisoning (as a contaminant in mouldy food) over a long or short period.
- Paraquat – a herbicide.
- Thallium – a rodenticide (little used now).
- Methimazole, and possibly carbimazole, used in treating hyperthyroidism in the cat.
- Propylthiouracil, also used to treat hyperthyroidism in cats.
- Paracetamol (acetaminophen), especially in the *cat*.
- Organic solvents, e.g. chloroform and carbon tetrachloride.

Many other drugs cause liver damage, with leakage of enzymes and/or liver dysfunction, but without obvious hyperbilirubinaemia.

Infectious diseases
The important primary infections are with canine adenovirus-1 and leptospirae, and hyperbilirubinaemia is associated with acute inflammation.

- Infectious canine hepatitis (systemic canine adenovirus-1 infection) – hyperbilirubinaemia, jaundice and bilirubinuria are less common than might be expected because the resultant centrilobular necrosis interferes less with bile drainage than does peripheral necrosis. However, 35% of severe cases show jaundice.
- Leptospirosis – overall about 15% of canine cases show jaundice. It is seen only occasionally with *L. canicola* which is much more common, but 70% of *L. icterohaemorrhagiae* cases show jaundice. Generally, the hyperbilirubinaemia is *not* due to haemolysis but to hepatocellular degeneration and particularly to intrahepatic cholestasis.

Hyperbilirubinaemia also occurs in:

- Feline infectious peritonitis – often mild to moderate increases in bilirubin occur, especially in the peritoneal (wet) form or with granulomatous hepatitis.
- Toxoplasmosis in cases of *acute* hepatic necrosis, especially in cats with cholangiohepatitis.
- Feline leukaemia virus infection – see 'Myeloproliferative disorders' below.
- Histoplasmosis, blastomycosis and coccidioidomycosis (none of which occurs in the UK). Bilirubinaemia in these chronic diseases is due primarily to cholestasis following dissemination of infection to the liver (pyogranulomatous hepatitis).
- Salmonellosis may *rarely* be a cause of jaundice.

Parasites
Liver flukes (although not in the UK) can cause biliary obstruction and hepatitis in cats.

Severe trauma

Impaired excretion of bilirubin persists after an initial episode of ischaemia and/or hypotension.

Feline liver disorders of uncertain aetiology

• Feline cholangiohepatitis.

CHECK for high ALP, prolonged BSP clearance, prominent inflammation.

• Feline hepatic lipidosis.

CHECK for massive increase in WBCs, neutrophilia, a shift-to-the-left; often associated with obesity.

• Feline lymphocytic cholangitis.

CHECK for increased WBC count with lymphopenia and a shift-to-the-left, liver enlargement with fibrosis and ascites.

Chronic active hepatitis

In its advanced stages this can result in hyperbilirubinaemia due to intrahepatic cholestasis with an associated increase in ALP, caused by inflammation and fibrosis (cirrhosis). It is characterized by a persistent elevation of ALP but there may be signs of liver dysfunction and failure, e.g. low albumin and urea levels, high ammonia and bile acid levels and prolonged BSP clearance, as well as a small liver (see Panel 6.1, p. 333).

It can be caused by:

• Excessive accumulation of copper in the liver, an inborn metabolic defect common in Bedlington Terriers and West Highland White Terriers (possibly also in Dobermann Pinschers in the USA).
• Infectious diseases such as leptospirosis and canine adenovirus-1 infection in *partially immune dogs.*
• Drug therapy, especially with primidone.
• Idiopathic causes, e.g. in Skye Terriers.

Myeloproliferative disorders

In the cat these are frequently associated with FeLV infection.

Jaundice is due:

• Primarily to the massive accumulation of haemopoietic cells in the liver sinusoids, causing atrophy of liver cells and intrahepatic cholestasis.
• In part (in certain cases) to extensive haemolysis (extravascular phagocytosis) within the spleen and lymph nodes.

Secondary liver damage

This is associated with *metabolic* disorders, e.g. diabetes mellitus, Cushing's syndrome and hypothyroidism. Secondary liver damage *rarely*, if ever, results in hyperbilirubinaemia in the dog but in the cat hyperbilirubinaemia is seen in:

• 10–20% of diabetes mellitus cases, possibly due to an associated pancreatitis and bile duct occlusion.
• 20% of hyperthyroid animals, associated with hepatic damage and increased enzyme activities (ALT, ALP, AST and LD).

Obstruction of the biliary tract [common]

Obstruction to the flow of bile (otherwise termed 'cholestasis') causes a damming back of conjugated bilirubin and its appearance in the plasma accompanied by an increase in ALP activity. It may be caused by one of the following.

Pressure of inflamed liver cells
This pressure occurs on the bile canaliculi in hepatocellular diseases (as mentioned above).

Presence of space-occupying lesions
These lesions (e.g. neoplasms or abscesses) can occur:

- Either within the liver.
- Or outside, in the biliary vessels (i.e. pressing upon the hepatic, cystic or bile ducts) or around the gall bladder (including a pancreatic adenocarcinoma).

Abnormal tissue deposition in liver
Obstruction can be caused by diffuse accumulation of abnormal tissue in the liver, e.g. neoplasia (lymphosarcoma or hepatocellular carcinoma), amyloidosis (uncommon) or fibrosis (cirrhosis), e.g. in chronic active hepatitis.

Pyogranulomatous hepatitis
This may be due to the dissemination of histoplasmosis, blastomycosis or coccidioidomycosis (none of which occurs in the UK).

Bile duct blockage [rare]
Obstruction can be caused by blockage of the bile duct by gall stones (usually jaundice is intermittent) or by the migration of ascarids up the duct (rare).

Biliary tract inflammation (cholangitis) and cholangiohepatitis
These conditions are due to ascending or haematogenously spread infection, irritation by retained bile or *especially* an associated acute pancreatitis (perhaps due to channels interconnecting with the pancreatic ducts), and can lead to inflammation sufficient to cause partial obstruction.

Right-sided heart failure
When present, for example due to congestive cardiomyopathy in large canine breeds and in cats, it may produce sufficient hepatic congestion to interfere with bile flow – however a more reliable guide than hyperbilirubinaemia is the increase in ALP activity.

Congenital cystic disease of the biliary tree in the dog [rare]

The most marked elevations in bilirubin are usually associated with extrahepatic cholestasis, up to $340\,\mu\text{mol/l}$ ($= 20\,\text{mg/dl}$); with intrahepatic obstructions levels usually do not exceed $70\,\mu\text{mol/l}$ ($= 4\,\text{mg/dl}$).

An extrahepatic lesion is probable if conjugated bilirubin accounts for more than 80% of the total bilirubin.

Rupture of the biliary tree [unusual]

This causes bile peritonitis.

It occurs mainly in the dog due to trauma – usually force applied to the abdomen, but sometimes to a penetrating wound.

Associated features with hyperbilirubinaemia:

- Obstruction to the flow of bile causes an increase in the activity of alkaline phosphatase (ALP), which is greater when the obstruction is extrahepatic.
- Damage to the liver cells causes an increase in the activity of alanine aminotransferase (and of other enzymes) – see p. 333.
- Obstruction, or liver cell damage, of sufficient severity causes bilirubin to appear in the urine (significant in the dog only if *more than* a one plus (+) reading) together with bile salts.
- Complete extrahepatic obstruction will produce pale, even white, fatty faeces because no bile will pass into the duodenum and there will be no conjugated bilirubin (to be converted ultimately to stercobilin, giving the brown colour) or bile salts (to assist fat digestion).

Causes of decreased plasma bilirubin levels (hypobilirubinaemia)

A low plasma level of bilirubin (*dog* <1.7 μmol/l (<0.1 mg/dl), *cat* <2 μmol/l (<0.12 mg/dl)) can be encountered in chronic diseases where there is depression of RBC formation that leads to *anaemia*. Due to the reduced number of RBCs subsequently phagocytosed the mononuclear phagocyte system produces less and less bilirubin and the plasma gradually loses its normal straw colour and *appears colourless*.

It occurs therefore in hypoproliferative anaemia attributable to

- Chronic infection and inflammation.
- Malignant neoplasia.
- End-stage renal disease.

Plasma bile acids

SI units of measurement are micromoles per litre (μmol/l). Other units have not been used routinely.

NORMAL REFERENCE RANGE (ADULTS)

Original RIA method

Dog: after 12-hour fast, 1–10 μmol/l (most <8 μmol/l).
    2 hours after feeding <16 μmol/l.
Cat: after 12-hour fast <2 μmol/l.
    2 hours after feeding <10 μmol/l.

Recent enzymatic method

This is widely adopted.

Dog: after 12-hour fast, <30 μmol/l.
    2 hours after feeding, <50 μmol/l.
Cat: after 12-hour fast, <25 μmol/l.
    2 hours after feeding, <30 μmol/l.

This is a comparatively new estimation; normal reference ranges are not well established and in any case should be *checked with individual laboratories*.

SOURCE

The liver synthesizes cholic acid and chenodeoxycholic acid (the primary bile acids) from cholesterol, conjugates them – principally with taurine in the dog and cat (to form taurocholic acid mainly, and taurochenodeoxycholic acid) – and to a much lesser extent with glycine. It then excretes these acids as their sodium salts (the bile salts) into the bile.

At the time of a meal they are discharged, contained in the bile, via the bile duct into the small intestine where they act principally as emulsifying agents in fat digestion and absorption.

In the large bowel bacteria:

- Deconjugate them to form free acids again.
- Convert a proportion of them to the secondary bile acids – deoxycholic and lithocholic acids.

The major part of the bile acids is reabsorbed in the distal small bowel and the large bowel and they pass, via the portal circulation, to the liver where they are extracted from the blood and recycled. The total pool of bile acids can recirculate up to five times per meal.

Only 2–5% of this total pool is lost in the faeces each day (mainly as the poorly soluble lithocholic acid), so that the need to synthesize entirely *new* bile acids is minimal.

A small proportion of the total bile acids, consisting of both primary and secondary, conjugated and unconjugated, is not extracted by the liver and reaches the circulating blood (in the ionized form, i.e. as bile salts) and it is *this* fraction which is measured. This amount in the blood normally increases transiently after feeding.

In cases of impaired liver function, extraction is poor and consequently the proportion reaching the peripheral circulation increases (Figure 5.4). Circulating bile acids can be used as a very *sensitive indicator of liver function*, and of the *integrity of the circulation* through the liver, biliary tract and intestines.

Higher values indicate impaired liver function and/or interference with the flow of bile (see 'Causes of increased bile acid levels', p. 265).

Lower values suggest intestinal obstruction or malabsorption (see 'Causes of decreased bile acid levels', p. 267).

However, care in interpretation is required because of the sensitivity of the test and its lack of specificity.

Notes

1. Bile acid measurement is
   (a) *more* sensitive than the bromsulphthalein (BSP) clearance test;
   (b) *equally as* sensitive as the ammonium tolerance test for detecting impaired liver function (e.g. hepatic failure, portosystemic shunts) and consequently more convenient in veterinary practice.
       Sensitivity is reported to be improved by measuring levels in samples collected after fasting and again 2 hours after feeding.
2. Bile acid measurement does *not* replace measurement of the activity of ALT (and other enzymes), e.g. arginase, SDH, OCT (see Chapter 6) as an indicator of liver *damage*.
3. Bile acid measurement *can* replace the measurement of bile salts in urine (Hay's test) as an indication that jaundice is due to hepatocellular disease or obstruction of the biliary tree rather than to haemolysis.

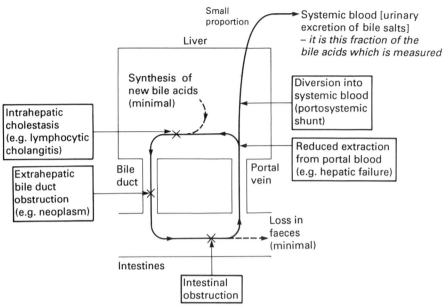

Figure 5.4 Circulation of bile acids. Intestinal obstruction will reduce reabsorption resulting in *lower* levels in the peripheral blood. The other interferences with circulation divert (either directly or by 'backing up') *more* bile acids into the peripheral blood

Causes of increased levels of bile acids

Summary
Impaired liver function
• Toxins – poisons and drugs
• Infectious diseases
• Other inflammatory disorders
Obstructed bile flow
• Intrahepatic
• Extrahepatic
Portosystemic shunt
Secondary liver damage
• Hyperthyroidism
• Hyperadrenocorticism
• Steroid dosage
• Diabetes mellitus

Important – see Notes 1–3 at the end of this section (p. 267).

IMPAIRED LIVER FUNCTION

There is a reduced ability of the liver cells to extract bile acids from the blood. The extensive loss of functional cells will result in *liver failure*.

Toxic degeneration due to poisons and drugs

This includes particularly phosphorus, phenols, oestrogens, aflatoxins and paraquat.

Infectious diseases

These may cause acute hepatic inflammation and necrosis, e.g. leptospirosis, infectious canine hepatitis and feline infectious peritonitis.

Other inflammatory disorders

These include:

- Cholangiohepatitis in the cat (bacterial infection ascending the biliary tree).
- Lymphocytic cholangitis in the cat (a possible autoimmune disorder).
- Secondary to acute pancreatitis or chronic colitis.
- Severe trauma.
- Chronic active hepatitis due to excessive copper storage (in Bedlington Terriers and West Highland White Terriers), drug therapy (e.g. with primidone), the effects of infectious diseases (e.g. leptospirosis and infectious canine hepatitis in partially immune dogs) and idiopathic causes.

In these diseases, as well as impaired function of the liver cells, there is interference with the flow of bile through the liver (intrahepatic cholestasis) caused by inflammatory swelling of the liver cells, infiltration of the liver by other types of cells and/or fibrosis.

OBSTRUCTION TO THE FLOW OF BILE

Intrahepatic

The free flow of bile through the liver can be hindered by:

- The inflammatory swelling of the liver cells in toxic and infectious liver diseases (as mentioned above).
- Fibrosis in cholangiohepatitis, lymphocytic cholangitis and especially chronic active hepatitis and chronic hepatitis; cirrhosis represents extensive replacement of functional liver cells by fibrous tissue.
- Neoplasia of the liver, e.g. lymphosarcoma or carcinoma.
- Amyloidosis of the liver (rare).
- Liver abscesses.

Extrahepatic

Flow of bile through the bile duct can be interfered with by such disorders as:

- Neoplasia in, or more often pressing on, the bile duct.
- Gall stones (choleliths) or ascarids blocking the duct; both of these are extremely rare.

PORTOSYSTEMIC SHUNTS

A major proportion of the liver cells are by-passed by anomalous blood vessels and therefore deprived of an adequate blood supply. This blood passes (together with the bile acids it is transporting) into the peripheral blood stream.

SECONDARY LIVER DAMAGE

This can be due to:

- Hyperthyroidism.
- Hyperadrenocorticism, i.e. Cushing's syndrome.
- Steroid administration (=steroid hepatopathy).
- Diabetes mellitus.

In general any increase in the level of bile acids in these disorders is only slight or moderate.

Notes

1. If there is coincidentally intestinal obstruction or malabsorption, values may be within the normal range.
2. Some fasted animals that might be expected to show elevated levels of bile acids *may* show bile acid levels that lie within or only slightly above the normal range (e.g. where there is obstruction due to small primary neoplasms and metastases) and other liver function tests may not produce abnormal results.

   In such cases a blood sample collected *2 hours after feeding* may show a significant increase in the bile acids.
   Occasionally low 'fasted' values are found in dogs with cirrhosis or portosystemic shunts; again *2 hours after feeding* the levels are substantially increased.
3. In general it is not possible to predict the nature or severity of the liver lesions from the bile acid level, although values are often particularly elevated with cirrhosis, and with lymphocytic cholangitis in the cat.

Liver biopsy has been recommended wherever levels exceed 30 µmol/l in the dog or 20 µmol/l in the cat.

Causes of decreased levels of bile acids

SIGNIFICANT INTESTINAL OBSTRUCTION OR SEVERE MALABSORPTION

These are the most likely causes of values which are low (e.g. <1 µmol/l) both after fasting and 2 hours after feeding, although in each case the lesion needs to be severe, i.e. the test will not detect lesser changes.

ERROR: TEST METHODS NOT VALIDATED FOR USE IN THE DOG OR CAT

Error appears to be particularly likely with methods based on radio-immunoassay (RIA).

Plasma triglycerides

SI units of measurement are millimoles per litre (mmol/l). Previous units were mg/dl (= mg/100 ml).

CONVERSION FACTORS

- To convert mg/dl to mmol/l multiply by 0.0114.
- To convert mmol/l to mg/dl multiply by 87.5.

NORMAL REFERENCE RANGE (ADULTS)

Dog and cat: 0.6–1.2 mmol/l (50–100 mg/dl).

Triglycerides are the most common form in which lipid is stored (in adipose tissue) and are a major energy source. Each molecule of triglyceride consists of three fatty acid molecules attached to a molecule of glycerol – hence their name.

They are synthesized:

- In the intestinal mucosa from the components of dietary lipids following fat digestion and absorption.
- Within the liver.

ACCURACY

Modern enzymatic determinations

These break down the triglycerides and measure the glycerol that is liberated. Consequently, if there is already a high level of glycerol in the plasma it will be added to that produced by the test and the total amount will be assumed to have been derived from triglyceride, i.e. the triglyceride level will be *falsely elevated*.

Vigorous exercise

This can result in an enormous (10- to 20-fold) increase in free glycerol in the plasma (Snow *et al.*, 1988); therefore for accurate readings triglyceride measurement should not be made within 2 hours of exercise.

High levels of vitamin C

These *may* be present in some dogs and cats and can inhibit triglyceride estimations although probably the effect is marginal.

Note

Lipaemia (hyperlipaemia = hyperlipidaemia = hyperlipoproteinaemia) denotes an abnormally high level of lipid in the blood plasma and the term encompasses high levels of triglyceride and/or cholesterol.

However, when applied to plasma (or serum or whole blood) samples the term 'lipaemia' implies *gross* lipaemia, i.e. an obvious turbidity of the sample due to an excess of lipid. This indicates that there is an increase in the triglyceride component, because cholesterol does not produce turbidity.

SOURCE

Triglyceride formed in the intestinal mucosal cells

This triglyceride is formed from the components of dietary long chain triglycerides and is transported, first in the intestinal lymph (chyle) and later in the blood, in the form of *chylomicrons*. These 'fat particles' consist almost solely of triglyceride (80–95%) with the addition of very small amounts of cholesterol, phospholipid and a plasma protein whose attachment is necessary to keep the lipid 'soluble'.

Chylomicrons are an example of lipoproteins and, because of their dietary origin, are referred to as *exogenous triglycerides*.

Triglyceride formed in the liver

This is transported in the blood in the form of very-low-density lipoproteins (VLDLs). These somewhat smaller particles consist mainly of triglyceride (approximately 60%) but the amounts of cholesterol, phospholipid and plasma protein are relatively greater than in the chylomicrons. The VLDLs are referred to as *endogenous triglycerides*.

In large quantities in the blood these triglyceride-rich lipoproteins will cause lipaemia (hyperlipaemia or hyperlipidaemia), i.e. a milkiness or turbidity of the plasma. After its collection whole blood has a 'strawberry milkshake' or 'cream of tomato soup' appearance (see 'Lipaemia', p. 20).

Chylomicrons appear in the blood after a fatty meal but clear within 12 hours.

The accuracy of many biochemical blood tests is impaired if performed on lipaemic plasma (or serum) and, consequently, it is preferable to fast an animal (e.g. overnight) before blood collection. If the sample is strongly lipaemic it will require dilution before testing.

The source of the excess triglyceride can be determined by placing the sample in the refrigerator for 4–8 hours (up to 12 hours). Chylomicrons (of dietary origin) will rise to the surface forming a fatty layer with clear plasma or serum beneath that can be used for testing.

VLDLs (of liver origin) will continue to cause turbidity in the sample, i.e. there is no separation into layers.

In contrast high levels of cholesterol (without triglycerides) do not produce turbidity.

The enzyme, lipoprotein lipase (LPL), situated in the endothelium of the capillaries, especially in adipose tissue and skeletal muscle, causes the breakdown (hydrolysis) of the triglycerides in the chylomicrons and VLDLs into free fatty acids and glycerol, so that the free fatty acids can be taken up by the fat cells. LPL therefore clears any lipaemic turbidity from the plasma. The activity of LPL is enhanced by a number of enzymes (insulin, glucagon, thyroid hormone) and by heparin. This is of practical value because plasma which is grossly lipaemic can usually be cleared within 15 minutes by giving the patient an intravenous injection of heparin (90–100 units/kg).

In summary then, triglycerides in the plasma are in the form of either chylomicrons or VLDLs.

The two other types of lipid particles which occur in the plasma (HDLs and LDLs) transport cholesterol primarily (see 'Cholesterol', p. 272) and contain much smaller amounts of triglyceride; they do not cause turbidity of the plasma.

Plasma levels of triglycerides are found to be *high*:

- After a fatty meal (for up to 12 hours) while LPL is acting (this is the most common cause).
- Where there is a deficiency of LPL activity secondary to some other disorder, e.g. diabetes mellitus.
- Where there is apparently an inherent (idiopathic) deficiency of LPL activity – a very rare occurrence.

Measurement of triglyceride levels forms the basis of the fat (LCT) absorption test in the diagnosis of defective fat digestion/absorption (see Appendix I, p. 472).

Causes of increased plasma triglyceride levels (hypertriglyceridaemia)

Summary

- Following a fatty meal [common]
- Diabetes mellitus
- Hypothyroidism
- Acute pancreatitis
- Hyperadrenocorticism
- Cholestasis [transient]
- Starvation (if obese)
- Nephrotic syndrome [possible?]
- Idiopathic hyperlipoproteinaemia [rare]
- Idiopathic hyperchylomicronaemia [rare]

Error: exercise

High levels of triglycerides can cause ocular disturbances (photophobia, 'cloudy eyes', blindness), CNS disturbances and acute pancreatitis.

POSTPRANDIAL HYPERLIPIDAEMIA [COMMON]

Chylomicron production following a fatty meal can result in a high plasma triglyceride level for up to 12 hours afterwards (although often for a much shorter time). If there is a high level of triglycerides *after a 12 hour fast* it has some other cause.

DIABETES MELLITUS

The hyperlipidaemia of diabetes mellitus is primarily a hypertriglyceridaemia with a less marked hypercholesterolaemia.

Type I (insulin dependent) diabetes mellitus

In this type of diabetes mellitus, the increase in triglycerides is due to the lack of insulin, since insulin is required to synthesize and activate lipoprotein lipase – the enzyme which hydrolyses the triglycerides in chylomicrons and VLDLs. The production of VLDLs by the liver is actually reduced, but since VLDL breakdown is decreased to an even greater degree the net effect is an increase in the concentration of VLDLs.

Type II (insulin resistant) diabetes mellitus

In this type of diabetes mellitus, the increase in triglycerides is due to an increase in the hepatic production of VLDLs.

Following insulin therapy triglycerides are metabolized and their concentration falls, but cholesterol, derived from the VLDLs and chylomicrons, can remain consistently high for a long period.

Lipaemia, with high levels of triglyceride and cholesterol, is common in the ketotic stage of diabetes mellitus resulting from an increased rate of lipolysis.

HYPOTHYROIDISM

The use and catabolism of lipids is reduced to a greater extent than is lipid synthesis, so that often there is an overall increase in plasma lipid levels.

Cholesterol is more frequently elevated than triglyceride, especially in severe cases, but the latter may also be raised.

ACUTE PANCREATITIS

An association has been noted between hyperlipidaemia (e.g. following the eating of a fatty meal) and the onset of an 'attack' of acute pancreatitis. It seems likely that the attack is due to the action of pancreatic lipase on the high concentration of triglycerides in the blood passing through the pancreatic capillaries which causes the release of large amounts of free fatty acids. When bound to albumin free fatty acids are not toxic, but if the binding capacity of albumin is exceeded the unbound free fatty acids could cause serious inflammation triggering further lipase release (Zerbe, 1986).

Hypertriglyceridaemia (denoted by lipaemic plasma) is a less frequent finding than hypercholesterolaemia.

HYPERADRENOCORTICISM

Hypertriglyceridaemia as well as hypercholesterolaemia can be the result of Cushing's syndrome *or* the administration of glucocorticoids. This is because the secretion of VLDLs by the liver is also increased as well as the activity of LPL being decreased.

CHOLESTASIS

Interference with the flow of bile is reported to cause a transient increase in the triglyceride level. Primary liver disease does not usually cause an increase in triglyceride, although it may result in an increase in the level of cholesterol.

Note

An increase in triglycerides is not a consistent feature of feline hepatic lipidosis (a chronic disease characterized by massive fat accumulation within the liver cells).

STARVATION

Starvation in obese animals can cause an increase in triglyceride levels following mobilization of fat stores.

NEPHROTIC SYNDROME (AND OTHER PROTEIN-LOSING RENAL DISORDERS)

It seems *likely* that with increasingly severe protein losses in the urine and the development of hypoproteinaemia, there would be an increase in the triglyceride level, in addition to that of cholesterol. This is the case in humans, but it is not well documented in small animals.

The following two idiopathic conditions are sometimes referred to as primary causes, all others being designated secondary. However, in the dog the term 'primary causes' is not a good one since the conditions are not proven to be inherited.

IDIOPATHIC HYPERLIPOPROTEINAEMIA (HYPERLIPIDAEMIA)

This disorder in the Miniature Schnauzer causes an increase in the concentration of triglyceride that may exceed 100 times the upper limit of normal and (usually) a lesser increase in the level of cholesterol. The underlying defect is not established but it can result in seizures, blindness and/or an apparent acute pancreatitis. A marked fall in triglyceride concentration follows the injection of heparin intravenously.

IDIOPATHIC HYPERCHLYOMICRONAEMIA

This reported disorder is characterized by marked lipaemia (triglyceride in the dog, triglyceride *and* cholesterol in the cat) that does *not* decrease appreciably in the usual way, i.e. following the intravenous administration of heparin. A familial inherited hyperchylomicronaemia in the cat has been established, that at times is associated with peripheral nerve paralysis (Jones et al., 1986).

ERROR: EXERCISE

Falsely elevated triglyceride concentrations are recorded in animals immediately after exercise. Most triglyceride assays actually measure the level of glycerol after releasing it from triglyceride by enzyme action. They will therefore assume that any glycerol present has been derived from triglycerides in the sample.

Glycerol is released in large amounts during exercise when free fatty acids are used as an energy source.

Note

There is no clear record of increases in plasma levels of triglycerides in *pregnancy* or *obesity* in small animals as *is* the case in humans (although obesity is often a *feature* of certain disorders, e.g. diabetes mellitus and acute pancreatitis, in which hypertriglyceridaemia occurs).

Plasma cholesterol

Cholesterol consists of both free cholesterol and cholesterol esters which are measured together as total cholesterol.

SI units of measurement are millimoles per litre (mmol/l). Previous units were mg/dl (= mg/100 ml).

CONVERSION FACTORS

- To convert mg/dl to mmol/l multiply by 0.026.
- To convert mmol/l to mg/dl multiply by 38.7.

NORMAL REFERENCE RANGE (ADULTS)

Dog: 2.5–8 mmol/l (100–300 mg/dl).
Values in racing Greyhounds are in the lower two-thirds of this range.

Cat: 2–6.5 mmol/l (75–250 mg/dl).

ACCURACY

Falsely high values

These can be due to:

- Haemolysis, interfering with the Liebermann–Burchard reaction.
- Phenytoin, which may cause a 15–20% increase in values.

Falsely low values

These may be due to high levels of vitamin C (which can be produced by some dogs and cats), although probably the effect is marginal.

Increased levels are mainly associated with feeding, endocrine disorders, acute pancreatitis and the renal loss of protein. Decreased levels can arise with hepatic failure, low fat diets and intestinal malabsorption.

SOURCE

Cholesterol is a major lipid in the body, being the precursor of all the steroid hormones (e.g. sex hormones and glucocorticoids) and the bile acids, and a component of the plasma membrane of cells.

It is both obtained from the diet and synthesized in the liver.

The lipoproteins richest in cholesterol are:

- The low-density lipoproteins (LDLs) derived from the breakdown of VLDLs (very-low-density lipoproteins, see 'Plasma triglycerides', p. 267).
- High-density lipoproteins (HDLs) – the smallest of the lipoprotein particles.

As with other lipoproteins, LDLs and HDLs also contain amounts of triglyceride and phospholipid in addition to cholesterol and the protein component needed for transport.

Essentially LDLs act as a source of cholesterol to peripheral cells (e.g. the adrenal gland) and HDLs convey cholesterol from the peripheral cells back to the liver.

Neither LDLs nor HDLs contribute to grossly visible lipaemia, i.e. hypercholesterolaemia does not result in the lipaemic turbidity of plasma samples.

Normally surplus cholesterol is excreted via the bile.

Causes of increased plasma cholesterol levels (hypercholesterolaemia)

Summary

- Following a fatty meal
- High fat diets
- Hypothyroidism
- Diabetes mellitus
- Acute pancreatitis
- Hyperadrenocorticism and steroid dosage
- Severe trauma
- Starvation (if obese)
- Primary liver damage
- Bile duct obstruction
- Renal loss of protein (nephrotic syndrome)
- Steatitis
- Familial renal diseases
- Idiopathic hyperlipidaemias

Error: haemolysis; phenytoin

POSTPRANDIAL HYPERLIPIDAEMIA

The cholesterol level will temporarily rise slightly following a fatty meal (the rise can be up to 3 mmol/l), but values should return to normal within 12 hours.

Consequently samples should always be obtained from fasted animals.

HIGH FAT DIETS

Evidence suggests that a high fat diet can result in even 'fasting' values being elevated above the normal reference range.

HYPOTHYROIDISM

Thyroid hormones both stimulate cholesterol synthesis and also cholesterol degradation to bile acids; a lack of them affects synthesis less than breakdown. Consequently, the cholesterol level usually rises above the normal range (in over three-quarters of hypothyroid dogs).

In general, the higher the cholesterol level the more likely it is that a raised level is due to hypothyroidism than to some other cause; values above 20 mmol/l (770 mg/dl) are probably only due to this disorder. At times levels may go much higher.

Reference should be made to specific tests (e.g. 'TSH stimulation test', p. 399) which are able to distinguish disorders that may present similarly, especially Cushing's syndrome (see p. 401).

Cholesterol levels can conveniently be monitored during therapy for hypothyroidism to assess the response.

DIABETES MELLITUS

Rises in the cholesterol level are usually seen in diabetes mellitus, subsequent to the great increase in triglycerides (VLDLs) which degrade to LDLs (both are relatively rich in cholesterol) and also to the decreased hepatic breakdown of cholesterol.

However, the increase in cholesterol is usually less than that of the triglycerides.

Increases in cholesterol are also common in the ketotic stage of diabetes mellitus.

ACUTE PANCREATITIS

Hypercholesterolaemia is a frequent feature, apparently due to increases in both LDLs and HDLs, and is more common than hypertriglyceridaemia.

HYPERADRENOCORTICISM (CUSHING'S SYNDROME) AND EXOGENOUS GLUCOCORTICOID ADMINISTRATION

Eighty to ninety per cent of both dogs and cats with Cushing's syndrome show increased cholesterol levels but they seldom reach, let alone exceed, 20 mmol/l (770 mg/dl).

Similar rises can result from prolonged high doses of glucocorticoids.

SEVERE TRAUMA

Lipolysis increases, under the influence of catecholamines, and insulin secretion is suppressed so that the cholesterol level may be elevated within 48 hours. Corticosteroids contribute to fat mobilization.

STARVATION

Starvation can cause hypercholesterolaemia chiefly in obese animals. Fat mobilization and degradation are responsible.

PRIMARY LIVER DAMAGE

See following entry.

OBSTRUCTIVE LESIONS OF THE BILE DUCT

Liver disease usually does not cause an increase in cholesterol but since surplus cholesterol is excreted in the bile, cholestasis (intrahepatic or extrahepatic), e.g. due to neoplasia, can result in its accumulation, and occasionally levels can be appreciably elevated.

The ratio of free cholesterol to esters has been measured and is less likely to be abnormal in cases of acute hepatitis, but there are much better indicators of liver damage and dysfunction.

RENAL LOSS OF PROTEIN

This is seen particularly with primary glomerular diseases (glomerulonephritis and renal amyloidosis) and leads to the nephrotic syndrome. Possibly other renal disorders, characterized by excessive protein losses in the urine, can produce the same effect, although because of losses being smaller this would necessarily take a longer period.

The development of severe hypoalbuminaemia is accompanied by a corresponding hypercholesterolaemia, and this is an essential feature of the nephrotic syndrome. Correction of the underlying disorder and restoration of albumin levels to normal results in the plasma cholesterol level also returning to normal.

Note

In contrast, cholesterol levels in protein-losing enteropathies tend to be *low*.

STEATITIS (PANSTEATITIS)

In cats this can result in an increased cholesterol level.

FAMILIAL NEPHROPATHIES IN STANDARD POODLES AND DOBERMANN PINSCHERS

These disorders in juvenile animals produce clinical signs of renal failure with azotaemia, and also hypercholesterolaemia. In Standard Poodles this arises despite normal plasma albumin values.

IDIOPATHIC HYPERLIPIDAEMIAS

In idiopathic hyperlipoproteinaemia in Miniature Schnauzers and in hyperchylomicro-naemia in the cat, there may be lesser increases in cholesterol that accompany the marked rises in triglyceride levels.

ERROR: FALSELY ELEVATED VALUES

These may be due to:

- Haemolysis which interferes with the Liebermann–Burchard reaction.
- Administration of phenytoin (which can increase levels 15–20%).

Causes of decreased plasma cholesterol levels

Summary

- Liver failure (acquired or congenital)
- Anticonvulsant therapy
- Low fat diets
- Intestinal malabsorption and exocrine pancreatic insufficiency
- Hyperthyroidism (cat)
- Hypoadrenocorticism (occasionally)
- Protein-losing enteropathy [possible?]

Error: high vitamin C level (minimal effect)

LIVER FAILURE

Both acquired (e.g. due to cirrhosis) and congenital liver failure (e.g. portosystemic shunts) will result in the reduced synthesis of cholesterol, accompanied by reduced albumin and (often) urea levels.

As hepatocellular disease progresses so the cholesterol level begins to fall, although any associated cholestasis will tend to increase the cholesterol level because of its reduced excretion in the bile.

ANTICONVULSANT THERAPY

Primidone therapy long term reduces cholesterol levels in 70% of dogs due to loss of hepatic function. Phenytoin therapy *long term* has a similar result.

LOW FAT DIETS

Reduced availability of fat lowers the cholesterol level.

INTESTINAL MALABSORPTION AND EXOCRINE PANCREATIC INSUFFICIENCY

A severe reduction in the availability of fat will lower the cholesterol level.

HYPERTHYROIDISM

Usually in hyperthyroid cats both the synthesis, and particularly the clearance, of cholesterol and triglycerides are increased so that overall modest falls *may* be seen. In general, however, cholesterol levels remain within the normal reference range.

Similarly in hyperthyroid dogs *marked* decreases are not evident.

HYPOADRENOCORTICISM

Hypocholesterolaemia has occasionally been recorded (Chastain and Ganjam, 1986).

PROTEIN-LOSING ENTEROPATHY

Low cholesterol levels have been recorded in association with protein-losing enteropathies in humans, but it is not clear whether this is the case in the dog and to what extent associated fat malabsorption might be responsible.

ERROR: FALSELY LOW VALUES

These can be due to high levels of vitamin C interfering with cholesterol estimation. Such high levels might be produced by dogs and cats, although in practice the effect is probably minimal.

Plasma glucose

Note

Blood samples usually need to be collected in a fluoride–oxalate tube (see 'Accuracy' below).

SI units of measurement are millimoles per litre (mmol/l). Previous units were mg/dl (= mg/100 ml).

CONVERSION FACTORS

- To convert mg/dl to mmol/l multiply by 0.056.
- To convert mmol/l to mg/dl multiply by 18.0.

NORMAL REFERENCE RANGE (ADULTS)

Dog and cat: 3.5–6 mmol/l (60–100 mg/dl).

Note

Measurements performed on whole blood (i.e. including the RBCs) are slightly lower (approximately 0.5 mmol/l = 10 mg/dl). The term 'blood glucose' can be confusing because it may (e.g. in older publications) refer to estimations performed on whole blood, *or* simply be used to distinguish the level in *blood* from the level in *urine*. In the latter case it is probably better to refer to plasma (or serum) glucose values.

ACCURACY

Lipaemia and/or haemolysis

These will interfere with photometric methods of glucose measurement giving falsely elevated values.

Metronidazole

The hexokinase method of determination is affected by the presence of metronidazole giving falsely higher values.

High level of vitamin C

This inhibits the glucose oxidase/peroxidase (GOD/POD) method of estimation resulting in falsely low values. Although such high levels of vitamin C can be produced by dogs and cats, probably in practice the effect is marginal.

Glycolytic enzymes in blood cells [important]

These enzymes will continue to utilize glucose in the blood, following its collection, if they remain in contact with the liquid portion, i.e. if cells remain in contact with the plasma (when heparin has been used as the anticoagulant) *or* if cells in a clot remain in contact with the serum (when no anticoagulant has been used).

The result is a glucose level that *falls* with time, and more rapidly at higher temperatures, until eventually no glucose is present. Approximately 5–10% of the glucose is converted into lactic acid each hour at room temperature – more if there is leucocytosis or bacterial contamination of the sample.

This progressive fall in glucose content can be avoided by:

- Either removing the plasma (or serum) from the cells as soon as possible (with plasma this can be done straight away; with serum it is necessary to wait 2 hours for full clotting and clot retraction to occur); however, if haemolysis has occurred enzymes from the cells will *still* be present in the plasma or serum sample.
- Or adding an enzyme inhibitor to stop enzyme action. Usually sodium fluoride is used in combination with the anticoagulant potassium oxalate. (Sample tubes containing fluoride–oxalate are usually colour coded yellow and, in the 'Vacutainer' system, grey.)

Note

The concentration of enzyme inhibitor will usually not affect enzyme-based photometric methods for glucose estimation, *but will* inhibit enzyme reactions on *strip tests* for glucose, which may be used as a rapid check on glucose levels in veterinary practice. The latter are generally intended to be used with 'fresh' blood, i.e. straight from a vein.

It is important to check the instructions given by a particular laboratory, or by the manufacturers of tests used in a practice, concerning the addition or otherwise of an enzyme inhibitor to the blood sample.

SOURCE

Glucose is continuously required as an energy source by all the body cells, and therefore it is essential to maintain an adequate level in the plasma.

After a meal much of the glucose in the blood is that which has been absorbed in the small intestine (the end product of carbohydrate digestion) and is on its way to be stored as glycogen in the liver and muscles. At other times glucose may be liberated from tissues to maintain a sufficient plasma concentration. The glucose to 'top up' the plasma glucose comes principally from the conversion of liver glycogen (glycogen-olysis), together with some which is derived from non-carbohydrate sources (by hepatic gluconeogenesis).

In starvation glucose is increasingly derived from the breakdown of fats and proteins, primarily from muscle tissue, through gluconeogenesis in the liver and the kidneys.

Regulation of the level of plasma glucose is normally achieved by the secretion of glucagon (to raise the glucose level) and of insulin (to lower it). Glucagon, glucocorticoids (e.g. cortisol), adrenaline (epinephrine), growth hormone and progesterone (which stimulates growth hormone output) all raise the plasma glucose level by increasing gluconeogenesis or glycogenolysis, or by interfering with the utilization of glucose. Insulin, by inhibiting gluconeogenesis and increasing the cellular uptake of glucose, lowers the plasma glucose concentration.

All of the plasma glucose is filtered from the blood through the renal glomeruli and then totally reabsorbed in the tubules. Only when an excess is present in the glomerular filtrate, so that complete reabsorption cannot be achieved (i.e. when the renal threshold is exceeded), does glucose (usually) appear in the urine (glycosuria). Exceptionally there are individuals with an abnormally low renal threshold for glucose, so that glycosuria occurs in the absence of hyperglycaemia (see p. 438).

Increases in plasma glucose levels are due to:

- Either increased glucose production or release, for example after meals, with excitement and stress and due to the effect of glucocorticoids.
- Or decreased glucose usage, as in diabetes mellitus.

Decreases in plasma glucose levels can be due to an excess of insulin (endogenous or administered), a deficiency of cortisol, hepatic dysfunction (including vascular shunts and glycogen storage diseases) and the impaired ability to produce glucose and/or its excessive utilization (as in neoplasia, sepsis, polycythaemia and in puppies and (rarely) pregnancy).

Causes of increased plasma glucose levels (= hyperglycaemia)

Summary

Fear, excitement, stress [common, especially cat]
Severe trauma
Following a meal
Diabetes mellitus
Dioestrus phase of oestrous cycle (bitch)
Other conditions of insulin resistance:
• Hyperadrenocorticism (especially cat)
• Acromegaly
• Hyperthyroidism (occasionally)
• Obesity
• Phaeochromocytoma
Hormones which can induce diabetes mellitus
Other drugs
Convulsions
Extreme exercise
Serious insulin overdose – Somogyi effect [rare]
Acute pancreatitis
Following insulinoma removal
Feline urological syndrome
Familial renal diseases [rare]
Addison's disease [rare]
Error:
• Injection of dextrose (or other carbohydrate), e.g. intravenous drip
• Lipaemia
• Haemolysis
• Metronidazole

To avoid the temporary increase following feeding, samples should be collected from animals fasted for 12 hours.

FEAR, EXCITEMENT AND STRESS [COMMON]

Fear and excitement

The short-term stress associated with collection of a blood sample, particularly if struggling occurs, can cause a mild/moderate increase in the plasma glucose level. Adrenaline and noradrenaline (epinephrine and norepinephrine) are released, stimulating hepatic glycogenolysis.

In *dogs* plasma levels seldom exceed 8 mmol/l (150 mg/dl) and glycosuria does not appear (because the renal threshold is 10 mmol/l = 180 mg/dl).

In *cats*, however, the effect can be more marked and exceptionally levels of 16.5–22 mmol/l or more (300–400 mg/dl or more) may arise. These can be accompanied by glycosuria (when the renal threshold of 16 mmol/l (290 mg/dl) is exceeded).

Often collecting a subsequent sample (when the animal is more familiar with its surroundings and more relaxed) will produce a much lower value.

CHECK for accompanying signs of fear/excitement, i.e.
* A marked transient lymphocytosis in cats, although *not* in dogs.
* A transient increase in neutrophil numbers; less marked in the dog.

Of course the same effects will follow an injection of adrenaline (epinephrine).

Longer-term stress

This is caused by a variety of medical and surgical illnesses (including feline urological syndrome) and results in increased glucocorticoid (cortisol) output and gluconeogenesis, raising the glucose level, although to a lesser extent than adrenaline – see following entry.

CHECK for a typical steroidal blood picture, i.e. increased numbers of neutrophils and monocytes (the latter less common in the cat) and decreases in the numbers of lymphocytes and eosinophils.

SEVERE TRAUMA

Hyperglycaemia and decreased glucose tolerance frequently appear within 12 hours, under the influence of catecholamines and glucocorticoids (increasing glycogenolysis and gluconeogenesis, and suppressing insulin production). The effect may persist for 3 days depending on the severity of the injury.

CHECK for steroidal blood picture (as above).

POSTPRANDIAL INCREASE

After a meal, there will be a temporary rise in the glucose level but it will not exceed the renal threshold, i.e. the plasma glucose level seldom will exceed 8 mmol/l (150 mg/dl). If it did it would suggest concurrent hypoinsulinism or insulin resistance.

DIABETES MELLITUS OF ALL TYPES

* Type I, due to hypoinsulinism (insulin-dependent diabetes mellitus) – a lack of insulin-secreting beta cells, caused by either primary idiopathic (juvenile) atrophy or, less often, destruction (e.g. by pancreatic carcinoma or acute pancreatitis).
* Type II – insulin-resistant diabetes mellitus.
* Ketoacidotic diabetes mellitus.
* Hyperosmolar non-ketotic (rarely), where as well as hyperosmolarity of the plasma the glucose level is extremely high (over 33 mmol/l (600 mg/dl) and can rise to four times that level).

Almost always in diabetes mellitus the glucose level exceeds 14 mmol/l (250 mg/dl) in *untreated* cases, but there is no real correlation between the plasma glucose level and the severity of diabetes mellitus (which is related more to the tendency to develop ketosis).

Frequently there is an associated lipaemia (the increase in the level of triglyceride is greater than that of cholesterol) and 50% of dogs show ketonuria at diagnosis. The glycosylated haemoglobin value is high.

DIOESTRUS PHASE OF THE OESTROUS CYCLE (BITCH)

Increased progesterone secretion during this phase stimulates the output of growth hormone, which in turn inhibits the action of insulin. The resistance to the effects of insulin, and the consequent increase in glucose levels which occurs, is temporary, disappearing when progesterone secretion is reduced. The situation will probably recur during the next dioestrus phase, and subsequently. Insulin levels during this time may be within or above the normal range. Eventually there is likely to be a dioestrus phase during which the increased demand for insulin results in exhaustion of the beta cells and consequent hypoinsulinism. The diabetes mellitus will then be *permanent*.

OTHER DISORDERS WHICH MAY LEAD TO DIABETES MELLITUS

Most of these act by inducing insulin resistance, including the following.

Hyperadrenocorticism (Cushing's syndrome)

Diabetes mellitus occurs in less than 10% of affected dogs but in all feline cases.

Acromegaly in bitches

This is due to increased progesterone production in dioestrus, or progestogen therapy.

Hyperthyroidism

Diabetes mellitus occurs in less than 10% of affected cats.

Obesity

Obese individuals have fewer insulin receptor sites than normal and, in dogs, increasing obesity is accompanied by progressive insulin resistance (Mattheeuws et al., 1984).
    The insulin resistance results in hyperglycaemia and may develop into type II diabetes mellitus in which plasma insulin levels are either within or above the normal range. Ultimately beta cell exhaustion may result with consequent hypoinsulinism.

Hyperglycaemia and (type I) diabetes mellitus

These can (rarely) result from a phaeochromocytoma (tumour of the adrenal medulla) producing adrenaline and noradrenaline (epinephrine and norepinephrine), which inhibit the secretion of insulin and stimulate hepatic glycogenolysis.

HORMONES WHICH CAN INDUCE DIABETES MELLITUS

Examples include:

- Glucocorticoids (and ACTH), by stimulating gluconeogenesis.
- Progestogens (e.g. megestrol acetate and medroxyprogesterone acetate) by stimulating the production of growth hormone which is an insulin antagonist.
- Adrenaline (epinephrine).
- Thyroxine (marginal effect).
- Glucagon.

OTHER DRUGS

- Drugs to destroy beta cells in hyperinsulinism, e.g. streptozotocin, diazoxide or alloxan.

- Xylazine as a sedative in cats (can raise glucose level 500%), and clonidine, which both inhibit insulin.
- Morphine.
- Ketamine.
- Alphaxalone/alphadolone acetate (Saffan) in cats – a steroidal anaesthetic.

Other drugs are reported to cause hyperglycaemia in humans, e.g. phenytoin, chlorpromazine, frusemide (furosemide) and thiazide derivatives.

CONVULSIONS (SEIZURES)

Convulsions, due to hypocalcaemia or primary CNS disturbance, can raise the plasma glucose level due to adrenaline (epinephrine) release.

EXTREME EXERCISE

Immedicately after extreme exercise, e.g. in Greyhounds, the plasma glucose level is raised due to release of adrenaline (epinephrine) causing hepatic glycogenolysis.

SERIOUS INSULIN OVERDOSAGE OF A DIABETIC

This may cause a transient hyperglycaemia subsequently (Somogyi effect). Initially hypoglycaemia develops, although insufficient to produce coma and therefore not obvious, and in response glycogenolysis is greatly increased. However, because insulin production is impaired the rising glucose level cannot be easily reduced and commonly reaches a value of 22 mmol/l (400 mg/dl).

ACUTE PANCREATITIS (RARELY)

Any rise in glucose level is usually transient – possibly the result of massive glucagon release. Occasionally it can lead to diabetes mellitus.

FOLLOWING SURGICAL REMOVAL OF AN INSULINOMA

Hyperglycaemia is due to the transient release of adrenaline (epinephrine).

FELINE UROLOGICAL SYNDROME (FUS)

Hyperglycaemia is due either to the induction of stress (with release of adrenaline and glucocorticoids, see above) or to the inhibition of insulin by uraemic toxins.

FAMILIAL RENAL DISEASES [RARE]

These occur in certain breeds, e.g. nephropathies in Shih Tsus and Lhasa Apsos, renal cortical hypoplasia in Cocker Spaniels and spontaneous amyloidosis in young Abyssinian cats. These familial renal diseases can result in mild hyperglycaemia as well as azotaemia.

ADDISON'S DISEASE [RARE]

In a small proportion of affected dogs, there is slight increase in the glucose level.

ERROR
Following parenteral administration of dextrose

Following dextrose administration, commonly as an intravenous fluid, or some other carbohydrate which is metabolized to glucose, plasma glucose values can be high (e.g. 20 mmol/l = 360 mg/dl) and this obvious cause may be overlooked.

Lipaemia

Haemolysis

Lipaemia and/or haemolysis may interfere with some laboratory methods causing markedly increased glucose values.

Metronidazole

This may falsely elevate glucose values obtained by the hexokinase method.

Glucose tolerance tests

The main reason in the past for employing a glucose tolerance test (GTT) has been doubt about the diagnosis of diabetes mellitus, for example where an animal has a fasting glucose level that is obviously high but not markedly so, i.e. between 6.7 and 9.7 mmol/l (120–175 mg/dl) in the dog. The test requires glucose to be administered by mouth or intravenously, and blood samples to be collected at intervals afterwards. Where there is a lack of insulin, or a failure to respond to it, glucose is not withdrawn from the blood as rapidly as usual. Consequently, following an initial rise the plasma level of glucose continues to remain high.

THE ORAL GLUCOSE TOLERANCE TEST

This requires the administration of 2 grams glucose/kg body weight by mouth (as a 25% solution) to a fasted animal and the collection of blood samples just before dosing and after ½, 1 and 2 hours (and possibly 3 hours).

In normal dogs the peak value (usually below 8.9 mmol/l (160 mg/dl)) is reached after ½–1 hour, and the level falls to near the fasting level (certainly <7 mmol/l (<125 mg/dl)) after 2 hours. In diabetics the level at 1 hour is usually above 8.3 mmol/l (150 mg/dl) and does not fall rapidly.

THE INTRAVENOUS GLUCOSE TOLERANCE TEST

This is used to overcome the effects of malabsorption or slow stomach emptying on the oral glucose tolerance test.

A slow intravenous injection (lasting 30 seconds) of 0.5 gram glucose/kg body weight is given as a 50% sterile solution. Blood samples are collected as for the oral test, plus one after 15 minutes. An immediate rise in the blood glucose level occurs (above 16.6 mmol/l (>300 mg/dl) at 15 minutes) which in the normal dog returns to the fasting level in approximately 1 hour, but in the diabetic dog may not do so for 2–3 hours. (An intravenous glucose tolerance test should not be performed in an anaesthetized dog, because the reduced blood flow through the pancreas decreases insulin release.)

However, glucose tolerance tests have fallen out of favour with clinicians in both human and veterinary medicine because (in addition to the influence of drugs, other diseases etc.) the *excitement and fear* engendered by the collection of a series of blood samples can in itself elevate the glucose level, thereby confusing the results.

In an attempt to minimize the effect of stress some clinicians have advocated collecting a *single* blood sample, i.e. after 2 hours in the case of the oral glucose tolerance test, which is the best time at which to distinguish between normal and diabetic animals. This modification may prove helpful, but of course some animals become very agitated on even a single occasion (and with a single result there is no opportunity to judge the validity of the value obtained by comparing it with those from other samples in a series).

Rather than performing a glucose tolerance test, it is now considered preferable to establish, from the history, clinical examination and the result of other laboratory tests whether a moderate rise in plasma glucose might be due to the effect of drugs, dioestrus, obesity or some other disorder, especially Cushing's syndrome (see 'Diabetes mellitus', p. 408). Measurement of the level of insulin can help in this assessment.

A glucose tolerance test has also been used to aid diagnosis:

- Where there is glycosuria without hyperglycaemia, i.e. a glucose level less than 10 mmol/l (= 180 mg/dl) in the dog; where this happens consistently a renal tubular defect is likely to be present (see 'Causes of glycosuria', p. 436) and there is hardly a need to perform the test (which should produce normal values).
- Where a strong familial history makes it likely that an individual is a latent (early) diabetic, but this is a very rare situation.
- Where there is suspected small intestinal malabsorption to test the animal's ability to absorb glucose following oral dosing. It is, however, inferior to many other tests (see Panel 6.3, p. 344). With impaired absorption instead of the normal early peak plasma value, followed by a swift reduction, the level of glucose increases and decreases much more slowly without ever reaching a very high value, i.e. glucose plotted against time produces a much flatter curve. However, other factors (such as delayed stomach emptying) and other disorders can produce a similar result, and it may appear even in apparently normal animals. It is preferable to have folate and vitamin B_{12} levels in the plasma (or serum) measured as indicators of absorption in the jejunum and ileum respectively.

Causes of decreased plasma glucose levels (= hypoglycaemia)

Summary

Hyperinsulinism
- Insulin overdose
- Insulin-secreting tumour in pancreas (insulinoma)
- Insulin-secreting tumour of non-pancreatic tissue

Hypoadrenocorticism
- Primary (Addison's disease)
- Secondary (ACTH deficiency)

Liver dysfunction
- Acquired disorders
- Congenital – portosystemic shunts
- Glycogen storage diseases
- Feline idiopathic hepatic lipidosis

Puppy hypoglycaemia
Ketotic hypoglycaemia of pregnancy [rare]
Severe sepsis
Increase in blood cells, RBCs or WBCs
Neoplasia
Chronic starvation [rare]
Chronic malabsorption
Status epilepticus
Error: failure to inhibit glycolytic enzymes

Usually hypoglycaemia is manifested by restlessness, weakness, disorientation and ataxia, progressing to CNS signs (e.g. uncontrolled barking in dogs, convulsions), and ultimately coma and death. Such signs are particularly likely to follow fasting, exercise or excitement.

It is important to collect fasting samples, otherwise despite this history glucose values may be within the 'normal' range.

HYPERINSULINISM [RELATIVELY COMMON]

Overdosage of insulin

Hyperinsulinism can be caused by overdosage of insulin (*or* of other hypoglycaemic drugs, sulphonylureas (e.g. tolbutamide, chlorpropamide) and biguanides).

Insulin overdosage may be due to such factors as miscalculation of the dose, misreading the syringe, accidentally repeating a dose, failure of the animal to eat, a considerable increase in exercise *or* an abnormally long interval between insulin injection and feeding (>12 hours). At times owners may fail to test the urine at all, or not do so accurately, and therefore misjudge the insulin requirement.

Insulin-secreting tumour of pancreatic beta cells (= insulinoma)

Signs often appear 2–8 hours after feeding due to the resultant excessive insulin output.

Diagnosis is best made by also measuring the insulin level and using it in the following expression (the amended insulin:glucose ratio):

$$\frac{\text{Plasma insulin in } \mu\text{U/ml} \times 100}{\text{Plasma glucose in mg/dl } (or \text{ mmol/l} \times 18) - 30}$$

If the plasma glucose level is 1.7 mmol/l (30 mg/dl) or less, then the divisor should be replaced by 1.

A value from this ratio of more than 30 µU insulin/mg glucose is obtained in almost all cases where there is an insulin-secreting tumour. However, other causes of hypoglycaemia may also produce the same result.

Tumour of non-pancreatic tissue secreting insulin, or an insulin-like substance [rare]

Occasional cases have been reported, chiefly involving carcinomas (e.g. of mammary glands, lungs or salivary glands), liver tumours (primary and secondary) and haemangiosarcomas.

The formula mentioned above may be used in diagnosis.

HYPOADRENOCORTICISM (DEFICIENCY OF CORTISOL)

Addison's disease (= primary hypoadrenocorticism)

Overall about a quarter of dogs with Addison's disease show hypoglycaemia, because the lack of cortisol reduces hepatic glucose production and increases responsiveness to insulin.

> **Note**
>
> A small proportion of dogs with Addison's disease show a slight *increase* in the glucose level.

Other features of the disease are summarized on p. 406.

Inadequate ACTH secretion (= secondary hypoadrenocorticism) [very rare]

Destructive lesions of the pituitary gland or hypothalamus can result in reduced ACTH secretion (i.e. as part of hypopituitarism) leading to reduced cortisol secretion (i.e. secondary hypoadrenocorticism), with the same effect on glucose levels as in Addison's disease.

Since mineralocorticoids are not involved, plasma electrolyte levels remain unaltered.

The production of growth hormone, another glucogenic hormone, may also be diminished which will serve to reduce further the plasma glucose levels.

HEPATIC DYSFUNCTION

CHECK – usually associated with increases in bile salts and ALT and ALP activity and a low level of albumin, and possibly urea.

Acquired disorders

These result in a lack of functional liver cells.

- Destruction of hepatocytes due to neoplasia (primary or secondary), trauma, toxic drugs and chemicals or infectious agents.
- Replacement of hepatocytes, e.g. by fibrous tissue (as in cirrhosis).
- By-passing of the hepatocytes caused by an acquired vascular shunt.

In each case there are insufficient functional cells to carry out efficient glycogen storage or gluconeogenesis.

Congenital portosystemic shunts

Inadequate glycogen storage and gluconeogenesis, due to the lack of functional hepatic tissue, results in hypoglycaemia in many cases.

Glycogen storage diseases

A congenital deficiency (absolute or relative) of one of the enzymes that are necessary to convert glycogen to glucose can result in hypoglycaemia, particularly during fasting or exercise (in common with most disorders giving rise to hypoglycaemia). A feature of *these* disorders is liver enlargement due to the continual accumulation of glycogen (Strombeck, 1979). They have been recorded in some puppies (von Gierke-like syndrome, a type I glycogen storage disease which is not outgrown), in hunting dogs (functional hypoglycaemia – a type III glycogen storage disease) and in German Shepherd Dogs (a type III glycogen storage disease) among others.

Diagnoses are confirmed using a glucagon tolerance test, which produces no rise in plasma glucose levels.

Glucagon (0.03 mg/kg body weight) is injected intravenously and blood samples collected for glucose estimation just before injection and after 5, 15 (30, 45), 60 and 120 minutes.

Feline idiopathic hepatic lipidosis

Although sometimes described as a separate entity this could also be included under 'Acquired disorders' above.

PUPPY HYPOGLYCAEMIA

Puppies of miniature and toy breeds under 6 months of age may develop hypoglycaemia, with appropriate clinical signs, usually under conditions of stress (e.g. a change of environment and/or gastrointestinal upset). They do not show hepatomegaly and the condition disappears as the animal grows older, presumed due to the reduced requirement for glucose. The condition appears to be associated with deficient alanine production, and it can be effectively treated by frequent feeding.

KETOTIC HYPOGLYCAEMIA OF PREGNANCY [RARE]

Hypoglycaemia and ketonaemia have been described in a bitch in late pregnancy. This may also be related to a deficiency of alanine.

SEVERE SEPSIS (ENDOTOXAEMIA OR URAEMIA) [UNCOMMON]

Sepsis and endotoxaemia (e.g. pyometra, pyothorax, internal abscessation and Gram-negative septicaemia) may occasionally result in hypoglycaemia, primarily by interfering with various liver functions, but possibly also by increasing glucose utilization (especially if the white blood cell count is high – $>30 \times 10^9$/l) and causing the release of insulin-like substances.

CHECK – such cases show fever (later hypothermia), injected sclera and shock.

Uraemia may (rarely) produce a similar inhibition of liver function.

CHECK – increased urea, creatinine and inorganic phosphate levels.

INCREASED NUMBER OF BLOOD CELLS

Polycythaemia vera [very rare]

Increased glucose consumption by the large numbers of RBCs lowers the plasma glucose level (see Panel 2.6, p. 123).

Leucocytosis

There may be the same result from an elevated WBC count ($>30 \times 10^9$/l) although the effect is usually marginal.

NEOPLASIA [VERY RARE]

Hypoglycaemia *may* be due to the excessive utilization of glucose by some tumours (usually large abdominal or mediastinal tumours, e.g. hepatomas, or generalized neoplasia), or alternatively to their production of substances which inhibit the release of glucose from the liver. Such cases are seldom recognized in dogs and cats.

(It should be distinguished from hypoglycaemia attributable to tumours of the pancreas, or other tissues which secrete insulin or insulin-like substances.)

CHRONIC STARVATION [RARE]

Plasma glucose levels within the normal range can be maintained for several weeks in dogs and cats totally deprived of food (unlike the situation in humans, whose requirement for glucose appears greater). The exception is puppies and small breeds of dog who may not withstand even a few hours of fasting (see under 'Hepatic dysfunction' and 'Puppy hypoglycaemia' above).

Therefore hypoglycaemia is not the result of starvation or anorexia in itself (unless carried to extreme lengths), although of course the *cause* of the anorexia might also be the cause of hypoglycaemia.

CHRONIC MALABSORPTION [RARE]

Long-standing malabsorption, resulting in starvation to the point of emaciation, *might* result in hypoglycaemia although this would be rare (see entry above).

STATUS EPILEPTICUS

This results in hypoglycaemia due to prolonged muscle activity.

ERROR: FAILURE TO INHIBIT GLYCOLYTIC ENZYMES [COMMON]

Glucose levels *will inevitably be low* in samples of blood despatched to laboratories:

- either unseparated, if no enzyme inhibitor is added (i.e. in tubes containing only EDTA or heparin, or no anticoagulant);
- or where plasma or serum (without an enzyme inhibitor added) has been separated but shows haemolysis.

This is because glycolytic enzymes from the RBCs continue to break down the glucose.

As mentioned previously (under 'Accuracy', p. 277), it is important to collect the blood sample into a tube containing an enzyme inhibitor (invariably sodium fluoride in combination with potassium oxalate), or alternatively to separate (non-haemolysed) plasma or serum as soon as possible after collection, preferably within 30–45 minutes.

Note

Some disorders in humans, e.g. functional hypoglycaemia and hypoglycaemia due to alcohol, are unlikely to appear in small animals.

Plasma ammonia

SI units of measurement are micromoles per litre (μmol/l). Previous units used were μg/dl (= μg/100 ml).

CONVERSION FACTORS

- To convert μg/dl to μmol/l multiply by 0.57.
- To convert μmol/l to μg/dl multiply by 1.7.

NORMAL REFERENCE RANGE

Dog: 25–70 μmol/l (45–120 μg/dl).
Cat: 60–100 μmol/l (100–170 μg/dl).

But check the normal range for each particular laboratory.

IMPORTANT NOTE

1. Estimations of ammonia levels will obviously be falsely elevated by the prior presence of ammonia. EDTA is often recommended as the anticoagulant to use when obtaining plasma samples because it avoids the possibility of ammonium contamination that may occur with other anticoagulants. For example, lithium heparin can be contaminated with ammonium heparinate, and only a small amount can introduce an appreciable error.
2. After blood collection ammonia can be released, possibly from urea (each 0.01 mmol/l urea produces 200 μmol/l ammonia) although its derivation from the breakdown of adenyl phosphate, adenylic acid and glutamic acid is suspected (Hitt and Jones, 1986). These workers found the effect of temperature to be variable, but generally it is believed that to avoid the false elevation of ammonia levels, samples should be received by the laboratory within $\frac{1}{2}$–1 hour of collection (2 hours if kept chilled in a vacuum flask). Then the plasma should be separated and *either* refrigerated for analysis shortly afterwards *or* deep frozen ($-20°$C) for estimation within the next 3 days.
3. It is often recommended that blood from a normal animal should be submitted at the same time to check the validity of the assay.

The need for samples to be dealt with quickly and effectively rules out the measurement of ammonia for veterinary practices situated a long distance from a laboratory, i.e. postal samples are quite unsuitable. *As an alternative* the finding of increased bile acid levels (see p. 266), although not specifically incriminating ammonia, will indicate the existence of a disorder which could result in hyperammonaemia.

SOURCE

Ammonia found in the blood is principally that absorbed from the intestines, especially the colon, although some is derived from peripheral tissue metabolism, particularly in the skeletal muscles. The intestinal ammonia is derived from bacterial degradation of residual dietary amino acids in the bowel and of the endogenous urea that is excreted into the bowel. (Ammonia is also produced in the liver from the catabolism of dietary and tissue amino acids, but immediately enters the urea cycle and is converted into urea – see p. 225.)

Normally the ammonia transported from the bowel is also converted into urea when it reaches the liver, and therefore the level of ammonia in the systemic blood is low.

However, high ammonia levels result if liver function is impaired or if portal blood by-passes the liver, i.e. in a portosystemic shunt.

These higher circulating levels of ammonia, especially likely following a meal, usually affect the brain; this may simply result in listlessness, but often a variety of CNS signs are evident (confusion, circling, head-pressing, convulsions etc.) – the resultant condition is referred to as *hepatic encephalopathy*.

Often the severity of the clinical signs does not correlate well with the level of ammonia, especially in the cat. This may be because the signs are also caused by other toxins derived from the gastrointestinal tract – mercaptans, skatoles, indoles and short-chain fatty acids.

AMMONIA TOLERANCE TEST

Some animals suspected of being unable successfully to convert ammonia to urea, because they demonstrate CNS signs, may be found to have a blood ammonia level within the normal range. This can be due to natural fluctuations in fasting blood ammonia levels.

In these animals the ability to remove ammonia is best assessed by performing an ammonia tolerance test.

This test is often performed in cases with a portosystemic shunt because affected individuals may show no increases in ALT, ALP or bilirubin levels. However, total protein, albumin, cholesterol and urea levels are often low (or low–normal) and the measurement of bile acids serves to check the integrity of the enterohepatic circulation.

Nevertheless the finding of high blood ammonia levels (with or without the performance of an ammonia tolerance test) is the only way to *confirm* that they do in fact occur and therefore could be responsible for the CNS signs.

Method

1. Ammonium chloride (100 mg/kg up to a *maximum* of 3 g) is dissolved in water (20 mg/ml) and administered orally to a fasted animal.
2. Blood samples are collected before, and 30 minutes after administration (into dipotassium EDTA).

Possible, although fortunately uncommon, complications of the test are: vomiting and/or the precipitation of CNS signs.

(Since much of the ammonia absorption is from the large bowel, vomiting, if a major problem, can be avoided by giving the dose rectally and collecting samples before, and 20 and 40 minutes after administration.)

The blood ammonia level at the end of the test in *normal* fasted animals is less than 120 μmol/l (= 200 μg/dl) in dogs, and less than 175 μmol/l (300 μg/dl) in cats.

In *affected* animals it is usually considerably higher, representing at least a doubling of the basal value.

Causes of increased plasma ammonia levels

Summary

- Loss of liver function
- Portosystemic shunt
- Primary hyperammonaemia [rare]
- Severe uraemia
- Severe exercise (immediate)
- Ammonia poisoning [rare]

Error: Exaggerated urea breakdown

LOSS OF LIVER FUNCTION

The liver is unable to convert ammonia to urea efficiently causing an accumulation of ammonia, and this high level of ammonia may affect the brain producing a variety of CNS signs (hepatic encephalopathy).

Severe loss of liver function is described as liver failure.

PORTOSYSTEMIC SHUNT

This includes portacaval shunt and acquired hepatocellular insufficiency. There are a number of possible congenital defects in the vasculature which can result in blood in the portal vein effectively by-passing the liver cells. The portal vein may empty directly into the posterior vena cava or the azygos vein or, alternatively, empty into a patent ductus venosus which opens into the posterior vena cava.

Ammonia being transported from the gut is not converted into blood urea. Consequently blood urea values remain low.

PRIMARY HYPERAMMONAEMIA [RARE]

This congenital defect in the urea cycle is due to the lack of an enzyme and prevents ammonia from being converted into urea. The blood supply to the liver is normal and, in contrast to hepatic failure and portosystemic shunt, no other liver functions are affected, i.e. there are normal levels of albumin, cholesterol and clotting factors, and the BSP clearance is normal.

SEVERE URAEMIA

This will result in an increase in the ammonia level because the balance of the urea cycle is disturbed.

AMMONIA POISONING [EXTREMELY RARE]

SEVERE EXERCISE

A marked increase in plasma ammonia occurs immediately after severe exercise in Greyhounds (Snow et al., 1988).

ERROR: EXAGGERATED UREA BREAKDOWN DUE TO DELAY IN PROCESSING

Delay in the laboratory processing of the sample (of more than 2 hours) will result in erroneously high levels of ammonia due to its production from the breakdown of urea or other substances.

See the 'Important note' at beginning of 'Ammonia' section (p. 290).

> **Note**
>
> - Do not give animals with a portosystemic shunt or severe liver disease, particularly if showing signs of hepatic encephalopathy, a blood transfusion using *stored* blood because its ammonia content rises with storage, e.g. after just 24 hours' storage it contains 100 μmol/l (170 μg/dl).
> - Ammonium urate (actually biurate) crystals in the urine are a feature of animals with hyperammonaemia (and also normal Dalmatians, see p. 462).

Bromsulphthalein (BSP) clearance test (sulfobromophthalein excretion test, bromsulfalein retention test)

BSP is a dye which after intravenous injection is removed almost exclusively by the liver, being taken up, conjugated and excreted in the bile in a very similar manner to bilirubin. Delay in its elimination from the plasma generally indicates reduced liver function, biliary obstruction or inadequate hepatic blood flow (e.g. intra- or extrahepatic vascular shunting or poor perfusion, as with cardiac failure or hypovolaemia).

In the dog with impaired liver function, increased BSP retention is evident before any increase in plasma bilirubin levels. In cases of haemolytic jaundice BSP clearance will be unaffected.

After injection of the BSP (5 mg/kg to *dog* or *cat*) either a single plasma sample is collected after 30 minutes or a series are collected after 10, 20 and 30 minutes (see Appendix I, p. 472).

NORMAL REFERENCE RANGE

In most normal dogs less than 5% of the injected dose will remain in the blood after 30 minutes; certainly if more than 10% remains the result is abnormal. In most normal cats, less than 2% of the dose remains after 30 minutes. Retention of abnormal amounts indicates impaired liver function *or* reduced hepatic blood flow.

The advantage of collecting three samples at intervals after injection is that the BSP concentration can be plotted against time on semilogarithmic paper and the half-life for BSP clearance can be determined. This removes such errors as incorrect calculation or preparation of the dose, incomplete injection (provided none goes elsewhere in the body) and disparities between body weight and blood volume (e.g. in cases of obesity or ascites).

The normal half-life in the dog should be less than *7 minutes* (corresponding to <5% remaining after 30 minutes), and a half-life greater than *9 minutes* (corresponding to >10% remaining after 30 minutes) indicates impaired liver function or poor hepatic perfusion.

Likewise, the normal half-life in the cat should be less than 5½ minutes (corresponding to less than 2% remaining after 30 minutes).

As an *alternative to the BSP clearance test*:

● Indocyanine green has been substituted for BSP; this avoids local reactions outside the vein and, because it has a slightly longer half-life, may give a more accurate assessment of clearance (especially in the cat), but otherwise has few advantages.
● Bile acids can be measured (e.g. after fasting and again 2 hours after feeding. This test provides a more sensitive indicator of liver function without the need for previous injection or repeat sampling (and the associated problems). Also bile acids are stable in postal samples. Bile acid determinations seem destined to replace the BSP clearance test as a measure of liver function.

Note

Other biochemical tests cannot be performed on samples containing BSP; blood samples for routine tests should therefore be collected *before* its administration to the patient.

Causes of increased retention of BSP in the circulation

Summary

● Reduced liver function
● Decreased hepatic blood flow
● Biliary obstruction
● Obesity
● Ascites
● Drugs binding to albumin
Error: extensive perivascular injection

Causes of increased retention (i.e. reduced clearance) include:

REDUCED LIVER FUNCTION

There is reduced uptake, conjugation and secretion by hepatocytes (which may be due to reduced liver mass, as in cirrhosis).

DECREASED HEPATIC BLOOD FLOW

This may result from intra- and extrahepatic vascular shunts, congestive heart failure, hypovolaemia (as with severe dehydration), fever and shock.

BILIARY OBSTRUCTION

BSP retention is especially marked with complete bile duct occlusion.

OBESITY AND ASCITES

In both obesity and ascites, BSP clearance is reduced because the blood volume is less per unit body weight than normal (normal=50 ml/kg), i.e. fat and ascitic fluid do not contribute to the blood volume. Consequently, excess BSP will be injected in such cases if it is given on a strictly weight-related basis. The effect on clearance is usually marginal however.

DRUGS THAT BIND TO ALBUMIN

Such drugs compete with BSP and reduce its clearance. There are reports that bilirubin also competes with BSP for clearance, which would mean reduced BSP clearance following an increase in plasma bilirubin from whatever cause, but other reports deny that there is such competition (Yeary and Wise, 1975).

ERROR: EXTENSIVE PERIVASCULAR INJECTION OF THE BSP

BSP appears to be retained because absorption from the injection site into the plasma continues throughout the test.

Note

Very rarely abnormal BSP retention is found in the dog without any accompanying signs of liver dysfunction and this may be due to a deficiency of one of the intracellular binding proteins concerned with BSP uptake, storage and conjugation.

Causes of decreased retention of BSP in the circulation

The causes of decreased retention (i.e. increased clearance) include the following.

HYPOALBUMINAEMIA

For details see 'Causes of decreased plasma albumin levels' (p. 252).

BSP in the plasma rapidly binds to albumin and lipoproteins. The amount of unbound BSP is increased when albumin levels are lower, and the liver removes it faster. Where hypoalbuminaemia is a consequence of impaired liver function (one decreasing, the other increasing, BSP retention) the *net* effect can be either normal BSP clearance or only a *slight* increase in retention.

BILE ACID SECRETION (AFTER FEEDING)

Bile salts stimulate BSP clearance (up to two to three times normal). Therefore prior fasting is *important*.

Panel 5.1 Gammopathies

Gammopathies (or gamma-globulinopathies) are disorders in which there is an abnormal increase in the level of proteins resembling one or more immunoglobulins.

Plasma cells synthesize these immunoglobulins, and the polypeptides from which they are constructed. Each of the types of immunoglobulins (i.e. IgG, IgM, IgA etc.) is characterized by a different arrangement of four polypeptides. The polypeptides are of two types:

- Long chain polypeptides, usually called *heavy* chains.
- Short chain polypeptides, usually called *light* chains.

Gammopathies can be divided into polyclonal gammopathies and monoclonal gammopathies.

Polyclonal gammopathies

In these the increase is in *more than one immunoglobulin*. These immunoglobulins are produced by a number of lines of plasma cells (i.e. many clones) that have begun to proliferate, generally benignly, following antigenic stimulation by:

- Chronic infections (pyoderma, abscesses, feline infectious peritonitis, fungal and parasitic infections).
- Chronic inflammatory diseases.
- Immune-mediated disorders, such as systemic lupus erythematosus and rheumatoid arthritis.
- Lymphosarcomas (occasionally).

Despite being called 'gammopathies', on an electrophoretic trace there is a broad (saw-tooth) elevation in both the γ- and β-globulin regions (rarely the α_2 region).

Monoclonal gammopathies

In these the increase is in a *single* immunoglobulin produced by a single clone of plasma cells that have undergone proliferation that is usually malignant, although sometimes benign. This produces a high peak of immunoglobulin on an electrophoretic trace – a spike or 'church spire' in the same regions (i.e. usually γ- and β-globulins).

Monoclonal gammopathies are associated with:

- Plasma cell myelomas (malignant tumours *almost always multiple* rather than solitary, i.e. multiple myelomas).
- Macroglobulinaemia.
- Lymphoproliferative disorders, i.e. lymphosarcoma and lymphocytic leukaemia. This is the most *common* cause of monoclonal gammopathy, developing in about 5% of lymphoproliferative disorders in the dog although only occasionally in the cat.
- Other tumours (exceptionally).
- Chronic inflammation, immune-mediated disease or very, very, rarely with feline infectious peritonitis (examples of benign proliferation).

These abnormal proteins, which have no immune activity, can be referred to as paraproteins or myeloma proteins (M components). As well as complete immunoglobulins (usually IgG, but in the case of macroglobulinaemia IgM) there may also be immunoglobulin components present, i.e. the light chain polypeptides and, although rarely, fragments of heavy chain polypeptides. Because of their smaller molecules light chains are rapidly filtered by the kidney and appear in the urine (where they are referred to as Bence-Jones protein), but they do not appear, or are not recognized, in electrophoretic traces.

The increase in immunoglobulins creates an increase in the total plasma protein level and a decrease in the albumin:globulin (A:G) ratio.

A high concentration of immunoglobulins (chiefly IgM, less often IgA and rarely IgG) can result in increased viscosity of the plasma, known as hyperviscosity syndrome (HVS).

MACROGLOBULINAEMIA

Macroglobulinaemia is a monoclonal increase in IgM, the immunoglobulin which has the largest molecule. After the lymphoproliferative disorders this is the next most common cause of a monoclonal gammopathy.

A specific disorder, Waldenström's macroglobulinaemia, has been recorded in the dog, having many features in common with plasma cell myeloma *except* that bone lesions are absent. It can occur secondary to lymphosarcoma and to infection.

PLASMA CELL MYELOMA (= MULTIPLE MYELOMA)

This disorder is rare in the cat and uncommon in the dog, chiefly/solely affecting large breeds, especially German Shepherd Dogs, and accounting for 3–4% of all canine bone tumours.

A myeloma is a bone marrow tumour and invariably the term refers to a *plasma cell myeloma*.

In *multiple myeloma* the bone marrow is infiltrated at several sites by a particular clone of plasma cells which then proliferates and in doing so:

* Destroys the bone marrow and lyses the bone.
* Overproduces the particular immunoglobulin or polypeptides (i.e the light or heavy chains) which it is able to synthesize.

Very rarely a solitary plasma cell tumour (plasmacytoma) arises at some other site, e.g. spleen, liver or lymph node, and may metastasize to the bone marrow later.

Although designated a leukaemia, multiple myeloma is most often diagnosed on the results of plasma protein measurements.

Other *clinical* consequences of a myeloma can be the following:

* Skeletal pain, lameness and pathological fractures due to osteolysis (with 'punched out' areas of bone often visible on radiographs).
* Compression of the spinal cord nerve roots or peripheral nerves, due to vertebral fracture or plasma cell infiltration, giving rise to other problems, e.g. incontinence.
* Enlargement of liver, spleen, and mediastinal lymph nodes (the latter causing dyspnoea).
* Hyperviscosity syndrome (HVS) due to excessive amounts of protein, chiefly IgM and less often IgA (rarely IgG). The increased viscosity impairs blood circulation causing a number of defects.
* Bleeding disorders (e.g. epistaxis) due to a number of abnormalities including interference with platelet activity (adhesiveness and release of platelet factor 3) and thrombocytopenia due to myelophthisis (replacement of platelet-forming tissue in the bone marrow).

- Damage to the kidneys caused by the infiltration of neoplastic cells and by Bence-Jones protein which can form casts and (rarely) initiate amyloidosis; these events can lead to renal failure and azotaemia.
- Tendency towards myelogenous or myelomonocytic leukaemia (as a progression of the disease) or to some other form of neoplasia.
- Increased susceptiblity to infections due to neutropenia and decreased formation of other immunoglobulins (these paraproteins have no immune activity).
- Cryoglobulinaemia, i.e. the plasma forms a gel when cooled, due to the abnormally high level of IgM, resulting in dermatitis.
- Cold agglutinin disease – a form of autoimmune haemolytic anaemia occurring when the blood is cooled, and therefore especially likely to involve the ear tips.

Other *laboratory* features that may appear include the following:

- *Proteinuria* up to 1.6 g/l (in around 20% of cases).

Note

- If there are losses of protein elsewhere (e.g. from haemorrhage), the level of urinary protein could be in the normal range.
- Bence-Jones protein (see below), if present (some cats, <10% dogs), will not be detected by commercial strip tests (sensitive mainly to albumin), but can be detected using 20% sulphosalicylic acid.

- Bence-Jones protein in blood/urine – this protein consists of the light chain polypeptides that are part of the immunoglobulins. They are readily filtered by the kidney and therefore often *do not* appear on a plasma electrophoretic trace. However, they will appear in the urine (see 'Note' above) and give a characteristic band in the globulin region following electrophoresis of the urine.
- Hypercalcaemia – in some cases this is due to increased bone lysis caused by an osteoclast-activating factor produced by the tumour cells (or due to pseudohyperparathyroidism).
- Hypocalcaemia – in many cases due to hypoalbuminaemia (see p. 374).
- Anaemia in *most* cases (usually just below the lower limit of normal); this is chiefly non-regenerative due to bone marrow destruction, but can also be due to haemorrhage and the anaemia of chronic disease.
- Leucopenia due to neutropenia in a third of cases.
- Thromobocytopenia – also in about one-third of cases.
- Small numbers of plasma cells (abnormal in appearance, i.e. large and immature) in 50% of canine cases.
- Increased rouleaux formation.
- Increased plasma viscosity.
- Increased ESR usually, until the viscosity increases to the point where the ESR decreases. (Increased rouleaux formation plus a decreased ESR denotes serum hyperviscosity.)
- Azotaemia due to renal damage.
- Decreased levels of other immunoglobulins due to a decreased immune response.
- Increased numbers of plasma cells (>5–10%) on bone marrow aspiration or biopsy. This alone is not diagnostic because increased numbers of plasma cells can occur in inflammation and immune disorders, but in multiple myeloma plasma cells appear in clusters with a high percentage of abnormal and immature forms.

- Alkaline phosphatase (ALP) activity is not usually increased because increases in the bone isoenzyme of ALP relate to increased osteoblast actitivy not to increased osteoclast activity, as occurs here. If the liver is infiltrated with plasma cells, there may be increased ALP activity due to increases in the *liver* isoenzyme of ALP.
- At times hypoalbuminaemia.

The *diagnosis* of a plasma cell myeloma is usually based on finding two out of the following four:

1. Monoclonal gammopathy.
2. An increased number of plasma cells in bone marrow.
3. Bence-Jones proteinuria.
4. Osteolytic lesions.

Panel 5.2 Renal disorders

Renal diseases of the dog and cat may be classified into three broad groups:

1. Primary glomerular diseases.
2. Acute renal failure.
3. Chronic renal failure (and either of the first two can lead eventually to this).

Note

Bear in mind that, in addition to the biochemical changes described for these conditions, there *may* be an increase in the plasma glucose level, mainly in the cat (even occasionally causing glycosuria), due to the accompanying stress.

Primary glomerular diseases

These consist of:

- Glomerulonephritis (or glomerulonephropathy).
- Renal amyloidosis.

GLOMERULONEPHRITIS

This is an autoimmune condition in which antibodies are formed against a variety of antigens, including *E. coli* in pyometra, heartworms (not in the UK), malignant tumours (in 40% of canine glomerulonephritis cases), the viruses of feline infectious peritonitis and feline respiratory diseases, feline leukaemia virus, host DNA in systemic lupus erythematosus and possibly pancreatic enzymes (see Panel 2.7, p. 125). Antigen–antibody complexes form on the glomerular basement membrane causing damage.

RENAL AMYLOIDOSIS

This is mostly initiated by an acute phase reactant in chronic disorders, e.g. neoplasia and sepsis and, in the cat, by hypervitaminosis A (although in the cat amyloid is more frequently deposited in the renal medulla than in the glomeruli). A much rarer cause in the dog is multiple myeloma, producing light chain polypeptides as a precursor of amyloid.

Usually renal amyloidosis is associated with amyloidosis elsewhere, e.g. the spleen or liver, which can cause these organs to enlarge.

Damage to the glomerulus in both these diseases (glomerulonephritis and renal amyloidosis) allows protein molecules (especially the smaller albumin molecules) to pass through in quantities too large to be completely reabsorbed and consequently they are lost in the urine (proteinuria). The consequent fall in plasma proteins (hypoproteinaemia) may be severe enough to permit the development of generalized oedema including ascites. The presence of proteinuria, hypoalbuminaemia (accompanied by hypercholesterolaemia) and generalized oedema constitutes the *nephrotic syndrome*. This syndrome is *not* an inevitable consequence of primary glomerular disease.

Laboratory findings

See also 'Causes of proteinuria' (p. 431).

Proteinuria
This is usually much less than 10 g/l (1 g/dl) but in advanced cases of membranous glomerulonephritis and renal amyloidosis that concentration may be exceeded. The protein concerned is primarily albumin. However, with increasing damage and increasing protein loss proportionately more globulins are lost.

With the development of chronic renal failure and increased polyuria, the urinary protein is more diluted and so its concentration usually does not remain quite as high as previously.

In *cats* with amyloidosis, proteinuria *may not* be prominent (because amyloid may be deposited primarily in the renal medulla).

Hypoproteinaemia
Values for total plasma protein are normally less than 40 g/l (<4 g/dl).

Hypoalbuminaemia
Usually plasma levels are less than 20 g/l (<2 g/dl). At times values may be much lower, e.g. 10 g/l (1 g/dl).

Decreased albumin:globulin ratio (A:G ratio)
This occurs because albumin is lost more readily. Also, frequently there are increases in α-, β- and γ-globulins.

Hypercholesterolaemia
This is probably part of a hyperlipidaemia, i.e. the level of triglycerides is probably also increased, but this is not well documented in small animals.

Plasma cholesterol level is inversely proportional to the plasma albumin level. It rises due to increased liver synthesis of cholesterol-rich lipoproteins.

Values in the dog are usually more than 8 mmol/l (>300 mg/dl) and in the cat more than 6.5 mmol/l (>250 mg/dl).

Hypocalcaemia (low plasma calcium level)
A fall in plasma albumin is accompanied by a corresponding fall in the fraction of calcium that is bound to it (protein-bound calcium). Ionized calcium may also fall because the binding protein for active vitamin D_3 is also lost.

Sodium
Sodium is retained giving higher plasma levels.

Hyperfibrinogenaemia
An increased plasma fibrinogen level is recognized with renal amyloidosis, contributing or predisposing to thrombosis.
    Fibrinogen levels are inversely proportional to the level of plasma albumin.

Urea, creatinine and inorganic phosphate levels
Initially these are not elevated (although they may be intermittently), but in the later stages, as chronic renal failure develops, persistent elevations will occur.

Haematuria
This arises in the early stages of glomerulonephritis.

Hyaline casts
These are common in the urine due to the heavy protein loss via the tubules; rarely there are RBC casts.

Urinary specific gravity
Specific gravity can be high in early glomerulonephritis (>1.040), but falls to the isosthenuric range (1.008–1.012) as chronic renal failure develops.
    As well as checking for the above changes examinations for autoimmune disorders could be carried out, i.e. examining for LE cells and performing antinuclear antibody tests (ANA tests), and in the cat testing for FeLV.

Acute renal failure

There is acute suppression of renal function and clinical signs appear quickly, including the diagnostic oliguria (urine production <7 ml/kg body weight per day). Later polyuria supervenes if the animal survives.
    Acute renal failure is subdivided into prerenal (comparatively mild and reversible), renal (intrarenal or primary renal) and postrenal (obstructive).

PRERENAL ACUTE RENAL FAILURE

Otherwise designated as prerenal azotaemia this involves decreased renal perfusion. The condition arises from a severe reduction in blood flow through the kidneys with an overall reduction in glomerular filtration rate (GFR).
    The causes can be dehydration, severe haemorrhage, shock, hypoadrenocorticism, both primary (Addison's disease) and secondary, reduced cardiac output, caused by congestive heart failure or cardiac arrhythmias, and hypoalbuminaemia (causing reduced plasma oncotic pressure).

Laboratory findings

Increased plasma urea level
Plasma urea is more than 7 mmol/l (>40 mg/dl; BUN >20 mg/dl) in the dog *or* more than 11 mmol/l (>65 mg/dl; BUN >32 mg/dl) in the cat. However, in both species the urea level is less than 35 mmol/l (<210 mg/dl; BUN <100 mg/dl). Values are usually much less than these upper limits (often 14–17 mmol/l).

Increased plasma creatinine level
Plasma creatinine is usually more than 130 μmol/l (>1.5 mg/dl) in both the dog and the cat. However, values are less than 250 μmol/l (<3 mg/dl) in both species, and at times *may* remain in the normal range.

An increased urea:creatinine value
This occurs because urea reabsorption is relatively increased:

- If creatinine is in μmol/l and urea in mmol/l, the ratio is >0.08.
- If creatinine is in mg/dl and urea is in mg/dl, the ratio is >43.
- If creatinine is in mg/dl and BUN is in mg/dl the ratio is >20. However, one should be aware that some UK laboratories allegedly report BUN (in mmol/l) when in fact they are reporting *urea* in mmol/l.

CHECK for this discrepancy by checking the laboratory's reported normal ranges (see p. 224).

PCV
This may be increased with dehydration or decreased with severe haemorrhage.

Total protein and albumin concentrations
These may similarly be increased with dehydration or decreased with severe haemorrhage.

RENAL ACUTE RENAL FAILURE

This condition is also designated as intrarenal acute renal failure or primary acute renal failure and may be due to acute interstitial nephritis (AIN) or acute tubular necrosis (ATN).

Acute interstitial nephritis (AIN)

AIN is due to infectious agents:

- In the dog: canine adenovirus-1, canine herpes virus, *Leptospira canicola* (causing acute leptospirosis) and *Klebsiella* infection.
- In both species organisms incriminated include *E. coli*, *Proteus*, staphylococci and streptococci.

Acute tubular necrosis (ATN)

This is principally due to nephrotoxins or ischaemia.

Nephrotoxins
These include compounds of lead, arsenic, mercury and bismuth, the rodenticide thallium, amphotericin B and the antibiotics of the polymyxin/bacitracin and aminoglycoside (streptomycin, neomycin, gentamicin etc.) groups plus the less soluble sulphonamides, organic compounds such as carbon tetrachloride, chloroform, methyl alcohol, phenol and ethylene glycol (in anti-freeze), the analgesics phenacetin and phenylbutazone, cyclophosphamide, methoxyflurane, chlorinated hydrocarbons and radio-opaque contrast media.

Also large amounts of myoglobin, as a result of muscle breakdown (rhabdomyolysis) or crush injuries, and of haemoglobin, following massive haemolysis, in the plasma produce similar effects by obstructing the tubules.

The effects of all of the above will be enhanced by dehydration and, in the case of drugs which are excreted via the kidney, by pre-existing renal damage.

The inherited disease of young cats, primary hyperoxaluria, causes acute renal failure by the deposition of calcium oxalate crystals in the tubules – which also occurs with ethylene glycol poisoning (McKerrell et al., 1989).

Ischaemia
This is due to a severe and irreversible lack of perfusion of the kidney associated with hypotension and/or hypovolaemia.

It may arise following prolonged surgery or anaesthesia, severe acute haemorrhage, disseminated intravascular coagulation (DIC), burns, heart failure, shock, trauma, incompatible blood transfusions, obstruction of the renal blood vessels by infarcts or thrombi, diffuse nephrocalcinosis (with hypercalcaemia) and following prolonged prerenal acute renal failure, i.e. decreased renal perfusion.

Laboratory features

Increased plasma urea level
In the dog plasma urea is more than 7 mmol/l (>40 mg/dl; BUN >20 mg/dl) and in the cat more than 11 mmol/l (>65 mg/dl; BUN >32 mg/dl).

Unlike prerenal ARF, values may exceed 35 mmol/l (>210 mg/dl; BUN >100 mg/dl).

Increased plasma creatinine level
In the dog and cat, plasma creatinine is more than 30 μmol/l (>1.5 mg/dl) and is especially significant when it exceeds 250 μmol/l (>3 mg/dl).

A normal value for the urea:creatinine ratio
This is 0.08 or less if creatinine is measured in μmol/l and urea in mmol/l (43 or less if creatinine and urea are measured in mg/dl, and 20 or less if creatinine and BUN are measured in mg/dl).

Urinary specific gravity
This is less than 1.029 in the dog and less than 1.034 in the cat, if two-thirds of the nephrons are non-functional, and generally less than 1.012 (although sometimes up to 1.015) in the dog and less than 1.025 in the cat if three-quarters of the nephrons are non-functional. A dilute urine cannot be formed (specific gravity <1.007) and with increasing nephron losses isosthenuria develops (i.e. classically a specific gravity between 1.008 and 1.012, although this may be stretched to 1.007–1.015).

Hyperphosphataemia
There is an accumulation of phosphate derived from protein, which rises progressively as renal function decreases.

It is more than 1.6 mmol/l (>5 mg/dl) in the dog and more than 2.6 mmol/l (>8 mg/dl) in the cat. (In puppies under 1 year of age the upper limit of normal is 3.2 mmol/l = 10 mg/dl.)

Low/low–normal calcium level
This often arises (i.e. around 2 mmol/l (=8 mg/dl)), although in some cases calcium may be elevated.

The sudden development of hyperphosphataemia often causes a significant fall in the calcium level.

Hyperkalaemia
This is an increased plasma potassium level, i.e. often more than 6 mmol/l in both the dog and cat (>6 mEq/l).

The situation becomes critical if potassium levels exceed 9 mmol/l (>9 mEq/l).

In the polyuric phase the potassium level falls.

Fall in total carbon dioxide content (bicarbonate)
Such a fall (with the development of acidosis) is proportional to the severity of the azotaemia.

Urinalysis
This reveals the presence of proteinuria, haematuria, casts and, in the case of ethylene glycol poisoning (anti-freeze poisoning), oxalate crystals.

POSTRENAL ACUTE RENAL FAILURE CAUSING POSTRENAL AZOTAEMIA

This can be due to complete obstruction to the outflow of urine, caused by calculi (the single most common cause), neoplasms or blood clots anywhere along the urinary tract (most commonly in the urethra; obstructions above the bladder need to be bilateral unless the kidney on the unobstructed side is already non-functional), feline urological syndrome (FUS), congenital urinary tract abnormalities, surgical ligation of both ureters (e.g. at spaying), herniation (perineal or inguinal) of the bladder, severe prostate gland enlargement or attempts at prostatectomy or drainage of an abscessed prostate gland.

Postrenal azotaemia, but *without* renal failure, is a consequence of rupture of the bladder, urethra or both ureters (or a single ureter if the non- ruptured ureter drains a non-functional kidney).

Laboratory findings

Increased plasma urea level
Values are often more than 60 mmol/l (>360 mg/dl; BUN >170 mg/dl).

Increased plasma creatinine level
Often values exceed 400 μmol/l (>4.5 mg/dl).

Normal value for the urea:creatinine ratio
The ratio is 0.08 or less if creatinine is measured in μmol/l and urea in mmol/l (43 or less if creatinine and urea are measured in mg/dl, and 20 or less if creatinine and BUN are measured in mg/dl).

Urinary specific gravity
This is variable; it can be less than 1.029 in the dog and less than 1.034 in the cat, if two-thirds of nephrons are non-functional and less than 1.012 (or at least <1.015) in the dog and less than 1.025 in the cat if three-quarters of the nephrons are non-functional.
    Animals cannot produce a dilute urine (i.e. specific gravity not usually <1.007) and progressively isosthenuria develops (specific gravity classically between 1.008 and 1.012 although it may extend to 1.007–1.015 and for a short time even be as low as 1.004).

Hyperphosphataemia
The phosphate level stays within normal limits until two-thirds of function is lost then rises, e.g. in dogs (over a year old) exceeding 1.6 mmol/l (>2.9 mEq/l). Values of more than 2.3 mmol/l (>4.1 mEq/l) in dogs more than 1 year old carry a guarded prognosis.

Potassium level
The plasma level may be elevated, i.e. >6 mmol/l (>6 mEq/l). The situation becomes critical if values exceed 9 mmol/l (>9 mEq/l).

Chronic renal failure

This condition is associated with polyuria (i.e. >50 ml urine/kg body weight per day) until the terminal oliguric phase. Causes include the following.

Chronic interstitial nephritis

This can be due to canine adenovirus-1 infection and leptospirosis.

Chronic glomerulonephritis

This condition is associated with FeLV infection, chronic viral respiratory infections, bacterial infections, systemic lupus erythematosus, pancreatitis and the dry form of feline infectious peritonitis causing granulomatous inflammation.

Chronic amyloidosis

Chronic pyelonephritis

This is associated with bacterial organisms commonly causing urinary tract infections, especially *E. coli*, *Proteus* spp., *Pseudomonas aeruginosa* and *Staphylococcus aureus*.

All of the above four conditions result in 'end-stage' kidneys.

Hypercalcaemic nephropathy

This is also known as diffuse nephrocalcinosis and results from hypercalcaemia.

Neoplasia

The most common tumours are carcinomas, nephroblastomas and lymphosarcomas (in association with FeLV infection).

Familial renal diseases

These diseases affect certain strains of certain breeds.

- The advanced stage of Fanconi's syndrome, especially in Basenjis.
- Renal cortical hypoplasia in Cocker Spaniels.
- Progressive renal diseases in Norwegian Elkhounds, Lhasa Apsos, Shih Tsus, Samoyeds, Dobermann Pinschers and Standard Poodles.
- Hydronephrosis and other lesions in Pembroke Welsh Corgis with telangiectasia.
- Renal dysplasia in Soft-coated Wheaten Terriers.
- Hereditary nephritis in Bull Terriers.
- Amyloidosis in Abyssinian cats.
- Polycystic kidneys, especially in long-haired cats, Beagles and Cairn Terriers.

Familial renal diseases are relatively rare as are the following remaining causes of CRF:

- Hydronephrosis.
- Pyonephrosis.
- Nephrolithiasis.
- Polyarteritis nodosa.
- Glomerulosclerosis due to diabetes mellitus.

Laboratory findings

Increased plasma urea level
In the dog plasma urea is more than 7 mmol/l (>40 mg/dl; BUN >20 mg/dl), and in the cat more than 11 mmol/l (>65 mg/dl; BUN >32 mg/dl).
    In both species the condition is significant when values exceed 35 mmol/l (>210 mg/dl; BUN >100 mg/dl).

Increased plasma creatinine level
In the dog and cat it is more than 130 μmol/l (>1.5 mg/dl) and is especially significant when it exceeds 250 μmol/l (>3 mg/dl).

Normal value for the urea:creatine ratio
The ratio is 0.08 or less if creatinine is measured in μmol/l and urea in mmol/l (43 or less if creatinine and urea are both measured in mg/dl, and 20 or less if creatinine and *BUN* are measured in mg/dl).

Urinary specific gravity
This is less than 1.029 in the dog and less than 1.034 in the cat if two-thirds of the nephrons are non-functional, and less than 1.012 (or at least <1.015) in the dog and often less than 1.025 in the cat if three-quarters of the nephrons are non-functional.

Animals cannot produce a dilute urine (i.e. specific gravity is not usually <1.007) and progressively isosthenuria develops (specific gravity is classically between 1.008 and 1.012, although it may extend to 1.007–1.015 and for a short time even be as low as 1.004).

Hyperphosphataemia
The phosphate level stays within normal limits until two-thirds of renal function is lost then rises, e.g. in dogs (over a year old) exceeding 1.6 mmol/l (>2.9 mEq/l). Values of more than 2.3 mmol/l (>4.1 mEq/l) in dogs more than 1 year old carries a guarded prognosis.

Calcium level
The calcium level in plasma is often maintained within the normal range but with terminal uraemia it may be increased or decreased. In renal secondary hyperparathyroidism, the increased parathyroid hormone secretion usually succeeds in keeping calcium levels normal although they may be low.

Remember

CRF can be the *result* of hypercalcaemia (see 'Causes of increased calcium', p. 368). Plasma calcium concentrations of more than 3 mmol/l (>12 mg/dl) in mature animals raise the possibility of hypercalcaemic nephropathy.

Potassium level
This is usually within normal limits in the plasma, but can be:

- Elevated with severe uraemia (<5–10% of nephrons functional) in late CRF, or with restricted sodium intake, increased gastric or intestinal losses of salt, the use of potassium-sparing diuretics or secondary to metabolic acidosis.
- Decreased in early CRF with reduced potassium intake (diet, anorexia) or excessive use of potassium-losing diuretics (e.g. frusemide=furosemide), or with prolonged vomiting.

Bicarbonate
The plasma bicarbonate (= total CO_2 capacity) is generally maintained above 19 mmol/l (= 19 mEq/l) in compensated cases, but falls with decompensation.

Sodium level
The level of plasma sodium is usually within normal limits, but there is reduced ability to modify reabsorption; *sudden* reductions in sodium intake or increased gastrointestinal losses will produce a decreased plasma sodium level; *sudden* increases in intake can cause transient hypernatraemia.

Mild–moderate non-regenerative anaemia
Normocytic/normochromic anaemia, seen in 70% of dogs (King et al., 1992), results from reduced erythropoietin secretion.

Lymphopenia
This arises from depressed lymphopoiesis.

Reduced platelet count
Thrombocytopenia is possibly due to the effect of uraemic toxins on the bone marrow.

Alkaline phosphatase activity
It can be elevated if there is renal secondary hyperparathyroidism with bone demineralization.

Amylase activity
This may be elevated because of reduced excretion and/or increased pancreatic secretion, consequent upon increased gastrin secretion.

Early warning of reduced renal function

By the time an appreciable rise in the urea and creatinine levels is evident severe renal failure is present. Earlier diagnosis of a reduction in renal function can be obtained by:

- Measuring the fractional excretion of phosphorus (Mikiciuk and Thornhill, 1989).
- Measuring the ratio of urea (or creatinine) in urine:plasma. A ratio in the range 30:1–10:1 needs further investigation; a ratio lower than 10:1 is frequently found in advanced CRF.
- Monitoring the mean daily water intake, since increased urinary output (and increased water intake) begins when approximately two-thirds of the nephrons have been lost, and at that stage the urine cannot be concentrated above a specific gravity of 1.029 in the dog or 1.034 in the cat (even following water deprivation or the injection of ADH).
- Measuring fibrinogen degradation products (FDPs) in urine, which may permit early glomerular damage to be detected (Steward and Macdougall, 1981).
- Assessing the GFR by measuring the rate of *clearance* of substances from the blood via the kidney. This technique is also valuable in monitoring the progress of cases.
- The phenolsulphonphthalein test – see below.
- Measurement of urinary γ-glutamyl transpeptidase activity – see below.

Assessing the GFR

Provided the substance chosen is neither reabsorbed nor secreted in the kidney the clearance rate (in ml/min per kg) = GFR:

$$GFR = \frac{\text{Urine concn (mg/ml)} \times \text{urine volume (ml/min)}}{\text{Plasma concn of substance (mg/ml)} \times \text{body weight (kg)}}$$

Appropriate substances are as follows.

Inulin
This is a polymer of fructose; the technique is time consuming.

Creatinine
There is very, very slight tubular secretion in the dog; it is the substance most often used in practice.

Sulphanilite
Sulphanilite clearance is an extremely sensitive test (able to detect unilateral nephrectomy) and is best suited where only a comparatively small reduction in renal function is suspected.

With inulin and creatinine a 24-hour clearance is common. All the urine for 24 hours is collected in a metabolism cage, with bladder washout before and after, and a blood sample is collected after 12 hours (i.e. at the mid-point). In normal dogs GFR ranges between 2.8 and 3.7 ml/min per kg.

Sulphanilite 10 mg/kg (5% solution) is injected intravenously and blood samples collected every 30 minutes for 1½ hours to allow the half-life of the drug to be determined (as for BSP clearance). Normal values are:

Dog: half-life = 50–80 minutes.
Cat: half-life = 30–60 minutes.

Longer times indicate a loss of renal function (Carlson and Kaneko, 1971; Greenwood and Finco, 1979).

Phenolsulphonphthalein (PSP) excretion test

The organic dye PSP is excreted via the proximal renal tubules but the test method essentially assesses renal blood flow and uses it as an index of renal function.

Table 5.2 Laboratory findings in renal disease

	Primary glomerular diseases	*Acute renal failure*			*Chronic renal failure*
		Prerenal (poor perfusion)	*Renal (primary)*	*Postrenal (obstructive)*	
Plasma					
Urea	N, ↑ later	↑	↑	↑	↑
Creatinine	N, ↑ later	↑	↑	↑	↑
Calcium	↓, N	N	↓, N, ↑	N	↓, N, ↑
Inorganic phosphate	N, ↑ later	N ↑	↑	↑	↑
Sodium	(↓), N, ↑	(↓), N, (↑)	↓, N, ↑	↓, N	N
Potassium	↓, N	N	↑, N later	↑, N later	(↓) N, ↑ later
Bicarbonate	N	↓, N	↓, N	↓, N	↓, N
Protein (total)	↓, N	(↓), N, ↑	N, ↑	N, ↑	N, ↑
Albumin	↓ [a]	(↓), N, ↑	N, ↑	N, ↑	N, ↑
Albumin:globulin ratio	↓	N	N	N	N
Plasma $\dfrac{\text{urea (mmol/l)}}{\text{creatinine (μmol/l)}}$	<0.08	>0.08	<0.08	<0.08	<0.08
Packed cell volume	N	(↓), N, ↑	(↓), N, ↑	N	↓, (N) [b]
Urine					
Specific gravity	D C } variable	D>1.025 C>1.035	D<1.029[c] C<1.034[c]	D C } variable	D<1.029[c] C<1.034[c]
Protein	++	±	±	±	±
Blood	± early	–	±	±	±
Casts	±	–	+	–	±
Urea, urine:plasma ratio	D and C >20:1 decreased later	D>30:1 C>20:1	D<10:1 C< 3:1	variable	D<10:1 C< 3:1
Creatinine, urine:plasma ratio		D>20:1 C>40:1	D< 5:1 C<15:1		D< 5:1 C<15:1

N = in normal range. ↑ = above normal range. ↓ = below normal range. ( ) = uncommon. ++ = present invariably. + = often present. ± = possibly present. D = dog. C = cat.

[a] Associated with increase in plasma cholesterol level.
[b] Often accompanied by lymphopenia, defective platelet production and abnormal platelet function.
[c] May reach isosthenuric range, 1.008–1.012.

In acute and chronic renal failure albumin and total protein levels may be raised due to dehydration, but with severe haemorrhage these (and PCV) *will* be low.

(Based on Polzin and Osborne (1986) and Ross (1986).)

The test requires the intravenous injection of PSP (6 mg in 0.1 ml of solution regardless of body weight) and collection of all the urine formed in the next 20 minutes. In normal dogs, around 45% of the PSP is excreted; less than 30% is abnormal (Finco, 1971). If the half-life of PSP is calculated in the dog, it is 18–24 minutes (Finco, 1980).

Note

The dye gives a red colour to the urine, which might be confused with haematuria.

Measurement of urinary γ-glutamyl transpeptidase (GGT) activity

The activity is used as an indicator of renal tubular damage, e.g. caused by heavy metals or aminoglycoside antibiotics.

With renal tubular necrosis (i.e. intrarenal acute renal failure) caused by gentamicin, significant increases in urinary GGT activity occurred 3–4 days before there were detectable changes in plasma creatinine, endogenous creatinine clearance, urinalysis or clinical status (Greco et al., 1985).

Chapter 6

Enzymes

Clinical enzymology

The cells of the different body organs contain particular enzymes to enable them to perform their specific functions. Some enzymes are widely distributed, others occur in high concentration only in the cells of a limited number of organs, sometimes a single one.

A small amount of all of these enzymes is normally present in the plasma, following their release from the cells either when the enzyme is being excreted or when cells are being replaced.

Finding that the plasma level of an enzyme is significantly higher than normal indicates a disorder of the organ, or organs, that contain it and to which the enzyme is normally confined. This might involve actual *destruction* (necrosis) of a substantial number of cells, resulting in their release of the enzyme, *or* a *sublethal injury* which has increased cell membrane permeability, allowing the enzyme to leak out.

At times the cells may have been induced to synthesize more enzyme than usual. Often, although not always, this occurs from the influence of a drug, and is termed 'enzyme induction'.

An increase in the amount of an enzyme is the most usual change from normal but sometimes a deficiency of cells in an organ results in a fall in the enzyme level in the plasma.

UNITS OF MEASUREMENT

Enzyme levels differ from those of other substances in that they are measured not in terms of molar concentrations or mass concentrations but rather as the amount of enzyme activity in a given volume (1 litre) of plasma (or serum). Essentially what is measured is the *rate* at which one substance (the substrate) is converted into another by the enzyme. Activity is expressed in international units (of enzyme activity) per litre, i.e. iu/l.

However, the definition of an international unit is somewhat loose; it is the amount of enzyme which will convert one micromole of substrate in one minute. If the substrate used in the method is changed, or if the incubation temperature, or the buffer, is changed then the numerical result changes also. So that what sounds like an absolutely cast iron set of units (international units/litre) turns out to vary depending upon how the estimation is performed. For some enzymes (e.g. alkaline phosphatase) many methods exist and the results obtained vary considerably (by a factor of 5 or more).

IMPORTANT NOTE

The variation in activity obtained with different methods means that in practice it is *not possible* to state 'normal' reference ranges for enzymes, because there are no absolute values; the range obtained by a particular laboratory depends entirely upon what method it uses. Consequently, in order to interpret an enzyme value from a particular laboratory it is necessary to know the normal reference range obtained by *that* laboratory using the same method (and of course for the species in question). A good laboratory, therefore, will print its normal reference range alongside the result.

For this reason *increases* in enzyme activity are best related to the upper limit of the 'normal' range (e.g. two to three times the upper limit of normal etc.)

Efforts to introduce a standard SI unit of enzyme activity, the catal, have not so far been very successful.

Some of the older enzyme methods, e.g. the King–Armstrong method for alkaline phosphatase, specified every factor involved so that *no* variation was possible and the results were expressed in specific units, e.g. King–Armstrong units (KA units). In these cases normal reference ranges *could* be stated because every laboratory would be performing the measurement in exactly the same way.

INTERFERENCE

In all photometric estimations the presence of strong colours (e.g. due to haemolysis or jaundice) or of turbidity (due to lipaemia) in the sample is unwelcome, because it can reduce light transmission leading to falsely elevated values (depending on the method). But in enzyme estimations haemolysis is *particularly undesirable* because some enzymes are present in high concentrations in the RBCs (e.g. aspartate aminotransferase (AST) and lactate dehydrogenase (LD)) and their release will cause misleadingly high values. Lipase activity, on the other hand, is severely inhibited by the presence of haemoglobin.

A good laboratory will inform the clinician about the presence of haemolysis or other features which need to be taken into account in interpreting results.

SPECIFICITY

Some enzymes are essentially organ-specific (i.e. they occur in high concentrations only in one organ, e.g. alanine aminotransferase (ALT) and ornithine carbamyltransferase (OCT) in the liver, and lipase in the pancreas) so that when high activity is found in the plasma there is no doubt about where the enzyme has come from. But some enzymes are present at a number of sites and there can be uncertainty about where they have been released. Three factors can prove helpful in coming to a decision about their site of origin.

1. The presence of clinical signs and other laboratory findings which suggest the involvement of one organ in particular.
2. Estimating the activity of other enzymes. The organs in which different enzymes are present, and enzyme concentrations within those organs, vary considerably. So, by examining a combination of enzymes, it is more likely that the organ concerned will be correctly identified.
3. Measuring the activity of a particular isoenzyme – some enzymes exist in slightly different molecular forms, although all the forms have exactly the same enzymatic effects, and these variants are known as isoenzymes. In some instances all forms of

the enzyme are present at each site (e.g. AST), but in the case of other enzymes each isoenzyme occurs at a different site, or the isoenzymes may be present in different combinations at different sites. Consequently measuring the activity of each isoenzyme separately may establish the origin of the enzyme.

Assay techniques for isoenzymes

These assays are complex, but usually involve:

- Either measurement of the individual fractions following electrophoresis or some other separation process.
- Or estimation of total enzyme activity before and after selectively inhibiting the activity of one isoenzyme so that its activity can be found by difference. This is an important area for development and one which promises to be of considerable assistance in diagnosis.

Enzymes important in small animals and which are known to exist in multiple molecular forms (isoenzymes) include aspartate aminotransferase (AST), alkaline phosphatase (ALP), creatine kinase (CK), lactate dehydrogenase (LD), γ-glutamyl transferase (GGT), acid phosphatase (ACP) and amylase.

Alanine aminotransferase (ALT)

This is also known as serum alanine aminotransferase (SALT) and was previously known as glutamic–pyruvic transaminase (GPT), or serum glutamic–pyruvic transaminase (SGPT).

NORMAL REFERENCE RANGE

This is totally dependent on the method used (see 'Important note', on p. 312).

This enzyme is essentially liver specific in the dog and cat and elevations generally indicate damage to the liver cells that has resulted in enzyme release. It is the best test to detect liver damage of those routinely available. *It is not a test of liver function.* There are no specific isoenzymes; concentrations of ALT in the heart and kidney are a quarter and a tenth of the liver concentration respectively.

Low activities have no known significance.

The degree of liver damage, causing increased ALT activity, can range from mild and reversible injury (sublethal cell injury), sufficient to permit leakage of cellular enzymes through the cell membrane but having no appreciable effect on cellular functions (as with hypoxia due to shock), to cell necrosis with a total loss of function (e.g. caused by infectious canine hepatitis). The increase in activity is roughly proportional to the *number* of cells injured and *not* to the *degree* of injury.

Slight increases in ALT activity are probably unimportant; since one of the liver's roles is detoxification it would not be unusual for it to suffer a mild degree of injury occasionally.

The half-life of ALT is variously reported both as 3 hours and as 3 days; the former seems most probable (Hall, 1985).

After an isolated incident which results in extensive liver necrosis (e.g. infectious canine hepatitis or carbon tetrachloride poisoning), ALT activity rises rapidly, peaking after 3–4 days and then declines to normal levels in 10–14 days. Consequently plasma activity can remain high for some days, despite the fact that the damage is being repaired. It seems likely that increased cell production during hepatic regeneration is responsible for this continued elevation of ALT activity. (Arginase activity on the other hand, peaks earlier and returns to normal in about 3–4 days, and therefore can provide a favourable prognosis following injury earlier than ALT activity can.)

Less extensive damage by hepatotoxins causes earlier peaking and a more rapid return to normal.

Persistent damage results in a persistence of the elevated plasma activity, as with primary neoplasia and chronic active hepatitis.

Causes of increased ALT activity

Summary

Liver damage
- Acute infectious hepatitis
- Toxic hepatitis
- Chronic active hepatitis
- Severe liver trauma
- Acute pancreatitis
- Lymphocytic cholangitis and idiopathic feline hepatic lipidosis (cat)
- Severe shock causing hypoxia
- Neoplasia
- Hepatic amyloidosis
- Secondary liver disease (mild/moderate effect)
- Portosystemic shunt (slight effect, if any)
Drug induction
Myocarditis
Fever (slight effect)

LIVER DAMAGE (HEPATOCELLULAR DAMAGE)

The extent of the rise does *not* correlate with the liver's ability to recover from the injury or to function normally. It does, however, reflect the number of hepatocytes involved in acute disease.

Persistence of high activity indicates persistence of the cause. Of course the value obtained from a single sample will not necessarily be the peak value; samples *may* have been collected when the activity was either rising or falling.

Significant rises in ALT activity are due to diseases causing inflammation or to primary neoplasia (see Panel 6.1, p. 333). A fall from a previously high level of activity may be due to depletion of the enzyme and/or a reduction in the number of cells, *rather than* to recovery.

ALT activity does *not* correlate with liver function; it indicates the number of cells affected by liver damage (both severe and irreversible, or mild and reversible) at any one time.

Acute infectious hepatitis

This can be due to viruses, bacteria, fungi and protozoa, including cholangiohepatitis and liver abscesses (see Panel 6.1, p. 333).

ALT activity is especially increased in infectious canine hepatitis and leptospirosis. Where there is necrosis the activity can increase up to 30 times the upper limit of normal.

Despite recovery values may not return to normal for 2–3 weeks.

Toxic hepatitis

This refers to hepatitis due to drugs, chemicals and biological toxins (e.g. aflatoxin and bacterial toxins in pyometra).

Examples of drugs which may be responsible include paracetamol (acetaminophen), glucocorticoids, phenytoin, phenobarbitone, primidone and mebendazole (see Table 6.2, p. 339).

Note

Drugs and chemicals can raise ALT activity by two biological effects: toxicity and enzyme induction (see 'Drug induction' later); it can be difficult to establish a clear-cut distinction between them.

In general, toxicity causes lesser increases than acute hepatic necrosis due to infection and, provided the injury does not continue, values return to normal sooner.

Chronic active hepatitis

Causes include autoimmune disorders, copper storage problems (in Bedlington Terriers and Dobermanns) and idiopathic causes.

It is characterized by persistently high ALT activities, of the order of 12 times the upper limit of normal.

Severe trauma to the liver

This occurs, for example, from road accidents or involvement in a diaphragmatic hernia.

Acute pancreatitis

Toxins from the pancreas are carried to the liver in the portal vein.

Lymphocytic cholangitis and idiopathic feline hepatic lipidosis

In both these disorders in the cat, there may be a considerable increase in activity.

Severe shock

The resultant hypoxia can affect many cells and markedly increase ALT activity, as with any other diffuse hepatocellular damage.

Neoplasia

- Primary neoplasia, e.g. carcinoma, hepatoma (and also nodular hyperplasia). Activities may be 10 times the upper limit of normal (or more), and this elevation remains fairly constant.
- Metastatic neoplasia – a rise in activity is an infrequent occurrence.

Hepatic amyloidosis

This causes progressive cell destruction with moderate/severe increases in ALT activity.

Secondary liver disease

Mild (i.e. two to three times the upper limit of normal) to moderate increases in ALT activity are associated with many endocrine disorders. The causes include:

- 'Steroid hepatopathy' (hepatomegaly and occasionally necrosis) in hyperadrenocorticism (Cushing's syndrome) and following glucocorticoid administration; some degree of enzyme induction is involved.
- Hepatic lipidosis, in hypothyroidism (although occurring inconsistently), acromegaly and diabetes mellitus in dogs and cats (especially in ketoacidotic diabetes mellitus where hypoxia and pancreatitis may, in part, be responsible).
- Hypoxia occurring in 75% of hyperthyroid cases in the cat (and in a third of cases of thyroid tumours in dogs) and ischaemia in primary hyperparathyroidism.

Increases can also be seen in cases of hyperinsulinism, phaeochromocytomas and Zollinger–Ellison syndrome.

Portosystemic shunt

Only slight, if any, increases in activity result. In the cat increases are rare.

Other non-inflammatory causes

Changes other than neoplasia and liver damage secondary to endocrine disease *seldom* produce changes in ALT activity, e.g. cirrhosis and chronic passive congestion.

Biliary obstruction causes elevations in activity only when there is associated hepatic inflammation.

DRUG INDUCTION

Drugs may induce ALT rather than cause its release by their toxicity, e.g. anticonvulsants (primidone and phenytoin), glucocorticoids, and mebendazole and thiacetarsamide.

It can, however, be difficult to distinguish the contributions made by induction and toxicity, respectively, in elevating ALT activity.

MYOCARDITIS

This can cause slight to moderate elevations in ALT activity (although cardiac muscle has a concentration of ALT only 25% of that of the liver).

FEVER [SLIGHT EFFECT]

Slight elevations in ALT activity are reported to be possible in any highly febrile condition.

Aspartate aminotransferase (AST)

Otherwise termed 'serum aspartate aminotransferase' (SAST), this was previously known as glutamic–oxaloacetic transaminase (GOT) or serum glutamic–oxaloacetic transaminase (SGOT).

NORMAL REFERENCE RANGE

This is totally dependent upon the method used (see 'Important note', p. 312).

AST occurs in a wide variety of tissues, but with high concentrations in skeletal and cardiac muscle and in the liver. The main use of the assay in dogs and cats is to assist in diagnosing muscular disorders. In the investigation of liver disease ALT is superior because it is virtually liver specific.

Damage to cells in any of the above organs causes the release of two isoenzymes, which increase plasma activity, i.e. increases in AST activity are attributable to damage to the liver, and to damage to cardiac and/or skeletal muscle.

No particular significance is attached to a low AST activity.

Causes of increased plasma AST activity

> **Summary**
> - Liver damage
> - Skeletal muscle damage
> - Cardiac muscle disorders
> - Severe exertion
>
> **Error**: haemolysis

A major problem with AST is its lack of specificity and, therefore, whenever possible other enzyme assays and/or other investigations should be performed to provide confirmation of presumptive diagnosis.

LIVER DAMAGE

All those liver disorders which result in an increased plasma ALT activity (see 'Causes of increased ALT activity', p. 313) will also raise AST activity, although the magnitude of the rise is often less. Again some drugs (e.g. anticonvulsants and oestrogens) may induce AST activity as well as increasing activity by a toxic action.

SKELETAL MUSCLE DAMAGE

All of those muscle disorders (see Panel 6.4, p. 347) which will produce increases in CK activity also increase AST activity, although usually the increase in activity is less than that of CK and is reached more slowly. Usually activity peaks after 12–24 hours and lasts for 5–6 days.

CARDIAC MUSCLE DISORDERS (CARDIOMYOPATHIES)

Cardiac ischaemia

Most cardiac diseases do not involve myocardial injury, but high levels of AST activity have been recorded with cardiac ischaemia due to:

- Bacterial endocarditis.
- Heartworm disease (dirofilariasis).
- Aortic thrombosis.
- Myocardial infarction.

Other cardiomyopathies

Lower levels of activity have been found with other cardiomyopathies, i.e. due to trauma, necrosis, degeneration or neoplasia.

Cardiac congestion

Where cardiac congestion is a feature the major contribution to the total AST activity may come from a congested liver.

SEVERE EXERTION

A doubling of AST activity immediately after racing occurs in Greyhounds (Snow et al., 1988).

ERROR: HAEMOLYSIS

There is a significant concentration of AST in the RBCs, and its release in haemolysis will therefore increase plasma AST activity.

Alkaline phosphatase (ALP)

This was previously known as serum alkaline phosphatase (SAP).

NORMAL REFERENCE RANGE

This is totally dependent upon the method used (see 'Important note', p. 312). Normal values in the cat are about a third of those in the dog.

ALP exists as a group of isoenzymes produced by the cells of a number of organs: liver (bile duct epithelial cells and hepatocytes), bone (osteoblasts), intestine, kidney and placenta. Increases in plasma activity are due to the isoenzymes derived from liver and bone; the others have half-lives of only 3–6 minutes and therefore they contribute little to the total activity.

Unlike many other enzymes, increased plasma ALP activity is the result of induction (i.e. increased synthesis) rather than increased release from damaged cells. Possibly only newly produced ALP can pass out of a cell. In the dog, two isoenzymes are derived from the liver, one of which is specifically induced by the presence of steroids and therefore termed 'steroid-induced ALP' (SIAP). However, this isoenzyme appears to be absent in cats.

In diagnosis it helps to know the source of an increase in ALP activity, and techniques are available to separate the isoenzymes and measure their individual activities, e.g. electrophoretic, immunological and chromatographic methods.

A technique for measurement of SIAP was developed at Glasgow University (Eckersall and Douglas, 1988).

Cholestasis (interference with the flow of bile), in particular, induces hepatic ALP, and a rise in ALP activity is the most sensitive indicator of cholestasis because it develops before there is any detectable increase in plasma bilirubin levels. Probably bile acids stimulate ALP synthesis.

Increases in hepatic ALP activity are also seen with hepatic necrosis and inflammation, and are induced by such drugs as barbiturates and anticonvulsants.

In the cat the half-life of this normal hepatic isoenzyme is only 6 hours – much less than in the dog (3 days), and consequently increases in activity are less marked in feline liver and biliary disorders.

The bone isoenzyme is induced by osteoblast activity and therefore the activity of ALP is greater in young, growing animals and in those disorders where growth or remodelling of bone is taking place.

AGE

In dogs and cats under 6 months of age, activity can be up to six times the upper limit of normal in adults.

Increased ALP activities are principally associated with biliary destruction and/or liver damage, the effects of steroids and certain other drugs, extensive bone disease, some cases of neoplasia and some endocrine diseases. However, increases are also seen in 'normal' animals, consistently in those that are growing, but also in pregnant queens and Greyhounds in training.

Causes of increased plasma ALP activity

Summary

Biliary obstruction (cholestasis), intra- or extrahepatic
Liver damage
Steroid induced (dog)
● Hyperadrenocorticism
● Steroid dosage
Growing animals
Extensive or generalized bone disease – hyperparathyroidism etc.
Other endocrine disorders
Neoplasia
Septicaemia/endotoxaemia
Induced by drugs other than glucocorticoids
Severe starvation
Liver regeneration
Pregnancy (cat)
Training (Greyhounds)
Diet (s/d)

The greatest increases are found with cholestasis and steroid induction.

BILIARY OBSTRUCTION

Biliary obstruction, both intra- or extrahepatic, causes cholestasis and can lead to obstructive jaundice (see 'Plasma bilirubin', p. 254).

Increases in activity relate to the degree of obstruction and can be up to 150 times the upper limit of normal in cases of complete obstruction in the dog, and up to 15 times the upper limit of normal in the cat.

Causes (which inevitably overlap) include:

- The pressure of inflamed liver cells upon the bile canaliculi.
- The pressure of space-occupying lesions such as neoplasms or abscesses (either intrahepatic or extrahepatic) upon the biliary vessels.
- Diffuse accumulation of abnormal tissue in the liver, e.g. amyloid, fibrous tissue or neoplastic tissue,
- Pyogranulomatous liver lesions with disseminated chronic infections, such as histoplasmosis (not found in the UK).
- Blockage of the bile duct by gall stones (or rarely by migrating ascarids).
- Congenital cystic disease of the biliary tree in the dog (very rare).

Bile duct rupture can also increase ALP activity.

LIVER DAMAGE (HEPATOCELLULAR DAMAGE)

CHECK – in general there will be increases in ALT, AST and GGT activities and other changes such as decreases in albumin, urea and (possibly) glucose.

In part increases in ALP activity are attributable to intrahepatic cholestasis caused by damage to the bile canaliculi, swelling of inflamed liver cells and/or fibrosis. Consequently *centrilobular* damage results in smaller rises in activity. However, increases are also due to hepatic lipidosis.

Increases are generally up to six times the upper limit of normal.

Damage may be due to the following.

Infectious diseases, including cholangiohepatitis

Rises in ALP activity are not consistent.

Toxic drugs and chemicals, and biological toxins

Those principally responsible are phosphorus, phenol, paraquat and organic solvents (see Table 6.2, p. 339). Increases in ALP activity may occur later than those of ALT and AST, and may continue to rise during recovery whilst ALT and AST activities fall.

Chronic active hepatitis

This can arise from autoimmune disease, copper storage problems (Bedlington Terriers and West Highland White Terriers) and idiopathic causes, e.g. in Skye Terriers.

Severe liver trauma

The most common cause is road accidents.

Acute pancreatitis

This results from toxins being carried to the liver in the portal vein.

Lymphocytic cholangitis and idiopathic feline hepatic lipidosis

Usually there is a considerable increase in ALP activity in these feline disorders.

Neoplasia

- Primary, e.g. with carcinomas increases are invariably present but in general they are less than 10 times the upper limit of normal, although exceptionally in the dog they can reach 50–100 times the upper limit of normal, but much less in cats.
- Metastatic – rises are not invariable and only modest.

Cirrhosis

The increase in ALP activity is due to interference with bile drainage.

Portosystemic shunts

These in general produce no, or only a slight, increase in ALP activity.

STEROID INDUCED IN DOGS

Values can take months to return to normal.

Cushing's syndrome (hyperadrenocorticism)

Increase arises both in pituitary-mediated cases and in those due to adrenal neoplasia. A marked increase is seen in 95% of dogs although *not* in cats. (See next entry.)

Glucocorticoid therapy

Ultimately, this may create iatrogenic Cushing's syndrome.

Glucocorticoids, whether endogenous (cortisol) or administered, will induce a specific isoenzyme of ALP in dogs, although not in cats (steroid-induced alkaline phosphatase – SIAP) which can now be measured separately. It is this isoenzyme which accounts for the tremendous increases in ALP activity in the dog – up to 200 times the upper limit of normal.

GROWING ANIMALS

The bone isoenzyme of ALP is found in the plasma of young growing puppies and kittens, especially the large canine breeds, and this isoenzyme makes the major contribution to total ALP activity.

Activities can reach six times the upper limit of normal due to increased osteoblastic activity (especially in the first 6–9 months of life), although usually they are much lower.

High values in young animals could therefore be normal *if* less than six times the upper limit of the normal range.

EXTENSIVE OR GENERALIZED BONE DISEASE

Increased osteoblastic activity causes mild increases in ALP activity in dogs and greater ones in cats, as in the following examples.

Hyperparathyroidism

ALP activity can be normal to increased, along with changes in calcium and inorganic phosphate levels (see Panel 7.1, p. 383). Causes include the following:

- Renal secondary hyperparathyroidism –

  CHECK   for increases in urea and creatinine levels.
- Nutritional secondary hyperparathyroidism.
- Primary hyperparathyroidism.
- Pseudohyperparathyroidism, due to non-parathyroid tumours producing parathyroid hormone or a similar secretion (chiefly lymphosarcomas and perianal/ perirectal adenocarcinomas).

Canine panosteitis

Bone tumours

Major examples are primary osteosarcomas and carcinomas metastasizing to bone from elsewhere.

Bone healing

ALP activity increases with extensive healing, e.g. of fractures.

Craniomandibular osteoarthropathy

Rickets (osteomalacia) [rare]

Radiography is important in diagnosis, along with calcium and inorganic phosphate estimations.

OTHER ENDOCRINE DISORDERS

Endocrine disorders other than hyperadrenocorticism (due to steroid-induced liver isoenzyme) and hyperparathyroidism (due to bone isoenzyme) can be associated with increased ALP activity.

Acromegaly

The increase is due to the effect of growth hormone on bone, hepatic lipidosis and/or the steroidal effect of progesterone and progestogens.

Hyperthyroidism

In over 90% of cases in cats, total ALP activity is elevated; this is probably due to an increase in the bone isoenzyme as in humans.

Thyroid tumours

Increases occur in some cases in dogs – possibly related to hypercalcaemia.

Diabetes mellitus

In diabetic dogs and cats (particularly ketoacidotic) there can be increased ALP activity related to hepatic lipidosis.

Mild increases may also be seen in hypothyroidism (inconsistent), hyperinsulinism and Zollinger–Ellison syndrome (excess gastrin secretion).

NEOPLASIA

Apart from neoplasms of the liver, biliary tree, bone and adrenal glands, increases in ALP activity are seen with mixed mammary tumours, lymphosarcomas (although these may be causing pseudohyperparathyroidism – see above), haemangiosarcomas, undifferentiated sarcomas, mast cell tumours (mastocytomas), malignant melanomas and oral carcinomas.

SEPTICAEMIA/ENDOTOXAEMIA

Mild increases in ALP activity may be seen, most probably due to liver damage (up to five times the upper limit of normal in dogs and three times the upper limit of normal in cats).

DRUG INDUCTION

An increase in ALP activity can be induced by drugs other than glucocorticoids. Such drugs include the following:

- Anticonvulsants – primidone and phenytoin – increases are 3–5 times the upper limit of normal.
- Barbiturates (e.g. with phenobarbitone increases are up to 30 times the upper limit of normal).
- Dieldrin, mebendazole, thiacetarsamide and certain antibiotics have also been reported to induce increases in activity.

There is doubt about whether drug induction occurs in the cat (Rogers and Cornelius, 1985).

SEVERE STARVATION

Any increase is associated with hepatic lipidosis.

LIVER REGENERATION

Increases in ALP activity have been reported for up to 6 weeks after partial hepatectomy.

PREGNANT QUEENS

Modest increases in ALP are probably of placental origin.

TRAINING GREYHOUNDS

ALP activity may reach twice the upper limit of normal.

PRESCRIPTION DIET s/d (HILL'S) IN DOGS

This is reported to increase ALP activity.

TRAUMA

The activity of ALP is often found to be elevated in cases of trauma (e.g. road traffic accidents).

Amylase (AMS)

This is also known as alpha-amylase (α-amylase). It is present in plasma as a number of isoenzymes (isoamylases) that are chiefly derived from the pancreas, liver and small intestine. Total plasma activity in the dog is normally much higher (5–10 times) than in humans, and most of it is of small intestinal origin. Although amylase is principally used for the diagnosis of pancreatic disorders in small animals, the activity of the pancreas-derived enzyme (pancreatic isoamylase) is normally swamped by that from other organs, principally the intestines. However, when there is massive enzyme leakage from the pancreas, due to acute inflamation, *total* activity is substantially increased.

Separation of isoenzymes by electrophoresis or selective inhibition will allow the measurement of pancreatic isoamylase alone. In humans, both the abnormally high level found in acute pancreatitis and the abnormally low level due to exocrine pancreatic insufficiency can be identified, but this is *not* the case in dogs.

NORMAL REFERENCE RANGE

This is totally dependent on the method used (see 'Important note', p. 312).

Increases in total activity are a feature of acute pancreatitis, and some cases of renal failure and intestinal obstruction.

ACCURACY

- Falsely elevated amylase levels in dogs can be obtained by using the older saccharogenic assays. The maltase normally present in canine plasma will increase the amount of glucose that is measured in the method. To avoid this error an amyloclastic method (measuring the disappearance of starch) should be used instead.
- Falsely elevated amylase levels may be due to marked haemolysis (>0.25 g haemoglobin/dl, >2.5 g haemoglobin/l) or jaundice (> 170 μmol bilirubin/l, >10 mg/dl).

Causes of increased plasma amylase activity

Summary
- Acute pancreatitis
- Renal failure (dog)
- Small intestinal obstruction
- Other alimentary disturbances
- Glucocorticoid dosage

Error: saccharogenic assay method

ACUTE PANCREATITIS

Acute pancreatitis in the dog, and also some cases of pancreatic neoplasia, abscess formation and pancreatic duct obstruction, cause an increase in amylase activity.

Values more than three times the upper limit of normal are almost certainly due to acute pancreatitis.

Values between two and three times the upper limit of normal are *likely* to be due to acute pancreatitis but could have some other cause.

Values less than twice the upper limit of normal are of uncertain origin and quite likely not to be due to acute pancreatitis.

Sometimes amylase activity is found not to be elevated (possibly because the sample is taken too late in the progress of the disease) and therefore values should be assessed in conjunction with the activity of lipase.

Increases in amylase activity have *not* been found in acute pancreatitis in the *cat*.

(Measurement of the activity of the pancreatic isoenzyme *alone* (currently not routinely available) is not valuable in confirming the origin of any increased amylase activity.)

RENAL FAILURE (i.e. URAEMIA) IN THE DOG

Hyperamylasaemia (of the order of twice the upper limit of normal) has been noted in some cases of renal failure, although by no means invariably. It may reflect reduced clearance of amylase (as for creatinine) and/or increased pancreatic secretion of amylase caused by the increased secretion of gastrin.

CHECK for increased urea and creatinine levels.

SMALL INTESTINAL OBSTRUCTION IN THE DOG

Hyperamylasaemia is a feature of dogs with small intestinal obstruction that are able to eat and subsequently vomit. Activities are usually less than twice (certainly less than three times) the upper limit of normal.

CHECK because the clinical signs of acute abdominal pain, vomiting and fever are similar to those of acute pancreatitis.

OTHER ALIMENTARY DISTURBANCES

Other conditions may possibly cause mild increases in amylase activity, e.g. perforating duodenal ulcers, intestinal infarction, intestinal torsion and abdominal trauma.

Intestinal amylase might also be responsible for unexplained increases found at times in *cats*, and previously attributed to macroamylasaemia.

GLUCOCORTICOID ADMINISTRATION

The rise in amylase activity is due to the induction of lipaemia, hyperplasia of the pancreatic ductal epithelium and the more viscous pancreatic sections. It is not a consistent feature, however, since there are also reports of *falls* in activity following corticosteroid administration.

ERROR: SACCHAROGENIC METHODS OF ASSAY

These methods will give a falsely elevated reading in the dog due to the normal presence of maltase in canine plasma.

Causes of decreased plasma amylase activity

Summary
- Exocrine pancreatic insufficiency
- Pancreatic necrosis
- Corticosteroids

EXOCRINE PANCREATIC INSUFFICIENCY (EPI) IN THE DOG

Reduced production of pancreatic isoamylase will *not* cause an appreciable decrease in the *total* activity of plasma amylase because its effect is overwhelmed by the much greater concentration of amylase from other sources, principally the small intestine. Even if the pancreatic isoamylase is measured separately the magnitude of the fall is not sufficiently consistent to allow dogs with EPI to be identified with certainty.

PANCREATIC NECROSIS [RARE]

This disorder is associated with thrombosis of pancreatic blood vessels.

CORTICOSTEROID ADMINISTRATION

However, *rises* in amylase activity have also been found to follow corticosteroid administration.

Overall, reductions in total amylase activity are of doubtful value in diagnosis.

Lipase

The major site of lipase production is the pancreas, with a smaller amount coming from the gastric mucosa. The kidney is involved in its degradation.

NORMAL REFERENCE RANGE

This is totally dependent upon the method used (see 'Important note', p. 312).

Increased levels are primarily associated with acute pancreatitis.

ACCURACY

The turbidometric method may give *falsely elevated* values where there is:

- Severe haemolysis (>0.2 g haemoglobin/dl plasma, >2.0 g/l).
- Hyperbilirubinaemia (>340 μmol bilirubin/l plasma, >20 mg/dl).

There are also reports that haemolysis *inhibits* lipase activity (Prasse, 1986) and that heparin as an anticoagulant, by activating lipoprotein lipase, will falsely elevate lipase activity (Strombeck, 1979), but neither has been substantiated. However, lipase activity *may* be *falsely elevated* by administration in vivo of heparin shortly before collection of the sample.

Causes of increased plasma lipase activity

Summary
- Acute pancreatitis and other pancreatic disorders
- Renal disorders
- Liver disease
- Glucocorticoid dosage
Error: jaundice or haemolysis

ACUTE PANCREATITIS

An increase in lipase activity occurs in some cases of pancreatic neoplasia (due to adenocarcinoma in dogs), pancreatic abscess formation and pancreatic duct obstruction.

Lipase is regarded as the better enzyme to diagnose acute pancreatitis being apparently less affected than amylase by other factors and more consistently elevated, although technically it is more difficult to estimate.

Usually increases in dogs are more than two to three times the upper limit of normal, sometimes much more. Acute pancreatitis is unlikely if lipase activity is not elevated, provided samples are collected sufficiently early in the course of the disorder.

Unlike amylase, the activity of lipase usually rises in *cats* with acute pancreatitis, although occasionally the activity may be found to be within the normal range.

RENAL DISORDERS [RARE]

Very occasionally a modest increase in lipase activity occurs with decreased renal clearance.

LIVER DISEASES [RARE]

Mild increases in activity are reported.

GLUCOCORTICOID ADMINISTRATION [RARE]

This can slightly increase lipase activity by causing induction of lipaemia, hyperplasia of the pancreatic ductal epithelium, and provoking more viscous pancreatic secretions.

ERROR: FALSE ELEVATIONS OF LIPASE ACTIVITY

These may be due to markedly icteric (jaundiced) or haemolysed samples (and possibly also if heparin has been given in vivo immediately prior to sample collection).

Creatine kinase (CK)

This is also known as creatine phosphokinase (CPK). Despite the similarity in names this enzyme has no connection with creatinine, and the presence of each is used to diagnose quite different disorders.

CK occurs as three isoenzymes located principally in skeletal muscle, cardiac muscle and the brain respectively (although each is not entirely confined to one tissue). It is used primarily for the diagnosis of skeletal muscle injuries. It has a comparatively short half-life and the modest rise in activity occurring in most cardiomyopathies goes unnoticed. There are some disorders (especially myocardial infarction) in which greater rises are customary, but these seldom develop in small animals.

NORMAL REFERENCE RANGE

This is totally dependent upon the method used (see 'Important note', p. 312). Increases are associated primarily with skeletal muscle damage and, to a lesser extent, with hypothyroidism.

ACCURACY

Falsely high values may arise due to:

- Haemolysis (>0.2 g haemoglobin/dl).
- The presence of hyperbilirubinaemia.
- The release of CK from muscle following intramuscular injection (especially with irritant drugs or solutions), difficulty in venepuncture or increased exercise (especially in untrained animals).

Increases are of the order of two to three times the upper limit of normal.

AGE

Activity in dogs under 6 months old is double that of adults. Generally, aged animals have lower values.

SEX

Male dogs are reported to have 50% more CK activity than females.

CK activity increases rapidly after muscle injury, peaking after 6–12 hours, and disappears equally quickly (within 2 days) unless the damage continues. Consequently, although CK is the most sensitive indicator of muscle damage available, delay in sample collection may result in there being no *apparent* change in activity. Persistent CK activity indicates persistence of the disorder.

The instability of CK may result in modest increases in activity not being detected in postal samples.

Causes of increased plasma CK activity

Summary
- Skeletal muscle damage
- Severe exertion
- Hypothyroidism
- CNS disorders

Error: haemolysis, jaundice, injection or (?) sample dilution

SKELETAL MUSCLE DAMAGE

Increased CK activity is a feature of skeletal muscle disorders as listed in Panel 6.4 (p. 347).

SEVERE EXERTION

A doubling of CK activity occurs *immediately* after racing in Greyhounds (Snow et al., 1988).

HYPOTHYROIDISM

A third of dogs with hypothyroidism show a *mild* increase in CK activity, because a lack of thyroid hormone reduces the rate of CK catabolism, *and* increased permeability and/or degenerative changes in the muscle fibres permit increased CK release.

CNS DISORDERS

These disorders, e.g. convulsions, can produce an increase in CK activity but as a *result* of trauma to skeletal muscles.

ERRONEOUS RESULTS

- Falsely high values may be the result of haemolysis, hyperbilirubinaemia (jaundice) or the excessive release of CK from muscle following intramuscular injections, or difficulty in venepuncture or increased exercise.
- It has been reported that dilution of plasma or serum samples during the assay reduces the concentration of natural inhibitors and can result in greatly increased CK activity.

Lactate dehydrogenase (LD or LDH)

This is also known as serum lactate dehydrogenase (SLDH). This enzyme comprises five isoenzymes, each of which occurs in a wide variety of tissues, in particular skeletal muscle, cardiac muscle, liver and RBCs, and also kidney, pancreas, bone and lung. LD_1 is also known as hydroxybutyrate dehydrogenase (HBD or HBDH).

Electrophoretic separation of the isoenzymes can help establish the source of increased activity but is seldom employed in veterinary laboratories.

Although unseparated LD is not organ specific, it has the advantage of a longer half-life than CK in the diagnosis of muscle disorders.

NORMAL REFERENCE RANGE

This is totally dependent upon the method used (see 'Important note', p. 312). Increases are chiefly associated with disorders of skeletal muscle, cardiac muscle and liver.

ACCURACY

Any haemolysis will severely distort the accuracy of results because the concentration of LD in RBCs is 150 times that in plasma. (It is possible that the RBCs are the source of 'normal' plasma LD activity, although it seems more likely that it is derived mainly from liver.) Even leaving RBCs in contact with serum or plasma for a long period is undesirable because the anoxic RBC membrane leaks LD; therefore separation of the sample is preferable.

Causes of increased plasma LD activity

Summary
- Skeletal muscle disorders
- Cardiac muscle disorders
- Liver disorders
Error: haemolysis

SKELETAL MUSCLE DISORDERS

Increased LD activity is a feature of skeletal muscle disorders, as listed in Panel 6.4 (p. 347).

CARDIAC MUSCLE DISORDERS (CARDIOMYOPATHIES)

Increased LD activity has been recorded in association with cardiac ischaemia due to such disorders as bacterial endocarditis, dirofilariasis (heartworm disease), aortic thrombosis and myocardial infarction. Lower levels of activity are associated with other types of cardiac muscle injury including trauma, necrosis, degeneration and neoplasia.

LIVER DISORDERS

Increased LD activity is a feature of liver disorders where there is damage to the cells, as listed in Table 6.1 (p. 333).

ERROR: HAEMOLYSIS

This will elevate plasma LD activity because of the high concentration of LD in the RBCs.

Since it is not organ specific LD is much less useful in diagnosis than more specific enzymes.

Other plasma enzymes

GAMMA-GLUTAMYLTRANSFERASE (GGT OR γGT)

This enzyme is also known as gamma-glutamyltranspeptidase (GTP). This enzyme has not been routinely measured in small animals. GGT has its highest concentration in the kidney (renal tubular cells) and then the liver (biliary endothelial cells and hepatocytes), but is also found in the pancreas and small intestine.

Activity seldom increases in renal disorders, probably because the enzyme is excreted in the urine, and elevations are almost solely due to liver disease and biliary obstruction (cholestasis).

A comparison of GGT with ALP and ALT shows the following.

Liver damage and biliary obstruction

In liver damage (including neoplasia) and biliary obstruction, GGT activity increases in a similar way to ALP and ALT, although:

- It is not responsive to acute toxicity (i.e. carbon tetrachloride poisoning).
- Its longer half-life means that it *may* be more valuable than ALP in the diagnosis of liver disorders in the cat.
- Some believe that it is more consistently elevated in portosystemic shunts than ALT or ALP.

A GGT/ALT ratio has been used to distinguish biliary tract disease from hepatocellular disease with a high ratio indicating the former.

Glucocorticoids and anticonvulsant drugs

It seems possible, despite some doubts, that in the dog both glucocorticoids and (as in humans) anticonvulsant drugs (phenobarbitone and primidone) induce GGT synthesis. However, any increase in GGT activity due to glucocorticoids is much less than the associated increase in ALP activity.

Bone disorders

GGT activity does not increase in bone disorders (unlike ALP); it is more specific for liver and biliary disorders.

Normal reference values

These are totally dependent upon the method used (see 'Important note', p. 312) but there is normally *zero activity* in the cat.

SORBITOL DEHYDROGENASE (SDH)

This is also known as iditol dehydrogenase. This enzyme has its highest activity in the liver and (although 50% lower) in the kidney. Increases in plasma activity appear to be liver specific, and therefore in the dog SDH could be a useful indicator of liver damage. (Its use so far has been mainly confined to horses and cattle.)

It is, however, a very unstable enzyme and not well suited to estimation in postal samples.

ARGINASE

This enzyme is liver specific in the dog but its measurement is not routinely used or readily available.

Following liver damage arginase activity peaks and returns to normal faster than that of ALT (within 3 days). Consequently, if more than 3 days after the injury both ALT and arginase activities are high the prognosis is poor, whereas if ALT activity remains high and that of arginase is normal it denotes that recovery is underway.

ORNITHINE CARBAMYLTRANSFERASE (OCT)

This is a virtually liver specific enzyme in the dog, and increases in its activity provide a sensitive measure of hepatocellular injury – at least equal to that of ALT.

However, technically the test has been more difficult to perform and therefore it has been little used in small animal medicine.

ACID PHOSPHATASE (ACP)

This enzyme consists of a number of isoenzymes in a variety of organs (spleen, kidney, liver, intestine, blood and bone) including the prostate gland. The activity of the prostatic isoenzyme is inhibited by tartrate, and therefore measurements of total activity before and after treatment of the plasma with tartrate allow the contribution from the prostate to be assessed.

Normal reference values

These are totally dependent on the method used (see 'Important note', p. 312).

Increased activity

There are indications that in the dog, as in humans, a large increase in the activity of the prostatic isoenzyme of ACP is attributable to a prostatic carcinoma, especially when it has metastasized to bone. Lesser increases have been associated with prostatitis, but either condition may be present *without* producing any alteration in ACP activity in the plasma.

The main use of ACP assays in humans is to assess the response of prostatic carcinomas to treatment in those patients in which ACP activity is initially high.

Measurements of *total* ACP activity in the dog appear unable to help in the diagnosis of prostatic disorders (Weaver, 1981).

Note

- Some prostatic carcinomas lose the ability to produce ACP; a complete absence of the prostatic isoenzyme would suggest this.
- Palpation of the prostate in the week prior to performing the assay could release enzyme, giving a slight rise in ACP activity.
- Prostatic hyperplasia causes *no* significant change in ACP activity, although levels are reported to fall after successful treatment of that condition.
- Because the enzyme is very labile, unless samples are acidified to pH 5.6–6.0 those posted are likely to give inaccurate results.

Overall ACP assay is of dubious value in small animals.

TRYPSIN

It is not easy to measure the activity of trypsin directly because anti-proteolytic substances are present in association with it to prevent autodigestion of the pancreas. But it has been possible to develop an immunological technique to assay trypsinogen, the antigenically similar precursor of trypsin found in plasma. Antibodies to canine trypsin are produced in rabbits, and then by radioimmunoassay the level of trypsinogen present in the plasma or serum of canine patients can be assessed.

Trypsin-like immunoreactivity (TLI)

Also called immunoreactive trypsin (IRT). In the dog a low concentration of plasma trypsinogen (<2.5 µg/l) has been found to correlate with the presence of exocrine pancreatic insufficiency (Williams and Batt, 1983) in *fasted* animals.

Values between 2.5 µg/l and 5.0 µg/l are not clearly low or clearly normal, and probably arise in the early stage of exocrine pancreatic insufficiency. To clarify the diagnosis in such a case the test is best repeated 3 months later.

High levels may be found in cases of acute pancreatitis (as in humans).

Panel 6.1 Liver disorders

Laboratory tests can provide information about three aspects of liver diseases:

1. Whether there has been damage to the hepatic cells (hepatocellular damage).
2. Whether there is obstruction to bile flow (cholestasis).
3. Whether there is impairment of liver function (see Table 6.1, p. 338).

Obviously these effects are interrelated, but damage does not necessarily result in a loss of function – only if a high proportion (e.g. 75%) of the liver cells are severely affected. And conversely there are diseases (e.g. portosystemic shunts, glycogen storage diseases) where liver function is abnormal but with little or no accompanying damage. Even when severe damage has taken place, provided the cause does not persist, the liver cells can usually regenerate.

Disorders producing damage most often involve inflammation; less frequently neoplasia is the cause. If extensive, both types of damage will significantly impede bile flow.

Laboratory tests involving the excretion of substances via the liver (e.g. bilirubin, BSP, bile acids) will be seriously affected by both biliary obstruction and a reduction in liver function. If such tests produce obviously abnormal results *in the absence* of evidence of liver damage (e.g. raised ALT activity), the possibility of extrahepatic obstruction should be considered (e.g. neoplasia involving the bile duct or gall bladder etc.). Complete bile duct obstruction will, of course, eventually lead to complete liver failure.

Damage to liver cells (hepatocellular damage)

This is best detected by the release of enzymes from the damaged cells. (For toxic causes see Table 6.2, p. 339.)

ALT, OCT, SDH AND ARGINASE

These enzymes are all virtually liver specific. Conventionally, ALT is the enzyme routinely measured in small animals giving relatively high peaks and persisting for a moderate amount of time (i.e. peaking after 3–4 days and remaining elevated for around 2 weeks).

Remember that high activities reflect the number of cells involved but not the severity of the damage (although often severe inflammation, for example, will involve most, if not all, cells).

GGT

This is fairly liver specific and any rise in activity persists for a long time, but it also rises with biliary obstruction.

AST

AST is less specific, although increases in activity occur in the same situations that increase ALT, but the rises are generally not so great.

ALP

This is much less specific, responding especially to biliary obstruction and, therefore, increases in activity (usually moderate) are especially related to disorders which cause cholestasis, e.g. inflammation, large tumours etc.

LD

Activity of LD increases with liver damage but is very non-specific.

Obstruction to bile flow (cholestasis)

Obstruction is chiefly intrahepatic and it may be either generalized (e.g. inflammation of the hepatocytes, or amyloidosis, causing liver swelling) or focal (e.g. tumours and abscesses).

ALP AND GGT

These are the two enzymes released in large amounts where there is interference to the flow of bile. Greater increases in activity are reported where the obstruction is *extrahepatic* rather than intrahepatic. Generally ALP is the enzyme measured, although the longer half-life of GGT in the cat may make it the preferred enzyme in that species.

TOTAL BILIRUBIN

The level increases with obstruction of the biliary tree. An equal, or more usually a higher, proportion of the total bilirubin is in the conjugated form. The greatest rises are found with extrahepatic causes, and conjugated bilirubin then accounts for more than 80% of the total.

BILE ACIDS

Both intrahepatic and extrahepatic obstruction will cause a 'damming back' of bile acids and more will appear in the plasma.

BSP CLEARANCE TEST

Obstruction will impede the excretion of BSP (sulfobromophthalein) so that in the dog more than 10% of the dose will persist after 30 minutes and the half-life will exceed 9 minutes (see Appendix I, p. 472).

URINE

This will show the presence of both:

- Bilirubin (more than a 1+ reaction in the dog, because normal dogs have a low renal threshold and small amounts of bilirubin may appear in the urine of dogs without liver disorders).
- Bile salts (Hay's test), due to failure to excrete them in the bile.

A decreased level of urinary urobilinogen would be expected, because of decreased transport of conjugated bilirubin to the duodenum for conversion to urobilinogen, but the reliability of urobilinogen testing is questionable in small animals.

FAECES

Complete obstruction will result in *pale* (white or creamy) *fatty faeces*, the consequence of inability to produce stercobilin or to digest and absorb fat.

Impaired liver function

An extensive loss of functional liver cells (>75%) will result in liver failure. This may be the consequence of severe, acute damage or simply a progressive reduction in total mass (e.g. as with cirrhosis). All functions are not necessarily impaired to the same degree and some, e.g. the failure to remove ammonia from the blood, are associated with specific disorders.

TOTAL PLASMA BILIRUBIN

With reduced hepatocellular function the total plasma bilirubin level increases, although the cells' ability to excrete bile is less affected than their ability to conjugate bilirubin. Most cases have a toxic or infectious cause and *more than 50%* of the bilirubin is conjugated. With a chronic disorder (e.g. chronic active hepatitis) conjugated and unconjugated bilirubin are often *roughly equal* in amounts.

Secondary liver damage (e.g. in endocrine disorders) rarely produces increases in plasma bilirubin, although it is a feature of up to 20% of feline cases of diabetes mellitus and hyperthyroidism.

BILE ACIDS

Reduced extraction of recirculated bile acids by the hepatocytes diverts a higher proportion of them into the circulating plasma.

BSP CLEARANCE TEST

As with bilirubin, there is reduced uptake, conjugation and secretion of BSP by the liver cells, i.e. a reduction in BSP clearance. Consequently, in the dog an increased proportion remains after 30 minutes (> 10%) and the half-life of BSP is prolonged (> 9 minutes). Likewise in the cat more than 2% of the dose remains after 30 minutes, and the half-life of BSP exceeds 5½ minutes.

PROTEIN LEVELS

Albumin

Albumin concentration may be low (<25 g/l) due to reduced synthesis and this can, if severe, also result in:

- A low total plasma protein level (<57 g/l).
- A low urea level due to reduced protein catabolism.
- A low calcium level due to reduced protein binding.

Globulins

Non-immunogenic globulins may be low, but overall globulin levels are normal or increased. Any increase represents immunoglobulin production as a response to antigens originating from the gut.

UREA

This may be low, not only due to a lowering of albumin (which in the absence of liver failure is only a marginal effect), but when there is:

- A portosystemic shunt.
- Primary hyperammonaemia (urea cycle enzyme deficiency).

Both of these defects result in an inability to convert ammonia to urea.

AMMONIA

The level will be high in cases of liver failure (i.e. acquired hepatocellular insufficiency, such as cirrhosis), portosystemic shunts and primary hyperammonaemia.

CHOLESTEROL

Cholesterol may be elevated very occasionally in primary liver disease.

Mostly increases in cholesterol are a feature of *secondary* liver diseases such as diabetes mellitus, hypothyroidism and particularly Cushing's syndrome. (Usually there is no increase in *triglycerides*, except in certain secondary liver disorders – again hypothyroidism and Cushing's syndrome, and in particular diabetes mellitus.)

In hepatic failure and with portosystemic shunts *decreased* cholesterol levels are common.

GLUCOSE

Plasma glucose levels may be low, especially after fasting or exercise, if there are:

- Congenital or acquired portosystemic shunts causing liver cells to be by-passed.
- Severe, generalized destruction of hepatocytes (e.g. as with infection, trauma, toxic drugs and chemicals or neoplasia).
- Replacement of hepatocytes by fibrous tissue.
- Glycogen storage diseases.
- Feline hepatic lipidosis (in idiopathic lipidosis, low glucose levels can follow anorexia, although becoming normal or raised later).

POTASSIUM

Hypokalaemia is common in chronic liver disease in association with respiratory and/or metabolic alkalosis.

PROTHROMBIN TIME (PT OR OSPT) AND CLOTTING TIME

Both can be increased, due to impaired synthesis of prothrombin (factor II), and deficiencies of coagulation factors I (fibrinogen), V, VII, IX and X, which are produced in the liver.

Prothrombin time can also be increased in cases of extrahepatic biliary obstruction because the lack of bile salts affects intestinal absorption of fat-soluble vitamin K.

HAEMATOLOGICAL CHANGES

Acute inflammatory conditions

The usual features of leucocytosis, neutrophilia and a shift-to-the-left are evident (and if associated with severe stress there may be a fall in eosinophils and, possibly, lymphocytes).

Chronic inflammation (cirrhosis) and chronic neoplasia

In these conditions a mild/moderate non-regenerative anaemia is common, and a frequent feature of chronic liver diseases is the presence of thin macrocytes, acanthocytes and target cells.

Other possible findings include the following.

Thrombocytopenia

This can result from increased usage of platelets (e.g. with DIC), reduced platelet production by the bone marrow (due to lack of folate and possibly vitamin B_{12}) and/or splenic sequestration, due to portal hypertension.

Table 6.1 Laboratory findings in liver disorders

Disorder	Feature*
INFLAMMATORY	
Infectious	
Infectious canine hepatitis	
Canine herpes virus infection (neonatal)	
Feline infectious peritonitis	
Pyogenic and granulomatous bacterial infection (may cause abscesses)	
Gram-negative bacterial sepsis (*Salmonella* or *Clostridium* spp.)	D predominates – especially marked with acute conditions causing necrosis
Leptospirosis	O
Tyzzer's disease (rare)	F
Cholangiohepatitis (? bacterial)	
Systemic fungal infection (e.g. histoplasmosis, blastomycosis and coccidioidomycosis)	
Parasitism (trematodes in cat, heartworms – neither in the UK)	
Non-infectious	
Toxins, drugs and chemicals (toxic hepatitis)	
Lymphocytic cholangitis (? autoimmune)	D especially marked with acute conditions
Secondary to acute pancreatitis	O
Trauma – severe	F
Copper storage disease	
Chronic active (and chronic) hepatitis	
Sequel to most of the disorders above, plus immune-mediated and idiopathic causes	D moderate/O/F
Cirrhosis (= end-stage of inflammation)	F severe/O/D seldom and mild
NON-INFLAMMATORY	
Portosystemic shunts	F severe
Primary hyperammonaemia (urea cycle deficiency)	Specific F (urea, ammonia)
Glycogen storage diseases	Specific F (glucose)
Amyloidosis	D mild/O diffuse/F
Neoplasia	D/O especially if large or diffuse/F
Idiopathic feline hepatic lipidosis	D/O/F
Hypoxia/anoxia (e.g. shock)	D mild but extensive/F
Secondary liver damage	
Endocrine (hyperthryoidism (cat), diabetes mellitus, hypothyroidism, Cushing's syndrome, hyperinsulinism)	D mild but extensive/F mild usually
Congestive heart failure	D mild/F

* The letters alongside the disorders indicate which of the three principal features of liver disorders are present: *D*amage to liver cells; *O*bstruction to bile flow; *F*unctional deficiencies (if extensive result in failure). The laboratory tests best able to diagnose these features have been described in Panel 6.1 (p. 333) but are listed below. Of necessity this table is a general summary and individual cases will be met which do not conform exactly.

Appropriate diagnostic tests

Damage to liver cells

Liver specific	⎧ ALT ⎪ OCT ⎨ SDH ⎩ Arginase	Less liver specific in order of descending specificity	↓	⎧ GGT ⎪ AST ⎨ ALP ⎩ LD

Table 6.1 (cont.)

Obstruction to bile flow

ALP	BSP clearance
GGT	Urinary bilirubin
Bilirubin	Urinary bile salts
Bile acids	

Functional deficiencies

Bilirubin	Glucose
Bile acids	Potassium
BSP clearance	Routine haematological tests
Total plasma protein	Prothrombin time
Albumin	Urinary bilirubin
Urea	Urinary bile salts
Ammonia	FDPs
Cholesterol	

Table 6.2 Substances toxic to the liver (hepatotoxins)

Drugs	*Chemicals and anaesthetics*
Phenytoin	Chloroform
Primidone	Halothane
Glucocorticoids	Methoxyflurane
Anabolic steroids	Carbon tetrachloride
Oestradiol	Phenols
Methyltestosterone	Tannic acid
Phenylbutazone	Metofane
Mebendazole	Chlorinated hydrocarbons, e.g.
Tolbutamide	chlordane, dieldrin,
Paracetamol (acetaminophen) (C)	gamma benzene hexachloride,
Phenazopyridine (C)	(BHC = lindane)
Aspirin (C)	
Thiacetarsamide	
(heartworm or lungworm therapy)	
Chlorpromazine	
Propylthiouracil	
Methimazole (C)	
Carbimazole (C)	
Tetracycline	
Erythromycin	
Trimethoprim/sulphonamide	
Flucytosine	
Antineoplastic drugs	
Cinchophen	
Dapsone	

Metals and non-metals	*Biological toxins*	*Pesticides and herbicides*
Compounds of mercury, copper, iron, arsenic, selenium, phosphorus	Aflatoxin	Paraquat
	Blue-green algae endotoxin	Chlorate
	Bacterial endotoxin	Fluoroacetate
	Amanita mushroom toxin	Metaldehyde
		Thallium
		Triazine herbicides
		Chlorphenoxy herbicides

(C) = toxic in the cat; cats are relatively deficient in the enzyme glucuronyl transferase whose function is to conjugate chemicals with glucuronic acid.

Haemorrhagic anaemia

This is consequent upon the haemorrhages due to the prolonged clotting time.

A macrocytic anaemia

This can result from folate deficiency.

URINE

Urine may show the presence of:

* Bilirubin and bile salts – inadequate removal of both in the bile results in their appearance in the urine.
* An increased level of urobilinogen would be *expected* with a *moderate* loss of liver function (i.e. not so great as to reduce the conjugation of bilirubin but severe enough to decrease its re-excretion into the bile), but unfortunately the test is *unreliable* in the dog and cat (see p. 444)
* Ammonium urate (biurate) crystals in a breed other than a Dalmatian suggests hyperammonaemia.
* Tyrosine or leucine crystals [rare] suggest grossly impaired liver function with resultant aminoaciduria.

FIBRINOGEN DEGRADATION PRODUCTS (FDPs)

These may accumulate in the blood due to their reduced clearance.

Panel 6.2 Exocrine pancreatic disorders

The three major disorders that are recognized are acute pancreatitis, exocrine pancreatic insufficiency and pancreatic neoplasia.

Acute pancreatitis

In the dog this condition usually presents as a number of recurrent 'attacks', referred to as chronic 'relapsing' pancreatitis.

LIPAEMIA

Often the sample appears markedly lipaemic, and consequently the triglyceride level is high.

AMYLASE AND LIPASE

The activity of both amylase and lipase would be expected to rise, usually to two or three times the upper limit of normal, often considerably more. Lesser increases in activity may be due to other causes (and it is valuable to check urea and creatinine levels so that renal failure can be ruled out as a possible reason). Both enzymes have short half-lives, although lipase activity stays high for longer, and the activity of both may be normal if sample collection is delayed (especially after treatment has begun or, less frequently, if samples are collected very early in the disease). Continuing high enzyme levels suggest persistent damage likely to result in chronic pancreatitis and exocrine pancreatic insufficiency.

In general lipase is regarded as the better assay to perform, and acute pancreatitis is unlikely to be present if lipase activity is not elevated in a sample collected sufficiently early.

Performing *both* enzyme tests allows more cases to be diagnosed than using either test alone (Mia et al., 1978).

Usually lipase, but *not* amylase, activity rises in cats suffering from acute pancreatitis.

Note

Severe acute pancreatitis can result in ascites. If the amylase and/or lipase activity in the ascitic fluid is greater than that in the plasma it indicates acute pancreatitis, although (more rarely) the amylase activity in ascitic fluid can be elevated due to small intestinal perforation.

TRYPSIN-LIKE IMMUNOREACTIVITY (TLI)

The TLI (= immunoreactive trypsin (IRT)) value is usually high for a short time (1–3 days), although the test will not generally be carried out to make this diagnosis.

ALANINE AMINOTRANSFERASE (ALT) AND ALKALINE PHOSPHATASE (ALP)

Activities of ALT and ALP are frequently elevated due to the effect of toxins carried to the liver in the portal vein, although often they are no more than doubled compared with the upper limit of normal.

HAEMATOLOGICAL TESTS

These will show typical responses to acute inflammation and to stress, i.e. leucocytosis (which can be very high if there is extensive infection and/or abscess formation) with a neutrophilia, shift-to-the-left, lymphopenia, eosinopenia and occasionally monocytosis (rare in the cat). Dehydration will result in an increase in PCV.

CHECK   for accompanying increases in protein levels.

If the inflammation is severe, peritonitis is a sequel. Then the demand for neutrophils can result in a low, or normal, total WBC count with a degenerative shift-to-the- left (i.e. more band forms than adult neutrophils).

GLUCOSE

The glucose level may be elevated, due to increased glucagon secretion and, in some cases, reduced insulin synthesis and release indicative of the onset of diabetes mellitus (a possible sequel to acute pancreatitis).

HYPOCALCAEMIA

This is a frequent feature of severe acute pancreatitis that appears 5–8 days after its onset; it is likely that fatty acids and calcium combine to form insoluble calcium soaps.

CHOLESTEROL

The cholesterol level is often elevated due to increases in the concentration of both high- and low-density lipoproteins.

PLASMA PROTEIN LEVELS

These may be raised due to dehydration.

CHECK   for increased PCV.

UREA

The level of urea may be mildly elevated, although without a comparable increase in creatinine, consequent upon poor renal perfusion due to dehydration.

CHECK   for increases in PCV and plasma proteins.

BILIRUBIN

Very occasionally the plasma bilirubin level rises due to bile duct obstruction associated with inflammation.

METHAEMOGLOBIN

Methaemoglobin concentration in the blood may be elevated if there is haemorrhage from the pancreas (rare), following the action of pancreatic proteases on haemoglobin and subsequent binding of haem to albumin.

Exocrine pancreatic insufficiency (EPI)

In this disorder there is a failure to secrete sufficient pancreatic enzymes for efficient digestion and absorption in the small intestine. This requires 90% or more of the normal number of acinar cells to have been destroyed or to be non-functional. This may be the consequence of repeated or persistent damage to the acinar cells (chronic pancreatitis) or, more commonly, it may follow idiopathic atrophy of the acinar cells (juvenile atrophy) – especially in German Shepherd Dogs.

TRYPSIN-LIKE IMMUNOREACTIVITY (TLI) TEST

The TLI (immunoreactive trypsin (IRT)) test produces low values, i.e. in that carried out at Liverpool and London Universities less than 2.5 μg/l in *fasted* dogs.

Values in the 'grey area' between clearly low and clearly normal values (2.5–5 μg/l) suggest an early stage of the disease and the test should be repeated 2–3 months later. (This test has replaced the PABA-peptide (= BT-PABA) test.)

PANCREATIC ISOAMYLASE ACTIVITY

Specific measurement of pancreatic isoamylase activity (i.e. the activity of that isoenzyme of amylase produced by the pancreas) in the dog appears unable to establish that there is reduced amylase secretion.

FREE FAECAL TRYPSIN [UNRELIABLE]

The activity of free faecal trypsin (as determined by the X-ray film emulsion digestion test) is useful *only* in as much as high levels indicate the *absence* of EPI.

A low level of activity, or a complete absence, *may* be due to EPI but could equally well occur in a *normal animal*, due to the rapid degradation of free faecal trypsin (producing a false negative result).

Occasionally falsely high levels of, what appears to be, trypsin are detected in dogs that have EPI. In these cases digestion of the X-ray film emulsion is attributed to bacterial proteases associated with bacterial overgrowth accompanying the EPI.

Recently, a radial enzyme diffusion method of assaying faecal proteolytic activity has been reported to be of value in the diagnosis of EPI in the cat, provided several faecal examples are examined (Williams et al., 1990).

STAINING OF A DIRECT FAECAL SMEAR

Followed by examination under the microscope, this may show evidence of undigested foodstuffs, *provided* that they are present in the diet, i.e.

- Fat globules (stained with Sudan III or IV in faeces boiled with acetic acid).
- Starch granules (stained with Lugol's iodine).
- Undigested muscle fibres, showing nuclei, striations and ragged ends.

The last requires the feeding of raw (not canned or otherwise processed) meat. The fibres are best stained with 1% eosin solution or new methylene blue stain.

THE ABSENCE OF LIPAEMIA

The absence of lipaemia in blood samples collected 1–3 hours after a fatty meal is very suspicious of exocrine pancreatic insufficiency.

IMPAIRED ABSORPTION OF FOODSTUFFS

Resultant upon impaired absorption severe cases of EPI may show *low levels* of:

- Albumin, which if severe can in turn lead to a low total plasma protein level, a low urea level (due to reduced protein catabolism) and a low calcium level (due to reduced protein binding).
- Cholesterol.
- Fat-soluble vitamins, due to impaired fat absorption, including vitamin K and in consequence leading to a prolonged prothrombin time.

OTHER TESTS

Measurements of starch digestion, oral glucose tolerance, fat (LCT) absorption (abnormal in all dogs with EPI), xylose absorption (abnormal in a quarter of dogs with

EPI) and faecal fat, generally have no advantages in the dog over those tests already described and are far more time-consuming and often subject to error. (Nonetheless, the two most useful tests, fat (LCT) absorption and xylose absorption, are described in Appendix I, p. 466.)

However, the 72-hour faecal fat assay can be helpful in *cats*, a species in which more specific tests are singularly lacking. (All the faeces passed during 72 hours on a normal commercial diet are collected, and should be stored frozen. The laboratory mixes the faeces and measures the fat content of an aliquot. The amount of fat excreted should be less than 5% of the dietary intake.)

Pancreatic neoplasia

ADENOCARCINOMAS

Adenocarcinomas are the most significant neoplasms of the acinar cells. They can produce the same clinical signs as acute pancreatitis, due to the release of enzymes causing autodigestion, although opinions are divided as to how often this occurs. Their incidence is only one-tenth that of acute pancreatitis in the dog and they are even rarer in the cat.

They *can* cause obstruction of the bile duct (leading to plasma increases in conjugated bilirubin, bile acids, ALP activity and GGT activity) and the duodenum (leading to plasma increases in bile acids and amylase). Metastasis to other organs, such as the liver and lymph nodes, will result in additional features. Signs of liver disease are reportedly very common, with the main laboratory features being increases in ALT, ALP and GGT activity, increased conjugated bilirubin and bile acid levels and, sometimes, moderate increases in amylase and lipase activity.

Also, plasma TLI concentrations are likely to be normal in dogs with exocrine pancreatic insufficiency secondary to obstruction of the pancreatic ducts by tumours.

INSULINOMAS

Insulin-secreting tumours of the beta cells ('insulinomas') are the most common neoplasms of the endocrine cells, usually resulting in a significant fall in the glucose level, a marked rise in the insulin level and an amended insulin:glucose ratio greater than 30 µU/mg (see p. 286). Other non-specific features are described in panel 8.3 (p.410).

Panel 6.3 Small intestinal disorders

Small intestinal obstruction

This can result in:

- A decreased level of *bile acids* (<1 µmol/l), if severe, both following a fast *and* 2 hours after feeding, due to reduced bile acid reabsorption.
- An increase in *amylase* activity, especially in dogs that vomit after eating.
- Also if the bile duct is obstructed at the same time the total and conjugated *bilirubin* levels and the activities of *ALP and GGT* will be elevated.

Small intestinal malabsorption

This is often, although not necessarily, accompanied by diarrhoea, one reason being that the increased osmotic pressure of the intestinal contents attracts and holds water.

ORAL GLUCOSE TOLERANCE TEST (OGTT)

This test can be used to measure absorptive capacity, but is influenced by levels of glucagon and insulin, stomach emptying and other variables which render results inconsistent. As with the xylose absorption test vomiting, or increased gut motility, alters the result. (See Appendix I, p. 470.)

XYLOSE ABSORPTION TEST

This is a better test to estimate intestinal absorption of carbohydrates, since xylose is passively absorbed in the jejunum. It is, however, also subject to error, in particular from delayed stomach emptying or the bacterial metabolism of xylose, both of which cause the xylose to enter the blood slowly and over a long period and/or to give a low peak value – just the picture also expected with malabsorption (see Appendix I, p. 471).

Xylose absorption provides a relatively crude assessment of small intestinal function; it offers *no advantages* over the simpler measurement of vitamin B_{12} and folate levels, and it is not uncommon for normal results to be obtained from dogs with intestinal disease.

In normal animals it is expected that the peak level in the plasma will occur 1–1½ hours after oral administration and will exceed 2.5 mmol/l (37.5 mg/dl). In cases of intestinal malabsorption xylose absorption occurs more slowly and the maximum value achieved is often less than 2 mmol/l (30 mg/dl).

Summary

Both the oral glucose tolerance test and the xylose absorption test are time consuming to undertake and subject to considerable error.

FOLATE AND VITAMIN B_{12} (COBALAMIN) LEVELS

The levels of these vitamins in plasma or serum are clinically much simpler to estimate.

Normal folate range is often 3.5–8.5 µg/l in the dog.
Normal cobalamin (vitamin B_{12}) range is often 200–500 ng/l in the dog.
However, these ranges can *vary* depending on the method used by the laboratory concerned.

Low concentrations indicate interference with the normal function and structure of:

- The proximal small intestine (jejunum) in the case of folate.
- The distal small intestine (ileum) in the case of cobalamin (vitamin B_{12}).

This is a feature of an enteropathy resembling chronic tropical sprue in humans.

In dogs with *bacterial overgrowth* problems (stagnant or blind loop syndrome) in the small intestine (especially German Shepherd Dogs), there is often a raised folate level due to bacterial production of folate, and/or reduced vitamin B_{12} concentration, due to its increased utilization by intestinal bacteria.

In cases of *wheat sensitivity* in dogs (Irish Setters) folate absorption, like xylose absorption, varies appreciably between individuals, being low in less than half, whilst vitamin B_{12} levels remain within normal limits.

It should be emphasized, therefore, that normal vitamin B_{12} and folate levels *do not* totally eliminate intestinal malabsorption as a diagnosis.

Note

Low plasma folate levels have been found in some cases of *colitis* in the dog, where the animal is *not* showing features that would indicate the simultaneous presence of small intestinal malabsorption.

OTHER LEVELS

Resultant upon the impaired absorption of foodstuffs severe cases may show low levels of:

- Albumin, which if severe can in turn lead to a low total plasma protein level, a low urea level (due to reduced protein catabolism) and a low calcium level (due to reduced protein binding).
- Cholesterol.
- Fat-soluble vitamins including vitamin K (due to impaired fat absorption), in consequence leading to a prolonged prothrombin time.

Note

Albumin and total plasma protein levels can be especially low with lymphosarcoma of the bowel or other protein-losing enteropathies.

HAEMATOLOGICAL FINDINGS

- Eosinophilia is seen in cases of eosinophilic enteritis.
- Lymphosarcoma of the small intestine can be associated with a non-regenerative anaemia (in half of affected dogs and a third of affected cats), an increased WBC count (in 40% of dogs and a quarter of cats), an altered number of lymphocytes (decreased in a quarter of dogs and half of cats, and increased in 20% of dogs and approximately 10% of cats), the presence of lymphoblasts (in half of dogs and a quarter of cats) and an increase in plasma calcium values (in many cases in the dog *despite* a lower total plasma protein level). (See Panel 3.1, p. 183.)
- Long-standing folate deficiency can result in a macrocytic/normochromic anaemia.
- Dehydration, with an increased PCV, may be associated with severe fluid loss due to diarrhoea if access to water is limited.

FAT (LCT) ABSORPTION TEST

This test has the potential to distinguish cases of steatorrhoea due to defective absorption of fat (long chain triglycerides, LCTs) from those due to exocrine pancreatic insufficiency or a deficiency of bile salts (see Appendix I, p. 472).

Small intestinal haemorrhage

If severe this will result in the following.

REGENERATIVE ANAEMIA

The typical features are seen of acute or, if long standing, chronic haemorrhage, i.e. a regenerative anaemia (showing polychromasia and reticulocytosis). Iron deficiency anaemia, ultimately microcytic/hypochromic, might develop long term.

Note

Gastric haemorrhage (due to ulceration or neoplasia) could produce the same effects although often a distinguishing feature is the presence of vomiting.

CHECK – gastric endoscopy would be a valuable diagnostic aid.

AN ELEVATED UREA LEVEL

This is due to increased protein catabolism, i.e. of the blood proteins.

MELAENA OR OCCULT BLOOD IN THE FAECES

Either melaena (dark sticky faeces, i.e. visible evidence of bleeding) or occult (hidden) blood may be present – the latter can be detected by a test for occult blood in faeces provided that:

- The animal is deprived of foods containing haemoglobin or myoglobin for at least 4 (preferably 7) days before testing otherwise a false positive result could occur.
- The test used is not one specific for human haemoglobin (which could cause a false negative result).

Panel 6.4 Muscular disorders

Skeletal muscle damage

Skeletal myopathies may be classified as follows.

INFLAMMATORY

- Bacterial myositis, due to pyogenic bacteria (or *Leptospira icterohaemorrhagiae* in the dog, although this organism causes mainly necrosis with little inflammation).
- Immune-mediated polymyositis (idiopathic polymyositis) in the dog.
- Toxoplasmal myositis.
- Idiopathic myositis of masticatory muscles (eosinophilic myositis) with a possible viral origin – seen especially in German Shepherd Dogs.
- Localized or generalized myositis ossificans in the cat.

TRAUMATIC

- Road accidents etc.
- Surgical procedures.
- Exertional rhabdomyolysis, especially in racing dogs and particularly those that are undertrained.
- CNS disturbances, especially convulsions.
- Intramuscular injection or difficult venepuncture, which may raise CK activity.

INHERITED OR CONGENITAL

- Irish Terrier myopathy (X-linked myopathy with myotonia).
- Hereditary myotonia in Chows.
- Myotonia and muscle hypertrophy in black Labrador Retrievers (autosomal recessive myopathy with type II fibre deficiency and myotonia in Retrievers).
- Possibly Greyhound cramp, although rhabdomyolysis is more related to trauma.

ENDOCRINE

- Cushing's syndrome (and corticosteroid administration) in the dog.
- Hypothyroidism in the dog.

METABOLIC

- Mitochondrial myopathy.
- Glycogen storage diseases.

NUTRITIONAL

Vitamin E deficiency causes a degenerative myopathy in dogs and cats.

AORTIC THROMBOEMBOLISM

This leads to ischaemia of the muscles of the hind limbs.

MYASTHENIA GRAVIS

The muscle weakness is due to an autoimmune disorder.

NEOPLASIA [RARE]

MYOPATHIES ASSOCIATED WITH INFLAMMATORY JOINT DISEASE

Damage to skeletal muscles from any of these causes results in the following changes.

Increased muscle enzyme activity

There is an increase in the activities of the three muscle enzymes AST (GOT), LD and (most specifically and dramatically) CK.

After an injury CK activity peaks after 6–12 hours and then, unless the damage persists, reverts to normal within 2 days. It is the most specific enzyme and therefore the best to measure, but being very labile activity can disappear from postal samples.

AST and LD give lower peaks rather later, but they persist longer. AST peaks after 12–24 hours and lasts for 5–6 days.

LD is much less specific, taking several days to reach peak levels and several weeks to return to normal.

Myoglobinuria

Muscle injury can result in the release of myoglobin into plasma (producing myoglobinaemia), and when its concentration there exceeds 9–12 µmol/l (= 15–20 mg/dl) it appears in the urine (myoglobinuria).

Myoglobin will react with urine test strips for blood, but can be distinguished from haemoglobin (see 'Myoglobinuria', p. 454).

Hyperkalaemia

Because of the much higher concentration of potassium in muscle cells compared with plasma, massive muscle degeneration or necrosis results in a substantial increase in the plasma potassium level.

Cardiac muscle damage

Cardiomyopathies known to produce increases in AST and LD activities are:

- particularly those which cause ischaemia, e.g. bacterial endocarditis, aortic thrombosis, myocardial infarction and heartworm disease (dirofilariasis);
- (although causing lesser increases in activity) trauma, necrosis, degeneration or neoplasia involving cardiac muscle.

However, since these enzymes are not specific for cardiomyopathies, diagnosis of particular conditions is usually made using other methods.

Chapter 7

Electrolytes and metals

Plasma sodium

SI units of measurements are millimoles per litre (mmol/l). Previous units used were milliequivalents per litre (mEq/l) or mg/dl (= mg/100 ml).

CONVERSION FACTORS

- Numerically, mmol/l are the same as mEq/l.
- To convert mg/dl to mmol/l (*or* mEq/l) multiply by 0.44.
- To convert mmol/l (*or* mEq/l) to mg/dl multiply by 2.3.

NORMAL REFERENCE RANGES

Dog: 140–155 mmol/l, *or* mEq/l (320–355 mg/dl).
Cat: 145–157 mmol/l, *or* mEq/l (335–360 mg/dl).

Sodium is present mainly in the extracellular fluid (ECF) and in large part determines the volume of the ECF and its osmotic pressure (osmolality). The level of sodium in the cells is kept low by having a cell membrane which is relatively impermeable to its entry and a 'sodium pump' which returns any sodium that does enter the ECF.

The amount of sodium in the body, and with it the amount of water, is regulated principally by the kidney, which normally maintains the plasma sodium concentration within narrow limits, despite fluctuations in dietary intake (Figure 7.1).

Increased plasma sodium levels result from increased sodium intake, excessive water loss or decreased water intake.

Conversely, decreased plasma sodium levels are due to increased sodium loss, overhydration or to the relative overhydration which follows a reduction in renal perfusion.

ACCURACY

Hyperlipidaemia and hyperproteinaemia will result in *falsely low* plasma sodium levels. This is because in these conditions a high proportion of the plasma is occupied by excessive amounts of lipid or protein respectively. Since the sodium is present only in the aqueous fraction, its concentration in the total plasma will appear to be lower, i.e. it will be diluted by the lipid or protein.

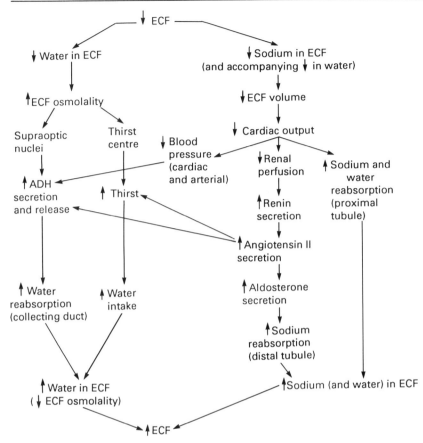

Figure 7.1 Mechanisms for regulating the osmolality and the volume of extracellular fluid (ECF). Exchanging ↑ and ↓ throughout will permit the converse of the above situations to be examined.

Causes of increased plasma sodium levels (hypernatraemia)

Summary

Increased sodium intake
Excessive fluid loss
- Vomiting, diarrhoea, evaporation giving moderate dehydration
- Diabetes mellitus (occasionally)
- Hyperadrenocorticism
- Other polyuric disorders (occasionally)
- Peritoneal dialysis with hypertonic solutions
- High protein diets
Inadequate water intake
- Water unavailable
- Inability to drink
- Osmoreceptor defects [rare]
Extreme exercise

> **Note**
>
> In the dog, a statistically significant increase in the sodium concentration of *serum* compared with that of *plasma* has been recorded (but did not correlate with the number of platelets or WBCs).

INCREASED SODIUM INTAKE

This will be exacerbated by inadequate water intake, including lack of access to water. It may arise from:

- A highly salted diet.
- Salt administration (e.g. to stimulate water intake, or to provoke vomiting in the treatment of poisoning).
- Drinking seawater.
- The administration of sodium-containing intravenous fluids (e.g. sodium bicarbonate solution or isotonic saline solution) where the need is to replace only a loss of water.
- Primary hypoaldosteronism [extremely rare].

EXCESSIVE FLUID LOSS

This is where fluid losses are in excess of sodium losses, which implies restricted water intake. This can result from the following.

Vomiting, diarrhoea and increased water evaporation

The latter is associated with panting (e.g. heatstroke, fever, hyperventilation) – sufficient to produce *moderate* dehydration.

Diabetes mellitus

Hypernatraemia is found, however, in only 8% of ketoacidotic dogs. In hyperosmolar non-ketotic diabetes mellitus [rare], the sodium concentration is variable but increases with developing hyperosmolality.

Hyperadrenocorticism (Cushing's syndrome)

A mild increase (i.e. usually *not* severe) occurs in 50% of canine cases (not due to the action of mineralocorticoids).

Other polyuric disorders

These occasionally result in hypernatraemia, especially diabetes insipidus, and also pyometra, where dehydration occurs because water intake cannot keep pace with water loss through the kidney; the effect may be compounded by vomiting etc.

Peritoneal dialysis

When hypertonic dextrose solutions are used, it causes a marked diuresis.

High protein diets

Their use causes a marked urea-induced diuresis.

INADEQUATE WATER INTAKE ALONE

Water not being provided or proving insufficient

Inability to drink

This may occur where animals are injured (including CNS damage and localized pharyngeal problems), comatosed, debilitated, or have protracted recovery from general anaesthesia.

Osmoreceptor defects[rare]

With such defects thirst is not manifest.

EXTREME MUSCULAR ACTIVITY

The plasma sodium level increases immediately after racing in Greyhounds. It is presumed that, in order to maintain membrane potential, sodium is actively transferred out of the muscle cells.

Causes of decreased plasma sodium levels (hyponatraemia)

Summary

Increased sodium loss
- Severe diarrhoea/vomiting giving severe dehydration
- End-stage chronic renal failure
- Addison's disease
- Diuretic therapy
- Osmotic diuresis

Overhydration
- Psychogenic polydipsia
- Acute renal failure (polyuric phase)
- Intravenous fluids (with low, or no, sodium)
- Inappropriate (i.e. increased) ADH secretion [rare]

Relative overhydration
- Increased blood pressure
- Decreased colloid osmotic pressure
- Following injury

Error: pseudohyponatraemia

A deficient intake of sodium alone, i.e. a low salt diet, is unlikely to result in hyponatraemia, but it is often a critical factor where there are increased sodium losses.

INCREASED LOSS OF SODIUM

Severe diarrhoea/vomiting

This results in severe dehydration (if sodium is not replaced).

Initially, a normal concentration of sodium in the ECF is maintained by allowing a corresponding loss of water to occur; consequently, the volume of the ECF falls.

However, this is not allowed to continue beyond a certain point; eventually the fall in ECF volume, cardiac output and blood pressure triggers increases in ADH secretion and in thirst, and water is replaced and conserved. Further sodium losses result in hyponatraemia at the expense of defending the ECF volume.

CHECK   for increases in PCV and total plasma protein.

End-stage chronic renal failure

Sodium excretion can be adjusted in response to its intake in moderate renal failure. But with the onset of the *terminal* stage of renal failure, sodium excretion tends to remain high and is less easily adapted to changes in the intake or loss of sodium. Consequently, relatively minor dehydration (caused by the accompanying vomiting and/or diarrhoea) is likely to result in hyponatraemia.

CHECK   for increased plasma levels of urea, creatinine and inorganic phosphate.

Primary hypoadrenocorticism (Addison's disease)

The reduced aldosterone secretion by the adrenal cortex adversely affects sodium and water conservation in the distal tubule. Whether ECF volume and sodium concentration can be maintained within the normal range depends upon whether sodium and water replacement is adequate.

In most instances the fall in ECF volume is relatively slight and successfully countered by increases in thirst and ADH secretion, but the plasma sodium level tends to fall. Sixty per cent of dogs and 100% of cats with this disorder show hyponatraemia.

A sodium:potassium ratio of less than 27:1 is considered indicative of this disorder, although it does *not* occur in *every* case.

If the water lost is not replaced the resultant dehydration can in part mask the fall in the sodium level.

CHECK   for eosinophilia, lymphocytosis and a mild increase in plasma urea without an associated increase in plasma creatinine, i.e. due to reduced renal perfusion.

Diuretic therapy

'Loop' diuretics (frusemide (furosemide) and ethacrynic acid) inhibit active reabsorption of sodium in the ascending limb of the loop of Henle. Benzothiadiazine derivatives (e.g. chlorothiazide) act mainly in the convoluted part of the distal tubule to block sodium reabsorption. Aldosterone antagonists (e.g. spironolactone) limit sodium in the distal tubule by competing with aldosterone for receptor sites.

Without adequate sodium replacement hyponatraemia can result.

Osmotic diuresis

Diabetes mellitus

In diabetes mellitus, especially the more advanced ketoacidotic stage, the hyperglycaemia draws water into the plasma from the cells and expands the ECF volume, diluting the sodium concentration.

Furthermore, the excess of glucose (and ketones) induces an osmotic diuresis resulting in increased urinary sodium losses.

Two-thirds of dogs with ketoacidotic diabetes mellitus show hyponatraemia.

Use of hypertonic dextrose and mannitol solutions

Following the use of hypertonic dextrose and mannitol solutions (10–20%) for the treatment of renal failure and of cerebral oedema, the same effects are seen as in diabetes mellitus (see above).

OVERHYDRATION

Pyschogenic polydipsia

Long term this *may* result in hyponatraemia following overdilution of the plasma due to the excessive water intake.

CHECK for very low urinary specific gravity (<1.007 and often much less), which can increase dramatically on water deprivation.

Polyuric phase

In the polyuric phase of acute renal failure an animal can drink excessively causing hyponatraemia and hypokalaemia.

Intravenous fluids

With intravenous fluids, i.e. with the administration of sodium-free or low sodium solutions (e.g. 0.45% saline solution *or* isotonic (5%) dextrose solution).

Inappropriate (i.e. increased) ADH secretion [rare]

This condition has been reported in the dog with heartworm disease (but might be anticipated in malignant neoplasia, as in humans). Uncontrolled ADH secretion induces excessive water retention with a consequent dilution of sodium.

RELATIVE OVERHYDRATION

This can follow decreased renal perfusion arising in association with oedema (including ascites and hydrothorax) due to the following effects.

Increased blood pressure

For example, from congestive cardiac failure.

Decreased colloid osmotic pressure

This is due to hypoalbuminaemia (see 'Causes of decreased plasma albumin levels', p. 252), e.g. with the nephrotic syndrome or cirrhosis.

The movement of fluid from the plasma to the extravascular compartment reduces blood volume and renal perfusion. The response is increased secretion of renin and then angiotensin II, which stimulates aldosterone output (causing retention of sodium and water) and also stimulates ADH secretion and thirst (which result in water retention).

Overall, both sodium and water levels are increased but there is a *relative excess of water* causing hyponatraemia.

Following injury

Salt retention is not as great as water retention, leading to dilutional hyponatraemia.

ERROR: PSEUDOHYPONATRAEMIA

This can be due to:

- Hyperlipidaemia (lipaemia).
- Hyperproteinaemia (extreme), e.g. due to multiple myeloma.

In these conditions a high proportion of the plasma (or serum) sample is occupied by the excess lipid or protein, but the sodium is only present in the aqueous fraction. Consequently, the level of sodium will appear lower than normal due to 'dilution' with the lipid or protein.

Plasma potassium

SI units of measurement are millimoles per litre (mmol/l). Previous units used were milliequivalents per litre (mEq/l) *or* mg/dl (= mg/100 ml).

CONVERSION FACTORS

- Numerically, mmol/l are the same as mEq/l.
- To convert mg/dl to mmol/l (or mEq/l) multiply by 0.26.
- To convert mmol/l (or mEq/l) to mg/dl multiply by 3.9.

NORMAL REFERENCE RANGE

Dog: 3.6–5.8 mmol/l or mEq/l (14–22.5 mg/dl).
Cat: 3.6–5.5 mmol/l or mEq/l (14–21.5 mg/dl).

Only 2% of the body's potassium is in the extracellular fluid (ECF), the rest being confined to the cells (intracellular fluid, ICF) and kept there by 'potassium pumps' in cell membranes.

The plasma level of potassium can change with:

- The intake of potassium.
- The loss of potassium (most of which takes place through the kidney, but which can also occur via the gastrointestinal tract).
- The movement of potassium between the cells and the ECF.

Any of these factors may be increased or decreased.

The hormone aldosterone promotes potassium excretion by the kidney, and insulin promotes a shift of potassium from the ECF into the cells.

The main causes of increased potassium levels are acidosis, hypoadrenocorticism, oliguric renal failure (essentially acute renal failure) and massive tissue damage. The main cause of decreased potassium levels is an increased loss by vomiting or diarrhoea, or through the kidney due to diuretics or a polyuric disorder.

Causes of increased plasma potassium levels (hyperkalaemia)

Summary

Reduced potassium excretion
- Hypoadrenocorticism
- Spironolactone dosage
- Low sodium intake
- Oliguric phase of renal failure (chiefly ARF)
- Bladder rupture

Redistribution of potassium from ICF to ECF
- Acidosis (especially metabolic)
- Hyperosmolality of plasma
- Extensive tissue damage
- Thrombocytosis (affecting *serum*)
- Drug action

Rapid/excessive potassium administration

Error: pseudohyperkalaemia (haemolysis)

In almost all cases hyperkalaemia arises from the *diminished ability to excrete potassium*.

ECG abnormalities usually become apparent above 7 mmol/l and death from cardiac arrest supervenes around 10–12 mmol/l.

REDUCED EXCRETION

Hypoadrenocorticism (e.g. Addison's disease)

Reduced aldosterone production is responsible for a decrease in the exchange of potassium for sodium in the distal tubule of the kidney and consequent potassium retention. In addition the reduced output of cortisol interferes with the efficiency of the 'potassium pump', allowing potassium to pass from the cells into the ECF.

These two factors may serve to increase the plasma potassium level to the point at which there is obvious interference with cardiac rhythm.

Combined with a fall in the plasma sodium level, this increase in potassium can produce a clinically significant sodium:potassium ratio of less than 27:1, although this is *not* an invariable finding.

Spironolactone

Prolonged use of the diuretic spironolactone, which is an aldosterone antagonist, results in potassium retention.

Low sodium intake

Animals on low sodium diets (e.g. for congestive cardiac failure) tend to be hyperkalaemic. This is probably due to insufficient sodium ions being delivered to the kidney distal tubule for ionic exchange.

The oliguric phase of renal failure

Chiefly this occurs in acute renal failure (ARF) (see Panel 5.2, p. 299) and the site of the problem may be:

- Intrarenal, i.e. tubular damage due to acute interstitial nephritis (e.g. leptospirosis) or acute tubular necrosis (due to nephrotoxins or ischaemia).
- Postrenal involving obstruction of the urinary outflow. Above the bladder such an obstruction must be bilateral (unusual), unless the unobstructed kidney is already severely diseased. Usually it affects the bladder neck or urethra, e.g. pressure of a tumour, obstruction by a calculus or the feline urological syndrome (FUS).
- In addition, the accompanying metabolic acidosis promotes movement of potassium out of cells into the ECF.

Potassium retention also occurs, although infrequently, in the terminal (oliguric) phase of *chronic* renal failure (CRF); in CRF it is almost always a *terminal* event.

Bladder rupture

This is usually due to road traffic accidents or other trauma.
   Renal failure does not develop but the animal is unable to eliminate waste products in the urine, including excess potassium.

REDISTRIBUTION OF POTASSIUM, i.e. FROM ICF TO ECF

Acidosis (especially metabolic acidosis) [most common cause]

The exchange of excess hydrogen ions in the ECF for potassium ions from the ICF inevitably raises the plasma potassium level. The effect is increased by dehydration.

CHECK   for increased PCV and plasma proteins.

Causes include:

- Acute and chronic renal failure.
- Respiratory acidosis due to decreased pulmonary ventilation or depression of the respiratory centre (e.g. by drugs).
- Lactic acidosis due to tissue hypoxia or liver failure.

Note

In chronic diarrhoea and diabetic ketoacidosis the increased renal loss of potassium is often *more* than the amount released from the ICF, so that the plasma potassium level generally stays *within* or falls *below* the 'normal' range.

Hyperosmolality of plasma

This can cause the passage of potassium from the cells to the ECF. This hyperosmolality can result from:

- Hypertonic mannitol or saline given intravenously.
- Hyperosmolar non-ketotic diabetes mellitus, thereby contributing to the elevated potassium levels seen in such cases.

Extensive tissue damage

Massive crush injuries or necrosis from some other cause – especially involving muscle – release a large amount of potassium from cells (see 'Pseudohyperkalaemia').

Thrombocytosis

This affects serum only. The release of intracellular fluid from platelets during blood clotting is believed to be the cause of the increased potassium content of *serum* found in dogs with thrombocytosis. (There is no similar increase in the level of potassium in plasma.)

Drug action

Some drugs release potassium from the cells into the ECF, e.g. digitalis and succinylcholine.

Note

Theoretically hypoinsulinism (type I diabetes mellitus) should cause a raised plasma potassium level because the lack of insulin limits the movement of potassium into cells, e.g. after a meal. In practice the renal loss of potassium more than outweighs this effect.

RAPID/EXCESSIVE POTASSIUM ADMINISTRATION

The rapid injection of a large dose of a potassium salt intravenously (e.g. potassium benzylpenicillin) will raise the plasma level suddenly, often to a dangerous degree.

Excessive oral administration of potassium may exceed the capacity of the kidneys to excrete it.

ERROR: PSEUDOHYPERKALAEMIA

In general, extensive haemolysis does *not* significantly raise the plasma potassium level in the dog and the cat, because the amount of potassium in their RBCs is similar to that in plasma. The situation is quite different in humans where haemolysis causes a marked elevation of the plasma (or serum) potassium level, referred to as *pseudohyperkalaemia*.

The exception to this rule is provided by some members of the Akita breed of dog which have a much higher RBC content (65–75 mmol/l) compared with normal (3.5–5.5 mmol/l). Consequently high plasma potassium levels result from haemolysis, or even leakage from the RBCs during prolonged blood storage. No link has been found between this trait and age or sex, or the presence of microcytosis – another RBC anomaly of Akitas.

Causes of decreased plasma potassium levels (hypokalaemia)

Summary

Decreased potassium intake
Increased potassium loss
- Chronic diarrhoea/vomiting
- Diuretic therapy
- Excess mineralocorticoid therapy
- Excess bicarbonate/lactate therapy
- Chronic liver disease
- Cushing's syndrome (and prolonged steroid dosage)
- Diabetes mellitus (occasionally)
- Polyuric phase of acute renal failure
- Fanconi's syndrome
- Other polyuric disorders
Shift of potassium from ECF to ICF
- Insulin therapy
- Alkalosis
- Recovery after severe trauma, e.g. crush injury
Error: pseudohypokalaemia

Hypokalaemia is a major cause of neuromuscular disorders in cats. It is characterized by persistent ventral flexion of the neck and referred to as feline hypokalaemic polymyopathy.

DECREASED INTAKE

This occurs, for example:

- In chronically anorexic animals that continue to drink, or are given low potassium intravenous fluids and maintain normal hydration, because potassium excretion continues normally for a time.
- In partially or totally anorexic cats receiving fluid therapy with potassium-free fluids after the relief of obstruction due to FUS.
- Possibly in association with malabsorption or intestinal obstruction.

INCREASED POTASSIUM LOSS

Chronic diarrhoea and chronic vomiting[common]

- With *diarrhoea* the loss of potassium in the faeces is considerable.
- With *vomiting* there is some loss of potassium in the gastric juice, but a greater amount is lost through the kidneys. This is because the loss of hydrogen ions creates an alkalosis, and a consequent exchange of potassium ions for hydrogen ions in the renal tubules. (In addition this metabolic alkalosis results in potassium being re-distributed from the ECF (including the plasma) to within the cells.)

In both conditions dehydration (hypovolaemia) will provoke aldosterone secretion and potassium losses via the kidney.

Diuretic therapy

The continued use of potassium-losing diuretics (e.g. frusemide (furosemide) and the benzothiadiazine derivatives, such as chlorothiazide) will result in hypokalaemia, but the contraction of the ECF produced by *any* diuretic stimulates aldosterone release and a resultant increase in potassium excretion.

Mineralocorticoid excess

Excessive mineralocorticoid therapy, e.g. with fludrocortisone, as well as the rare disorder hyperaldosteronism (*or* primary mineralocorticoid excess), promotes potassium excretion and will cause hypokalaemia.

Excessive bicarbonate/lactate therapy

This will produce a metabolic alkalosis, resulting in increased excretion of potassium because of the exchange of potassium and hydrogen ions in the renal tubules, plus redistribution of the potassium from the ECF to the ICF.

Chronic liver disease

There is often an associated alkalosis producing low potassium levels by the mechanisms described above. It may consist of a respiratory alkalosis (resulting from hyperventilation, probably due to stimulation of the respiratory centre) and a metabolic alkalosis caused by an accumulation of bicarbonate or a loss of acid, plus hyperaldosteronism following reduction of the ECF volume.

Cushing's syndrome (and prolonged, high-dose glucocorticoid administration)

A mild decrease in potassium is seen in about one-half of dogs with Cushing's syndrome, and is made worse by anorexia, vomiting or diarrhoea.

Diabetes mellitus

Dehydration, by stimulating aldosterone secretion, can result in increased potassium losses, and this is compounded by the diuresis caused by incomplete glucose reabsorption.

In addition, in ketoacidotic diabetes mellitus the metabolic acidosis, lack of insulin and increased plasma osmolality conspire to cause a shift of potassium from ICF to ECF with accelerated losses via the kidney.

Plasma potassium levels can *occasionally* be high in diabetes mellitus, but are more often normal or low.

Polyuric phase of acute renal failure

In this phase an animal can drink excessively causing hypokalaemia and hyponatraemia.

Fanconi's syndrome

This can result in hypokalaemia due to defective (i.e. reduced) renal tubular reabsorption, and also amino acids, glucose and inorganic phosphate are imperfectly reabsorbed.

Other polyuric disorders

These may produce potassium depletion due to hypovolaemia triggering increased aldosterone secretion and increasing renal losses of potassium, e.g. with diabetes mellitus or chronic renal failure.

SHIFT OF POTASSIUM FROM ECF TO ICF

Insulin therapy

Insulin stimulates the rapid uptake of potassium by cells and can cause hypokalaemia.

Alkalosis

This can be metabolic or respiratory.

Metabolic
Chronic vomiting, chronic liver disease and excessive bicarbonate therapy can cause the redistribution of potassium as well as increased losses (see above).

Respiratory
This can arise, for example, in pneumonia, pleural effusion and with hyperventilation (e.g. associated with chronic liver disease).

Recovery after severe trauma, e.g. crush injury

Restoration of cell function following a moderately severe crush injury can quickly deplete the ECF of potassium, reversing hyperkalaemia, and lead to hypokalaemia.

> **Note**
>
> Paradoxically, hypokalaemia may be noted immediately after trauma in some cases. The effect has been attributed to collagen taking up the released potassium.

ERROR: PSEUDOHYPOKALAEMIA

This can be due to:

- Hyperlipidaemia (lipaemia).
- Hyperproteinaemia (extreme), e.g. due to multiple myeloma.

In these conditions, a high proportion of the plasma (or serum) is occupied by the excess of lipid or protein, but the potassium is only present in the aqueous fraction. The level of potassium appears lower because of this 'dilution'.

Plasma chloride

SI units of measurement are millimoles per litre (mmol/l), which are *numerically equal* to those of the previously used units, milliequivalents per litre (mEq/l).
Some previous values were measured in mg/dl (=mg/100 ml).

CONVERSION FACTORS

- To convert mg/dl to mmol/l (or mEq/l) multiply by 0.29.
- To convert mmol/l (or mEq/l) to mg/dl multiply by 3.5.

In general *relative* increases in the concentrations of the two major anions, chloride and bicarbonate, occur at the expense of each other. Consequently high chloride concentrations are associated with bicarbonate lack (as in metabolic acidosis) and low chloride concentrations are associated with bicarbonate excess (as in metabolic alkalosis).

If there is no change in acid–base balance chloride concentrations generally reflect those of sodium.

NORMAL REFERENCE RANGE

Dog: 100–120 mmol/l (100–120 mEq/l = 350–420 mg/dl).
Cat: 115–130 mmol/l (115–130 mEq/l = 405–455 mg/dl).

Causes of increased plasma chloride levels (hyperchloraemia)

> **Summary**
>
> - Metabolic acidosis (uncompensated or partially compensated)
> - Conditions causing increased sodium levels
> - Ammonium chloride therapy

METABOLIC ACIDOSIS (UNCOMPENSATED OR PARTIALLY COMPENSATED)

- Diarrhoea.
- Shock.
- Renal failure.
- Fanconi's syndrome [rare].
- Ketoacidotic diabetes mellitus.
- Poisoning with ethylene glycol or metaldehyde.
- Excessive use of carbonic anhydrase inhibitors.
- Severe muscular exertion.

CONDITIONS WHICH INCREASE PLASMA SODIUM LEVELS

For these see 'Causes of increased plasma sodium levels', p. 351. Examples are:

- Increased sodium intake, e.g. in the diet or in intravenous fluid therapy.
- Excessive loss of water relative to loss of sodium.
- Reduced intake of water, e.g. water deprivation or inability to drink.

THERAPY WITH AMMONIUM CHLORIDE

For example, as a urinary acidifier.

Causes of decreased plasma chloride levels (hypochloraemia)

Summary
- Metabolic alkalosis
- Conditions causing decreased sodium levels
- Chloride-losing diuretics

METABOLIC ALKALOSIS

This is caused especially by vomiting immediately following eating – a loss of hydrochloric acid occurs and produces a loss of chloride without significant sodium loss.

CONDITIONS WHICH GIVE RISE TO DECREASED SODIUM LEVELS

For these see 'Causes of decreased plasma sodium levels', p. 353. These comprise:
- Increased sodium loss.
- Absolute overhydration.
- Relative overhydration.

DIURETICS WHICH INCREASE CHLORIDE LOSSES THROUGH THE KIDNEY

Examples are chlorothiazide, frusemide (furosemide) and ethacrynic acid.

Total carbon dioxide content (bicarbonate) in plasma

SI units of measurements are millimoles per litre (mmol/l), which are *numerically equal* to the previously used units, milliequivalents per litre (mEq/l).

NORMAL REFERENCE RANGE

Dog and cat: 17–24 mmol/l (17–24 mEq/l).

Essentially the total carbon dioxide content is the same as the *bicarbonate* content. The technique for measurement involves mixing the sample with a strong acid and measuring the carbon dioxide released. Most of it is derived from bicarbonate, a small amount coming from dissolved carbonic and carbamino acids.

Total carbon dioxide content is a stable constituent which can be measured quite satisfactorily in serum or plasma without the need for special collection or storage of the sample.

It is a useful measurement in establishing whether or not acidosis or alkalosis is present and, if so, how severe it is.

Causes of increased total carbon dioxide content (bicarbonate) in plasma

Summary
- Metabolic alkalosis
- Respiratory acidosis (partially compensated)
- Bicarbonate therapy

METABOLIC ALKALOSIS

Uncompensated or partially compensated metabolic alkalosis can both produce significant increases; moderate 27–32 mmol/l and severe >32 mmol/l.

Vomiting

This leads to a loss of hydrochloric acid which is almost invariably the cause of a metabolic alkalosis. Loss of hydrochloric acid results in a net increase in bicarbonate ions.

Excessive potassium loss associated with hypovolaemia

See 'Causes of decreased plasma potassium levels', p. 360.

Diuretics causing increased chloride losses

Examples are chlorothiazide, frusemide (furosemide) and ethacrynic acid.

RESPIRATORY ACIDOSIS (PARTIALLY COMPENSATED)

There is a mild increase in total carbon dioxide content, i.e. 24–29 mmol/l. If uncompensated, values are in the normal range.

Respiratory acidosis occurs with hypoventilation, e.g. anaesthesia, sedation, trauma to the head, severe pneumonia, pneumothorax, airway obstruction, severe pleural effusion and muscle weakness (myasthenia gravis, tetanus and the use of muscle relaxants, e.g. succinylcholine), i.e. there is interference with the control of ventilation and with the mechanics of getting gases to and from the lungs.

BICARBONATE THERAPY

Increased bicarbonate results from excessive use of antacids.

Causes of decreased total carbon dioxide content (bicarbonate) in plasma

Summary
- Metabolic acidosis
- Hydrogen ion intake
- Respiratory alkalosis (partially compensated)
Error: delay in processing

METABOLIC ACIDOSIS

Both uncompensated and partially compensated metabolic acidosis produce significant decreases in total carbon dioxide content, e.g. moderate = 12–17 mmol/l, severe <12 mmol/l. It may be the result of:

- Diarrhoea – fluids rich in bicarbonate are lost.
- Shock due to reduced tissue perfusion (e.g. following severe haemorrhage).
- Renal failure due to accumulation of uraemic acids; likely to occur earlier in chronic renal failure in the cat than in the dog.
- Fanconi's syndrome [rare].
- Ketoacidotic diabetes mellitus, with accumulation of acidic ketones (although acidosis is absent or only moderate in hyperosmolar non-ketotic diabetes mellitus).
- Poisoning with ethylene glycol or metaldehyde, because their metabolites are acidic.
- Excessive use of carbonic anhydrase inhibitors; these cause excessive bicarbonate losses.
- Severe muscular exertion. e.g. in status epilepticus. Immediately after racing, Greyhounds show a marked fall in plasma bicarbonate because it moves intracellularly to buffer the hydrogen ions formed from lactic acid.
- Addison's disease – mild to moderate acidosis is due to impaired hydrogen ion excretion.

HYDROGEN ION INTAKE [RARE]

This includes dosing with acidic compounds such as vinegar, or corrosive poisoning with strong acids (e.g. battery acid).

RESPIRATORY ALKALOSIS [UNUSUAL]

This can occur if partially compensated (which is unlikely). It results from hyperventilation, e.g. in heatstroke, fever, hepatic encephalopathy, fear/anxiety, convulsions, the use of a ventilator and too rapid correction of metabolic acidosis.

Compensated respiratory alkalosis will produce normal values.

ERROR: MARKED DELAY IN SAMPLE PROCESSING

This is an artefact.

Plasma calcium

Calcium is usually measured and reported as *total* calcium, which consists of three fractions:

1. Ionized calcium – the biologically active portion (50% of the total).
2. Protein-bound calcium, bound mainly to albumin (40%).
3. Calcium chelated with anions, e.g. phosphate and citrate (10%).

The last two fractions (above) are biologically inactive and they may be reduced in amount, reducing the total calcium level, without producing any ill effect.

SI units of measurement are millimoles per litre (mmol/l). Previous units used were milliequivalents per litre (mEq/l) *or* mg/dl (= mg/100 ml).

CONVERSION FACTORS

To make the following conversions multiply by the appropriate number.

To convert to	From mmol/l	From mEq/l	From mg/dl
mmol/l	–	0.5	0.25
mEq/l	2	–	0.5
mg/dl	4	2	–

NORMAL REFERENCE RANGE

Dog: 2–3 mmol/l (= 4–6 mEq/l = 8–12 mg/dl), and most frequently within the range 2.2–2.7 mmol/l. Values in the upper part of the range are usual in young dogs.

Cat: 1.8–3 mmol/l (= 3.6–6 mEq/l = 7.2–12 mg/dl).

ACCURACY

Falsely elevated calcium values can occur with lipaemia because the turbidity interferes with its measurement. Acidosis increases the ionized plasma calcium value, and alkalosis decreases it. Low plasma protein values (especially those of albumin) will reduce the protein-bound fraction and the total calcium level *without* reducing the ionized fraction.

With hyperproteinaemia and hyperalbuminaemia (and therefore with dehydration) the total calcium level *may* increase because the calcium-carrying capacity of the plasma (i.e. the protein-bound fraction) can increase.

Detergent residues on analytical glassware may increase or decrease calcium values.

SOURCE

As a major constituent of bone (and teeth) calcium plays a vital role in the the structure of the body, but also has important physiological functions involving the transmission of nerve impulses, the permeability and excitability of all membranes and the activation of enzyme systems, e.g. blood clotting (calcium is clotting factor IV). Calcium is absorbed from the small intestine and excreted by the kidney with bone acting as a reservoir.

Its concentration in the plasma is regulated by:

- Parathyroid hormone, which exercises fine control, increasing calcium levels.
- Calcitonin, which exercises coarse control to reduce high calcium levels, e.g. after meals.
- Vitamin D_3 required (in any form) for the reabsorption of calcium from bone and (as active D_3) for the absorption of calcium from the small intestine.

Causes of increased plasma calcium levels (hypercalcaemia)

Summary

- Pseudohyperparathyroidism [most common] – due to non-parathyroid malignant tumours
- Primary hyperparathyroidism – usually parathyroid tumours
- Osteolytic bone tumours
- Non-neoplastic lysis of bone
- Hypervitaminosis D
- Chronic renal failure
- Acute renal failure
- Hypoadrenocorticism [occasionally]
- Diffuse osteoporosis
- Hyperproteinaemia and/or hyperalbuminaemia
- Dehydration
- Status epilepticus
- Rare causes – hypothermia, hypocalcitoninism, hypervitaminosis A, hypothyroidism, hyperthyroidism, reaction to vitamin D

Errors:
- Administration of calcium intravenously
- Lipaemia
- Detergent residues
- EDTA effect [rare]

Increased plasma calcium levels, in both the dog and cat, are those that are more than 3 mmol/l (>6 mEq/l, >12 mg/dl).

Signs of hypercalcaemia include anorexia, depression, vomiting, generalized muscle weakness, polyuria and polydipsia. Dehydration and damage to the renal tubules (nephrocalcinosis) can lead to renal failure and cardiac arrhythmias.

A hypercalcaemic *crisis* develops with calcium levels above 3.75–5 mmol/l (7.5–10 mEq/l = 15–20 mg/dl) which can prove fatal.

Note

A high total calcium level can overcome the effect of anticoagulants, e.g. EDTA, and result in the clotting of blood samples.

PSEUDOHYPERPARATHYROIDISM [MOST COMMON]

This is due to non-parathyroid malignant neoplasms that produce a variety of secretions, in particular parathyroid hormone (parathormone), a parathormone-like polypeptide, prostaglandin E_2 and an osteoclast-activating factor. These substances cause osteolysis, resulting in a marked rise in the plasma calcium level and a reciprocal fall in the plasma inorganic phosphate level. There is no metastasis to bony tissue in this condition.

The tumours involved are:

- Lymphosarcomas, responsible for the majority of cases in the dog; in fact many dogs with lymphosarcomas show an elevated calcium level, whereas few cats do (see Panel 3.1, p. 183).

- Apocrine gland adenocarcinomas of the anal sacs.
- Adenocarcinomas elsewhere, e.g. the mammary gland, stomach, thyroid gland, nasal chambers and pancreas etc.
- Possibly prostatic adenocarcinomas, as in humans.
- Myleoproliferative disorders [unusual].

Where there is difficulty in establishing the presence of a lymphosarcoma, or other tumour, to account for hypercalcaemia (e.g. by radiography, biopsy etc.), the effect of glucocorticoids in high dosage should be assessed; a fall in the calcium level to within the normal range strongly suggests that neoplasia *is* responsible.

PRIMARY HYPERPARATHYROIDISM

This is more likely in older animals. The parathyroid glands are:

- Either hyperplastic (more than two of them).
- Or one or more must have developed a functional adenoma or, less often, an adenocarcinoma, of the chief cells.

There is a marked increase in the level of calcium and a fall in that of inorganic phosphate.

OSTEOLYTIC BONE TUMOURS

Osteolysis results from disruption of the bone by the invading neoplastic cells and the release of factors which stimulate osteoclast activity. Tumours can be either primary, i.e. osteosarcoma [uncommon], or metastatic, with extensive bone infiltration, e.g. metastasis from:

- Mammary adenocarcinoma [most common].
- Prostatic adenocarcinoma.
- Squamous cell carcinoma.
- Fibrosarcoma.
- Lymphosarcoma (plasma calcium level is high but plasma inorganic phosphate ranges from normal to elevated).
- Multiple myeloma – in addition to increased amounts of ionized calcium there may be extensive calcium binding to the increased quantity of globulin, producing a high total calcium value.

NON-NEOPLASTIC LYSIS OF BONE

The most common cause is osteomyelitis due to the septic infection of bone, usually with staphylococci. This may be associated with puppy septicaemia (part of the fading puppy syndrome).

Rarely fungal osteomyelitis occurs, e.g. associated with blastomycosis.

HYPERVITAMINOSIS D

This can result from:

- Calciferol poisoning (a rodenticide).
- Excessive supplementation of the diet with calcium.
- Plant toxicity, e.g. eating jasmine *Cestrum diurum*, which contains the active metabolite of vitamin D in high concentration.

With hypervitaminosis D *both* calcium and phosphate levels are increased.

CHRONIC RENAL FAILURE

Five to ten per cent of canine cases of chronic renal failure show increased calcium levels, due to decreased renal excretion, failure of the renal tubules to break down parathyroid hormone, increased calcium–citrate complexing and an exaggerated response to vitamin D increasing calcium absorption in the intestines.

Hypercalcaemia is a variable feature of familial nephropathies (e.g. in Cocker Spaniels, Lhasa Apsos, Shih Tsus, Standard Poodles and Norwegian Elkhounds).

Hypercalcaemia may also arise following the rapid lowering of phosphate levels using aluminium hydroxide therapy.

ACUTE RENAL FAILURE (PRIMARY RENAL DISEASE)

Hypercalcaemia has been noted at the start of the diuretic phase, presumed due to the sudden mobilization of calcium deposited in the soft tissues during the oliguric phase. The phenomenon is temporary and resolves spontaneously.

HYPOADRENOCORTICISM [OCCASIONALLY]

Hypercalcaemia is especially likely in an addisonian crisis. Indications are that the increase is in the non-ionized fraction of the plasma calcium and that ionized calcium remains within normal limits.

It is thought to follow increased tubular reabsorption of calcium and it is noted in 25–60% of canine cases of hypoadrenocorticism.

DIFFUSE OSTEOPOROSIS

This may follow long-term immobilization, resulting from neurological or musculoskeletal damage. There is continual bone resorption with the laying down of only minimal amounts of new bone.

HYPERPROTEINAEMIA AND/OR HYPERALBUMINAEMIA

These conditions increase the calcium-carrying capacity of the plasma, and so the protein-bound calcium fraction may increase and thereby increase the total calcium concentration slightly.

DEHYDRATION (HAEMOCONCENTRATION)

Most dehydrated animals *do not* develop hypercalcaemia, but the relative increase in protein levels can increase the calcium-carrying capacity (see above) and produce a slight increase in total values.

STATUS EPILEPTICUS

This disorder raises the plasma calcium level.

OTHER [RARE] CAUSES

- Severe hypothermia – the cause is unknown.
- Hypocalcitoninism – associated with extensive thyroid gland destruction.
- Exaggerated reaction to vitamin D in chronic granulomatous disorders, e.g. blastomycosis.
- Hypervitaminosis A.

- Hypothyroidism.
- Hyperthryoidism.

ERRORS

Administration of intravenous calcium salts

The administration of, for example, calcium gluconate or calcium borogluconate, during or just prior to collecting the blood sample, particularly if blood samples are taken from the same intravenous cannula or from the same vein at some other point.

Lipaemia

The increased turbidity of the sample can elevate the value obtained by autoanalysers.

Detergents

Residues of some detergents on glassware or plasticware falsely increase the calcium value (although other detergents decrease it).

EDTA [UNLIKELY]

EDTA can falsely elevate calcium values obtained by atomic absorption spectro-photometry.

Causes of decreased total plasma calcium levels (hypocalcaemia)

Summary

Severe hypocalcaemia (with clinical signs)
- Eclampsia
- Hypoparathyroidism
- Ethylene glycol (anti-freeze) poisoning

Mild hypocalcaemia
- Renal secondary hyperparathyroidism
- Nutritional secondary hyperparathyroidism
- Phosphate-containing enemas
- Acute pancreatitis
- Decreased plasma albumin
- Malabsorption
- Calcium-deficient diets
- Acute renal failure (especially postrenal)
- Medullary carcinoma of the thyroid
- Neoplasia
- Soft tissue trauma
- Glucocorticold therapy

Errors:
- Calcium-binding anticoagulants
- Haemolysis
- Intravenous fluid expansion of vascular space
- Detergent residues

Decreased plasma calcium levels are those in the dog that are less than 2 mmol/l (<4 mEq/l, <8 mg/dl) and in the cat less than 1.8 mmol/l (<3.6 mEq/l, <7.2 mg/dl).

A fall in total plasma calcium will not be clinically significant (resulting in hypocalcaemic signs) unless it involves a fall in the ionized (biologically active) fraction. It may simply represent a reduction in the protein-bound fraction (e.g. in conditions with low albumin levels). Since the ionized fraction is seldom measured independently, it is generally not possible to know for certain whether the ionized fraction *is* abnormally low. However, in the dog hypocalcaemic signs do not arise until the total calcium level is less than 1.7 mmol/l and often not above 1.25 mmol/l unless the ionized calcium level is disproportionately low. (Formulae have been devised to correct for low albumin levels – see below.)

Early, milder signs of hypocalcaemia include anorexia, weakness, vomiting, polyuria/polydipsia, hyperaesthesia and (in dogs) aggressiveness. Later there are muscle tremors (focal or generalized) causing ataxia and progressing to tetanic spasms and seizures. Significant hypocalcaemia results in bradycardia (and a prolonged Q–T interval on an ECG trace).

SEVERE HYPOCALCAEMIA WITH CLINICAL SIGNS

Eclampsia (puerperal tetany) [common]

This occurs in bitches (particularly small breeds and especially those with large litters) from late pregnancy to a month after weaning, usually 3 weeks after parturition.

The demand for calcium for lactation on top of the requirements for fetal bone formation exceeds the amount which can be supplied by the diet plus that mobilized from bone. Other factors (e.g. systemic alkalosis, stress etc.) probably also play a part.

The condition also occurs, although less often, in lactating queens.

Hypoparathyroidism [uncommon]

The causes include the following.

Idiopathic
This is probably due to:

* Either an autoimmune reaction (most cases) resulting in lymphocytic parathyroiditis.
* Or the lack of an enzyme required in parathyroid hormone synthesis.

Extensive parathyroidectomy
Parathyroidectomy generally needs to be bilateral; the same effect is produced by removal of the parathyroid blood supply. Such damage usually occurs inadvertently when performing a thyroidectomy (e.g. in treatment of feline hyperthyroidism); clinical signs usually appear within 3 days of surgery and generally hypertrophy of accessory parathyroid tissue occurs later and assumes the parathyroid's role (so calcium therapy is usually needed for only 2–6 weeks).

Extensive parathyroid destruction
This occurs, for example, with neoplasia, or following canine distemper (with virus particles in the chief cells).

Atrophy
This can be the result of previous prolonged *hyper*calcaemia arising from the increased dietary intake of calcium.

Ethylene glycol (anti-freeze) poisoning

Ethylene glycol is metabolized to oxalate which combines with calcium ions to form calcium oxalate monohydrate, the crystals of which are responsible for acute tubular necrosis (intrarenal acute renal failure). The hypocalcaemia can give rise to tetany.

CHECK for increases in urea and creatinine, calcium oxalate monohydrate crystals in the urine, oliguria and isosthenuria.

MILD HYPOCALCAEMIA

Renal secondary hyperparathyroidism in chronic renal failure

See Panel 5.2 (p. 299) for more detail.

The reduced glomerular filtration rate, combined with continual phosphate release from protein catabolism, produces an elevated plasma inorganic phosphate level and a reciprocal fall in calcium concentration. Renal damage also decreases the conversion of vitamin D_3 to its active form, reducing the intestinal absorption of calcium.

The consequent increase in parathormone secretion, provoked by the hypocalcaemia, is an attempt to restore the calcium level, chiefly by demineralization of bone, and it is frequently able to return the plasma calcium to within, or just below, the normal range. Acidosis raises the level of ionized calcium thus mitigating the fall.

CHECK for increased urea and creatinine levels, increased inorganic phosphate, a mild fall in PCV and isosthenuria.

Nutritional secondary hyperparathyroidism (juvenile osteoporosis)

This condition is seen in puppies and kittens during the period of rapid bone growth (3–12 months in puppies), and especially in the larger canine breeds. It is due to a marked relative imbalance of calcium (low) and phosphorus (high) in the diet caused by feeding large quantities of meat and/or offal. It is also especially common in Siamese and Burmese kittens, because they tend to be fed on high meat diets with little or no milk, and they also have large litters so that individual kittens have poor calcium reserves.

As the plasma inorganic phosphate level rises so that of calcium falls, stimulating the release of parathyroid hormone, which is usually effective in restoring the calcium level to just within, or just below, the lower limit of normal.

Phosphate-containing enemas (especially in cats)

These enemas are hypertonic sodium phosphate solutions and, following colonic absorption of the phosphate, there is a reciprocal fall in the level of calcium and the development of hypocalcaemic signs, including tetany, in cats and small dogs (and children). Signs appear within ½–1 hour of giving the enema.

Acute pancreatitis (in about half of the dogs with that disorder)

Fatty acids, released following the liberation of lipase, combine with calcium to form insoluble calcium soaps. The calcium depletion of the plasma can create a hypocalcaemia.

CHECK for increased amylase and lipase activities, increased WBC count with neutrophilia and shift-to-the-left.

Decreased plasma albumin level

This can occur, for example, due to impaired liver function, primary glomerular disease, severe malabsorption etc. (see 'Causes of decreased plasma albumin levels', p. 252).

A lack of albumin reduces the amount of calcium that can be protein bound. This has no clinical significance, since the biologically active fraction (ionized calcium) is unaffected, but it will give a low *total* calcium level. Typically, signs of hypocalcaemia are *absent*.

However, in some disorders characterized by a loss of albumin (principally primary glomerular diseases), there may be a fall in the level of ionized calcium also, due to an accompanying loss of the binding protein for active vitamin D_3.

Formulae have been proposed which will correct for low protein levels; one employs the albumin value and the other the total protein value (Finco, 1983).

Using albumin value

$$\text{Corrected Ca}^{2+} \text{ (mmol/l)} = \text{Measured Ca}^{2+} \text{ (mmol/l)} - \frac{\text{Albumin (g/l)}}{40} + 0.875$$

or

$$\text{Corrected Ca}^{2+} \text{ (mg/dl)} = \text{Measured Ca}^{2+} \text{ (mg/dl)} - \text{Albumin (g/dl)} + 3.5$$

Using total plasma protein (TPP) value

$$\text{Corrected Ca}^{2+} \text{ (mmol/l)} = \text{Measured Ca}^{2+} \text{ (mmol/l)} - [0.01 \times \text{TPP(g/l)}] + 0.825$$

or

$$\text{Corrected Ca}^{2+} \text{ (mg/dl)} = \text{Measured Ca}^{2+} \text{ (mg/dl)} - [0.4 \times \text{TPP(g/dl)}] + 3.3$$

Malabsorption

Hypocalcaemia could follow:

* Reduced absorption of protein, causing hypoalbuminaemia (see above).
* Malabsorption of vitamin D.
* Malabsorption of calcium that is complexed in the lumen of the intestine with fatty acids and proteins.

All of the above may occur in malabsorptive disorders, e.g. in lymphangiectasia, and conspire to produce hypocalcaemia.

Also cereal diets high in phytates interfere with calcium absorption, and calcium absorption is poor in cases of prolonged diarrhoea with increased gut motility.

Calcium-deficient diets

Some foodstuffs, e.g. meat, offal, grain, fruit, nuts, are deficient in calcium but normally a low calcium diet *alone* would not cause hypocalcaemia, unless given long term. Calcium loss might then exceed calcium absorption.

Calcium/phosphate imbalance usually results in borderline calcium values (see above).

Acute renal failure

Decreased plasma calcium levels may occur especially when the failure is postrenal (urethral obstruction), e.g. hypocalcaemia is present in half the cats with feline urological syndrome.

The sudden inability to excrete phosphate that follows the onset of acute renal failure, particularly urethral obstruction, causes a substantial rise in plasma inorganic phosphate leading, as in other disorders, to a corresponding fall in the level of calcium. However, the acidosis of renal failure raises the level of ionized calcium and therefore the overall fall in calcium level causes no adverse clinical signs.

Medullary (C cell) carcinoma of the thyroid [rare]

This results in secretion of excessive amounts of calcitonin (hypercalcitoninism) and lowering of the plasma calcium level.

Neoplasia

The following types of neoplasia may be associated with hypocalcaemia.

Parathyroid neoplasms

- Malignant neoplasia may cause extensive parathyroid destruction causing hypocalcaemia.
- There may be single or multiple adenomas causing oversecretion of parathyroid hormone and *hypercalcaemia*. Subsequent surgical removal of these provokes a rapid fall in the parathyroid hormone level (its half-life is 20 minutes) and in the calcium level; within 12–24 hours in animals with overt bone disease there may be hypocalcaemic tetany.
- Also excessive palpation of a functional chief cell adenoma responsible for primary hyperparathyroidism has resulted in infarction of the tumour and consequent hypocalcaemia.

Thyroid tumours causing hyperthyroidism

These are especially likely to occur in the cat. Hypocalcaemia develops because:

- Higher thyroid hormone levels can increase bone resorption inducing a decrease in parathyroid hormone secretion. As a result, the gastrointestinal absorption of calcium is reduced and excretion of calcium in urine and faeces can increase producing normal or low calcium levels.
- There may be increased calcitonin secretion by the thyroid.

Around one in five of hyperthyroid cats is hypocalcaemic.

Osteoblastic metastases of a bone tumour

In humans such tumours have caused hypocalcaemia by rapidly depleting the plasma of calcium in order to utilize it in bone formation.

Gastrinomas

In the Zollinger–Ellison syndrome in dogs, a hypocalcaemia may result either from the excessive gastrin secretion, stimulating C cell hyperplasia and calcitonin secretion, *or* from a concurrent hypoalbuminaemia.

Soft tissue trauma [rare] (Chew and Meuten, 1982)

Glucocorticoid therapy

This increases calcium excretion by the kidney and inhibits vitamin D_3 thereby inhibiting calcium absorption. Calcium levels fall rapidly following the administration of glucocorticoids.

ERRORS

Calcium-binding anticoagulants

EDTA, citrate and oxalate (in the fluoride–oxalate mixture used for glucose estimations) are all anticoagulants that work by combining with calcium, thereby preventing its essential participation in the clotting process.

Calcium levels measured in blood samples collected using one of these anticoagulants, rather than heparin, will be *abnormally low*. (A blood donation containing an excessive amount of citrate might conceivably result in hypocalcaemia in the recipient of the transfusion.)

Haemolysis

This can occur, for example, due to delayed separation of serum or plasma, and may produce an artefactual hypocalcaemia.

Expansion of the total vascular space

Expansion by large amounts of intravenous fluid can lower the total plasma calcium level.

Residues of some detergents

Such residues on glass or plastic vessels can falsely decrease calcium levels (although other detergents can cause an increase).

Note

1. *Alkalosis* decreases the ionized fraction of the plasma calcium and animals may show signs of hypocalcaemia *although* the *total* calcium remains within normal limits. This may follow the intravenous administration of excessive amounts of bicarbonate.
2. Conditions in humans known to result in hypocalcaemia but which have not so far been recorded in dogs or cats include:
   (a) pseudohypoparathyroidism – a familial disease in which target tissues are resistant to parathyroid hormone;
   (b) hypomagnesaemia – by reducing the production or release of parathyroid hormone or causing resistance to its actions;
   (c) chemotherapy for leukaemia, by releasing large amounts of inorganic phosphate from damaged cells;
   (d) anticonvulsant therapy;
   (e) *some* metastatic bone tumours (with marked osteoblastic activity) which deplete the plasma of calcium by incorporating it in bone.

Plasma inorganic phosphate

SI units of measurement are millimoles per litre (mmol/l). Previous units used were mEq/l, or mg/dl (= mg/100 ml).

Conversion factors

To convert from one set of units to another multiply by the figures below:

To convert to	From mmol/l	From mEq/l	From mg/dl
mmol/l	–	0.56	0.32
mEq/l	1.8	–	0.58
mg/dl	3.1	1.7	–

NORMAL REFERENCE RANGE

Dog: 0.8–1.6 mmol/l (= 1.4–2.9 mEq/l = 2.5–5 mg/dl). In dogs under 1 year of age
   the 'normal' range is doubled, i.e. 1.6–3.2 mmol/l (= 2.9–5.8 mEq/l =
   5–10 mg/dl).
Cat: 1.3–2.6 mmol/l (= 2.3–4.7 mEq/l = 4–8 mg/dl). In cats under 1 year of age the
   range is the same.

SOURCE

Inorganic phosphate is derived from the diet, especially meat and dairy products. It is
a major constituent of bone and teeth, and a vital cellular constituent, playing
important roles in the storage, release and transfer of energy and in acid–base
metabolism.
   Phosphate homoeostasis is regulated largely by parathyroid hormone which
promotes phosphate release from bone and phosphate excretion by the kidney.

ACCURACY

Haemolysis will falsely elevate phosphate values. Low phosphate levels may be due to
the use of oral phosphate-binding agents, primary or pseudohyperparathyroidism, or
glucocorticoids (either endogenous or administered).
   Increased phosphate values occur in young dogs. Otherwise chronic renal failure or
an osteolytic bone tumour are probable causes and, less commonly, hypoparathyroidism or hypervitaminosis D.
   Feline hyperthyroidism is also an important cause of hyperphosphataemia.

Causes of increased plasma inorganic phosphate levels (hyperphosphataemia)

> **Summary**
>
> - Age (dogs under 1 year old)
> - High phosphate diets
> - Renal failure
> - Bladder rupture
> - Hypervitaminosis D
> - Hypoparathyroidism
> - Osteolytic bone tumours
> - Hyperthyroidism (cats)
> - Hypoadrenocorticism in cats [rare]
> - Acromegaly in bitches [mild]
>
> **Error**: haemolysis

In adult animals with a clearly low calcium level hypoparathyroidism is strongly
suggested.
   With normal to slightly low calcium levels chronic renal failure is probable or, in the
cat, hyperthyroidism.
   With elevated calcium levels and increased urea/creatinine values hypercalcaemia as
either the cause or the consequence of chronic renal failure is probable.
   Where the calcium level is elevated and urea/creatinine levels are 'normal' an
osteolytic bone tumour, or (less often) hypervitaminosis D, should be considered.

AGE

Values in young dogs (<1 year old) are higher. In puppies phosphate concentrations can be up to 3.2 mmol/l (= 5.8 mEq/l = 10 mg/dl). The average level at 6 months of age is 2.3 mmol/l (= 4.1 mEq/l = 7.3 mg/dl).

Levels gradually fall with age reaching adult values at 9–12 months old.

In kittens the effect of age is less, and the normal range is essentially the same as for adults.

HIGH PHOSPHATE DIETS

These include a diet rich in meat and offal. There is a serious relative lack of calcium and excess phosphate in these foods which leads to nutritional secondary hyperparathyroidism in kittens and puppies.

However, the consequent release of increased amounts of parathyroid hormone results in the phosphate level being adjusted to within or near the normal range, provided renal function is normal, i.e. phosphate values are usually just above or just below the upper limit of normal. With some renal dysfunction they will be higher.

RENAL FAILURE [COMMON]

The reduced ability of the kidney to excrete phosphate in cases of chronic renal failure and acute renal failure (especially intrarenal and postrenal, e.g. feline urological syndrome) inevitably results in its accumulation in the plasma. It is a feature of familial renal diseases, e.g. Fanconi's syndrome in the Basenji, renal cortical hypoplasia in Cocker Spaniels and nephropathies in Dobermann Pinschers, Soft-coated Wheaten Terriers and Abyssinian cats.

One long-term consequence seen in chronic renal failure is a reciprocal fall in the plasma calcium concentration in most cases, which stimulates parathyroid hormone secretion and thereby the demineralization of bone (renal secondary hyperparathyroidism). This mechanism often successfully restores calcium levels to normal (or near normal) but also releases yet more phosphate into the plasma. However, in 5–10% of renal failure cases calcium levels are *elevated* (see 'Causes of increased plasma calcium levels', p. 368).

BLADDER RUPTURE

This results in the retention of urine, and the waste products it contains, within the peritoneal cavity. The consequent failure to excrete phosphate ions causes an elevated plasma inorganic phosphate level.

HYPERVITAMINOSIS D

As well as increasing the calcium level, that of phosphate is also raised. Possible causes are:

• Excessive dietary supplementation.
• Calciferol poisoning.
• Plant toxicity, increasing vitamin D uptake (e.g. eating jasmine).

HYPOPARATHYROIDISM (= PRIMARY HYPOPARATHYROIDISM)

Deficient parathyroid hormone production results in increased tubular reabsorption of phosphate and a consequent high plasma phosphate level.

OSTEOLYTIC BONE TUMOURS

The invading neoplastic cells, and the release of factors stimulating osteoclast activity, result in osteolysis. The tumours may be:

- Primary, i.e. osteosarcoma (uncommon).
- Metastatic with extensive bone infiltration, e.g. mammary adenocarcinoma (the most common), prostatic adenocarcinoma, squamous cell carcinoma, fibrosarcoma, lymphosarcoma or multiple myeloma.

HYPERTHYROIDISM (IN CATS)

Fifty per cent of cats show an increased plasma phosphate concentration, probably involving increased calcium release from bone (due to the effect of thyroid hormone) with consequent decreased parathyroid hormone production and increased renal reabsorption of phosphate.

HYPOADRENOCORTICISM (IN CATS)

A vast majority of the small number of reported cases showed an elevated plasma phosphate concentration.

ACROMEGALY IN THE BITCH

This can cause a mild increase in inorganic phosphate.

ERROR: HAEMOLYSIS

Haemolysis will falsely elevate plasma phosphate values.

Causes of decreased plasma inorganic phosphate levels (hypophosphataemia)

Summary

- Malabsorption (oral phosphate binding agents)
- Hypovitaminosis D [unusual]
- Primary hyperparathyroidism
- Pseudohyperparathyroidism
- Diuresis
- Fanconi's syndrome
- Glucocorticoid therapy
- Cushing's syndrome
- Rickets and osteomalacia
- Diabetes mellitus [rare]
- Severe liver disease [rare]
- Pituitary dwarfism [rare]

This is an unusual laboratory finding, being most probably due to the administration of oral phosphate binding agents, the administration or endogenous release of glucocorticoids, or primary or pseudohyperparathyroidism.

Hypophosphataemia can result in extravascular haemolytic anaemia (see p. 106).

MALABSORPTION

Poor absorption of phosphate is generally due to the use of oral phosphate binding agents (e.g. aluminium hydroxide); less commonly it is due to low phosphate diets or general starvation.

HYPOVITAMINOSIS D [UNUSUAL]

Hypovitaminosis D (impairing calcium absorption) or low dietary calcium levels can result in an unusual form of nutritional secondary hyperparathyroidism where the calcium level is normal or slightly raised, and the phosphate level is normal or slightly low.

PRIMARY HYPERPARATHYROIDISM AND PSEUDOHYPERPARATHYROIDISM

In both of these disorders, pseudohyperparathyroidism being far more common, the increased production of parathyroid hormone results in lower plasma phosphate levels due to its increased excretion (assuming unimpaired renal tubular function). Parathyroid hormone inhibits tubular phosphate reabsorption.

However, if there is also renal insufficiency, the plasma phosphate levels can remain within the normal range or even appear elevated.

DIURESIS

The increased excretion of water may lower plasma phosphate values.

FANCONI'S SYNDROME (IN DOGS) [RARE]

Extreme reductions in the renal tubular ability to reabsorb *can* result in low phosphate levels, although often values remain in the normal range. Later in the syndrome it is usual for acute renal failure to develop suddenly with *hyper*phosphataemia.

THE ADMINISTRATION OF GLUCOCORTICOIDS

Glucocorticoids stimulate the urinary excretion of phosphate.

CUSHING'S SYNDROME

Due to the effect of cortisol (see above) a third of dogs with Cushing's syndrome show hypophosphataemia.

RICKETS AND OSTEOMALACIA

In the (nowadays) rare disease of *rickets* (with the failure of osteoid and cartilaginous mineralization) in *growing* animals, there may be a low plasma level of calcium and/or phosphate (i.e. calcium <2.2 mmol/l, inorganic phosphate <1.2 mmol/l, plus a marked increase in alkaline phosphatase activity).

The cause is a lack of either of these minerals; a lack of vitamin D is only important if calcium and phosphate levels are low. Low phosphate levels are unusual in dogs and cats but may arise within unusual diets.

In mature animals the same deficiency can be the cause of osteomalacia (skeletal demineralization).

DIABETES MELLITUS [RARE]

This has been associated with hypophosphataemia in the dog (Perman, 1974) and, in humans, low phosphate levels are a *consequence* of treating ketoacidotic diabetes mellitus.

SEVERE LIVER DISEASE [RARE]

Hypophosphataemia can sometimes develop (Feldman, 1986).

PITUITARY DWARFISM [RARE]

In this disorder, hypophosphataemia may arise due to reduced renal tubular reabsorption.

Trace metals

IRON

Iron is an essential constituent of the haem portion of haemoglobin, and, as the haemoglobin in aged RBCs is broken down and fresh haemoglobin synthesized, so the iron in the body is continually re-cycled. Its transport within the body is in the plasma, attached to a β_1-globulin known as transferrin.

Iron derived from the degradation of haemoglobin by the mononuclear phagocyte system (MPS) – akin to the reticuloendothelial system – may be stored in the MPS (liver, spleen and bone marrow) in the form of ferritin or haemosiderin. However, most of the iron passes into the plasma, becomes bound to transferrin and is transported to the bone marrow. There it is incorporated into new haemoglobin, placed within newly formed RBCs and released into the circulation.

Inevitably there are losses of iron, chiefly in epithelial cells shed from the gastrointestinal tract, and replacement iron is absorbed from the diet, derived especially from meat. The rate of absorption is determined by:

- The amount of iron in storage (and therefore absorption increases when stores are low).
- The rate of RBC production, increasing as erythropoiesis increases.

Iron deficiency

In checking for a deficiency of iron in the body (as a possible cause of anaemia), it is important to determine not only the concentration of iron in the plasma but also the capacity of the plasma to carry iron.

Transferrin is usually measured in terms of the *total* amount of iron it can transport, and this is referred to as the 'total iron-binding capacity' (TIBC) of the plasma. Usually about a third of the transferrin binding sites are occupied by iron, so that the iron concentration is usually about a third that of the TIBC (Table 7.1).

In *true iron deficiency* the concentration of iron falls but the TIBC is unchanged, whereas in the anaemia due to chronic inflammation (or chronic infection or necrotizing inflammation) both iron concentration *and* TIBC may show modest falls.

In *haemolytic anaemia* the liberation of iron causes the iron content of the plasma to rise (especially with intravascular haemolysis) although the TIBC remains constant (Table 7.1).

Table 7.1 Levels of iron and iron-binding capacity

Levels in plasma	Normal dog	Iron deficiency	Anaemia due to inflammation	Haemolytic anaemia
Iron	15–42 μmol/l (= 84–233 μg/dl)	↓↓	Modest ↓	↑
Total iron binding capacity (TIBC)	51–103 μmol/l (= 284–572 μg/dl)	N	Modest ↓	N

N	= values in normal range.
Modest ↓	= value at bottom of normal range or below.
↓↓	= substantial fall.
↑	= rise.

Conversion factors:
- To convert μg/dl to μmol/l multiply by 0.179.
- To convert μmol/l to μg/dl multiply by 5.58.

When it occurs, *true* iron deficiency (as opposed to impaired transfer) is usually due to a severe and chronic loss of blood (e.g. gastrointestinal or urinary haemorrhages arising from ulcers or neoplasms). Rarely, it is due to a dietary deficiency (usually in young animals on a milk diet – a food notoriously low in iron content) and rarely to impaired iron uptake and utilization in dogs with portosystemic shunts.

The features of iron deficiency anaemia have been summarized in Panel 2.1 (p. 75) but essentially:

- The MCV and MCHC are normal in the early stages but one or both are later decreased.
- The RBCs show microcytosis, hypochromasia and poikilocytosis.
- A bone marrow biopsy shows the absence of an erythroid response.

COPPER

Although it is an essential trace metal the liver normally only maintains sufficient reserves of copper for routine metabolic purposes. Copper is a component of several major enzymes and plays a vital role in haemopoiesis. It is involved in the absorption and transfer of iron and its utilization for haemoglobin synthesis. In the plasma 90–95% copper is bound to ceruloplasmin, a glycoprotein which appears in the α_2-globulin zone on electrophoresis.

Excessive amounts of copper are toxic. In small animals abnormally high levels are unlikely to be due to an excess of copper in the diet, but in the dog an inherited disorder of copper metabolism occurs that leads to increased storage. In this disorder the biliary excretion of copper is impaired and this leads to its progressive accumulation in the lysosomes of the liver cells. Eventually hepatitis and cirrhosis supervene.

This copper storage disease has long been recognized as an inherited disorder of Bedlington Terriers ('Bedlington Terrier liver disease'), and more recently it has been found to occur in West Highland White Terriers, Dobermann Pinschers and Cocker Spaniels.

In both dog and cat, severe bile duct obstruction will impair biliary excretion of copper leading to higher plasma levels and its accumulation in the liver.

Normal plasma copper levels

These are around 15.7–19 μmol/l (100–120 μg/dl) in the *dog* and around 13.3–16.5 μmol/l(85–105 μg/dl) in the *cat*.

Conversion factors

- To convert μg/dl to μmol/l multiply by 0.157.
- To convert μmol/l to μg/dl multiply by 6.35.

Plasma levels in canine copper storage disease rise above this normal range, *only temporarily*, when the damaged liver cells release their stored copper into the circulation. Most of the time plasma copper levels stay *within the normal range*. Therefore, measuring the level of copper in the plasma may not establish the presence of defective copper storage. Measurement of ceruloplasmin has also been unrewarding in improving diagnosis.

Currently diagnosis is best made by liver biopsy to allow:

- Histopathological examination, including specific staining for copper in the cells.
- Estimation of copper levels in the liver using atomic absorption spectrophotometry.

In normal dogs tissue levels are less than 300 μg/g dry tissue. In severely affected animals levels can rise to 10 000 μg/g dry tissue. In addition there is an increase in the activity of ALT in acute cases (with liver damage), and of ALP and GGT (in chronic cases), plus increases in the levels of bile acids and bilirubin, and decreases in the albumin level and in BSP clearance – indicators of deteriorating liver function.

In the cat, increased concentrations of copper have been found in serum, liver and kidney after 12 weeks' treatment with phenytoin.

Panel 7.1 Parathyroid disorders

Hyperparathyroidism

In the dog and cat four major hyperparathyroid disorders are recognized: primary hyperparathyroidism, pseudohyperparathyroidism, renal secondary hyperparathyroidism and nutritional secondary hyperparathyroidism.

The secondary disorders occur most frequently. They are characterized by an increase in parathyroid hormone (parathormone) output in response to a low plasma calcium level, resultant upon a high inorganic phosphate level. Usually this succeeds in raising the calcium level to within, or just below, the normal reference range.

Of the other two disorders, pseudohyperparathyroidism occurs more frequently than primary hyperparathyroidism. In both, parathyroid hormone (or a secretion having identical effects) is produced autonomously, resulting in elevated calcium levels (highest in pseudohyperparathyroidism) and a low inorganic phosphate level (unless there is concurrent renal dysfunction which limits phosphate excretion, keeping it within, or even above, the normal reference range – Table 7.2).

Table 7.2 Laboratory findings in parathyroid disorders

	Plasma calcium	*Plasma inorganic phosphate*	*Alkaline phosphatase activity*
Hyperparathyroidism			
Primary	↑	↓ (to N)[a]	N to ↑
Pseudo-	↑	↓ (to N)[a]	N to ↑
Renal secondary	↓ to N[b]	↑	N to ↑
Nutritional secondary	(↓ to) N	N (to ↑)	↑[c]
Hypoparathyroidism			
Primary	↓	↑	N

N = normal, ↑ = increased, ↓ = decreased.

[a] If associated with uraemia, phosphate will be normal or increased.
[b] Not all cases of chronic renal failure result in renal secondary hyperparathyroidism; in 5–10% in the dog calcium levels are elevated due to decreased excretion and other effects.
[c] High ALP activity is usual in growing dogs, which are the group affected with nutritional secondary hyperparathyroidism; therefore it may not assist diagnosis.

PRIMARY HYPERPARATHYROIDISM

The autonomous hypersecretion of parathyroid hormone is most commonly due to a single adenoma in the dog, which may at times arise in ectopic parathyroid tissue in the anterior mediastinum. Parathyroid carcinomas are extremely rare in dogs and cats. The alternative cause of hypersecretion is hyperplasia of more than one parathyroid gland, although this accounts for less than 10% of canine cases.

The plasma calcium level is invariably raised, and that of inorganic phosphate is low (or low–normal), providing that there is not an accompanying azotaemia, in which case the phosphate level may be within the normal range or elevated. The alkaline phosphatase (ALP) activity may lie in the normal range (in approximately 50% of cases) or show a modest increase.

Other laboratory estimations, including haematological, show no consistent abnormal features. The detection of acute pancreatitis, which may be associated with primary hyperparathyroidism, can be made on the basis of WBC findings and lipase (and amylase) activity.

PSEUDOHYPERPARATHYROIDISM

This disorder results from the excessive production of bone-resorbing substances by a malignant tumour of non-parathyroid tissue including lymphosarcomas and solid tumours without bone metastasis (particularly apocrine gland adenocarcinomas of the anal sacs but also adenocarcinomas elsewhere, e.g. mammary gland, stomach, nasal chambers, pancreas, thyroid and possibly prostate gland) and in addition interstitial cell tumours, squamous cell carcinomas and (rarely) myeloproliferative disorders.

In the majority of cases, hypercalcaemia is present and (consequent upon hyperphosphaturia) a low or low–normal plasma inorganic phosphate level. ALP activity may be elevated.

Radiography is important in diagnosis.

Currently, pseudohyperparathyroidism forms part of the syndrome of *hypercalcaemia of malignancy*, which also includes solid tumours that metastasize to bone, causing osteolysis. The latter result in a normal or elevated plasma inorganic phosphate level as well as hypercalcaemia.

RENAL SECONDARY HYPERPARATHYROIDISM

In chronic renal failure the progressive destruction of nephrons causes both increased phosphate retention (due to a reduced glomerular filtration rate) and decreased conversion of vitamin D_3 to its active form which reduces the intestinal absorption of calcium. Both of these features induce hypocalcaemia, which in turn provokes parathyroid hormone secretion, resulting in osteolysis and, often, modest increases in ALP activity.

CHECK – increases in urea and creatinine levels, a mild non-regenerative (normocytic/normochromic) anaemia, lymphopenia and isosthenuric urine are diagnostically valuable.

Note

Despite the above, around 5–10% of dogs with chronic renal failure show elevated blood calcium levels, due to a number of possible mechanisms, including decreased renal excretion.

NUTRITIONAL SECONDARY HYPERPARATHYROIDISM

The optimum ratio of dietary calcium to inorganic phosphate is 1.1:1. However, a high meat diet typically has a calcium to phosphate ratio of 1:20, and this imbalance causes a considerable elevation of plasma inorganic phosphate and a reciprocal decrease in the plasma calcium level. This may be accentuated by the increased excretion of calcium that occurs on high protein diets.

This hypocalcaemia stimulates parathyroid hormone secretion with a resultant demineralization of bone, a decrease in calcium excretion and an increase in phosphate excretion. These effects are usually successful in restoring the calcium level to within, or just below, the lower limit of normal, and the inorganic phosphate level to within, or just above, the upper limit of normal.

Signs of nutritional hyperparathyroidism are most dramatic in growing animals (especially between 6–7 months in puppies and 4–5 months in kittens), with deformation of the skeleton and fractures arising from trivial injuries, following the withdrawal of supportive mineral from bone. The decreased density of bone is evident on radiography.

Although alkaline phosphatase activity is increased in this condition, it is also normally increased in growing animals, and therefore this feature usually does not help to make a distinction. Otherwise there are no consistent laboratory features.

Hypoparathyroidism (primary hypoparathyroidism)

Hypoparathyroidism is characterized by hypocalcaemia and hyperphosphataemia (the only other disorder where these changes are pronounced is renal failure – easily distinguished by high plasma urea and creatinine levels.) Other routine laboratory tests produce no significant alterations from normal reference values.

The causes of primary hypoparathyroidism consist of lymphocytic parathyroiditis (believed to be an autoimmune process and previously described as idiopathic hypoparathyroidism – a rare disorder), removal of the parathyroids or their blood supply during surgery (usually thyroidectomy in the treatment of hyperthyroidism in cats), extensive destruction due to neoplasia of structures within the neck, trauma to the neck, irradiation of the thyroid, toxic damage due to aminoglycoside antibiotics and atrophy following previous prolonged hypercalcaemia. Atrophy may also follow damage to the chief cells by the virus of canine distemper. (The condition can also be a temporary consequence of excising a parathyroid tumour that, as a result of its hypersecretion of parathyroid hormone, had caused the other parathyroid glands to atrophy. It persists until the other glands regain normal function.)

The removal of, or damage to, the glands results in reduced parathyroid hormone production, increasing the tubular reabsorption of phosphate and decreasing that of calcium, and also a failure to mobilize calcium and phosphate from bone. The low calcium level increases neuromuscular excitement which may progress to generalized tetany and convulsions. Only eclampsia and ethylene glycol poisoning are believed likely to give rise to hypocalcaemia of comparable severity.

Chapter 8

Hormones

Thyroxine (T$_4$)

SI units of measurement are nanomoles per litre (nmol/l). Previous units used were µg/dl and ng/ml.

Conversion factors

- To convert µg/dl to nmol/l multiply by 12.87.
- To convert ng/ml to nmol/l multiply by 1.287.
- To convert nmol/l to µg/dl multiply by 0.078.
- To convert nmol/l to ng/ml multiply by 0.78.

NORMAL REFERENCE RANGE FOR BASAL TOTAL THYROXINE LEVELS (BY RIA)

Dog: 17–46 nmol/l (= 1.3–3.6 µg/dl = 13–36 ng/ml).
Cat: 12–52 nmol/l (= 0.9–4.0 µg/dl = 9–40 ng/ml).

However, the precise range will vary slightly with each laboratory, depending upon the method employed, and the laboratory concerned should be consulted about its normal reference range.

AGE

Dog

Up to 3½ months of age thyroxine values are two to five times those of adult dogs (with the peak value at 1 month old); they then gradually reduce to adult levels.
Older dogs generally exhibit lower total (although *not* free) thyroxine values.

BREED

Dog

It has been postulated, although not proven, that thyroxine levels may be lower in the Labrador Retriever, German Shepherd Dog, Boxer, Cocker Spaniel, Beagle, Greyhound, Alaskan Malamute, Siberian Husky and other large and giant breeds. They *may* be higher in smaller breeds of dog.

ACCURACY

- A number of drugs may give false thyroxine levels. Oestrogens and insulin may *elevate* the values; anticonvulsants (primidone, phenytoin and phenobarbitone), mitotane, phenylbutazone, penicillin, diazepam, propylthiouracil, salicylates, sulphonylureas, androgens and, particularly, glucocorticoids may be responsible for *reduced* thyroxine levels.
- Simultaneous or recent therapy with thyroxine or tri-iodothyronine is likely to produce low thyroxine values due to the temporary suppression of TSH secretion. It is advisable to discontinue such therapy for 1–2 months before estimating the thyroxine level.
- Tests designed to measure levels of thyroxine in humans are not sufficiently sensitive to distinguish accurately the comparatively low level of thyroxine normally present in the dog (approximately a quarter of that in humans) from the even lower level found in canine hypothyroidism.

SOURCE

Thyroxine is the major metabolic hormone produced by the follicular cells of the thyroid gland, the other being tri-iodothyronine (T_3). Its production and release are regulated by thyroid-stimulating hormone (TSH or thyrotrophin) secreted by the adenohypophysis (anterior pituitary lobe), and the output of TSH is in turn regulated by the level of thyrotrophin-releasing hormone (TRH or thyrotrophin-releasing factor (TRF)) derived from the hypothalamus.

Most (>99%) of the circulating thyroxine is protein bound and metabolically inactive, with only the remaining unbound portion, known as *free thyroxine*, being biologically active.

A *low level* of (total) thyroxine can be due to primary hypothyroidism (i.e. where there is a deficit in the thyroid gland) or, much less often, to secondary or tertiary hypothyroidism (where the defect is within the pituitary gland or hypothalamus respectively). However, low total (although *not* free) thyroxine levels can be due to other factors, including other illnesses and drug therapy. The distinction between disorders producing low values is best made using a TSH stimulation test (or TRH stimulation test).

An *elevated level* of thyroxine is indicative of hyperthyroidism, and is almost always the result of thyroid neoplasia.

Causes of increased plasma thyroxine (T_4) levels

> **Summary**
> - Age
> - Hyperthyroidism
> - Oestrus, pregnancy and hyperoestrogenism
> - Drug therapy
>
> **Error:** autoantibodies

AGE

In dogs up to 3½ months old the thyroxine values are two to five times those of adult dogs; after this time they progressively fall to adult levels. The peak value is around 1 month of age.

HYPERTHYROIDISM

The increased output of thyroxine and tri-iodothyronine by thyroid neoplasms is responsible for virtually identical clinical signs in both the dog and cat (see Panel 8.1, p. 396). In the cat, in particular, T_4 levels may be markedly elevated, e.g. >650 nmol/l (>50 μg/dl, >500 ng/ml), although a *small* proportion of feline cases exhibit values just within the normal range. Likewise in the dog levels can be near normal.

OESTRUS, PREGNANCY AND HYPEROESTROGENISM

Some studies have shown increases in canine thyroxine values during pro-oestrus, oestrus and hyperoestrogenism, *and* during dioestrus and pregnancy. These have been attributed to higher levels of oestrogen and progesterone (respectively) at these times, which enhance the binding of thyroxine to plasma proteins.

DRUGS

Some drugs *may* elevate T_4 values, notably oestrogens and insulin (and possibly halothane and pethidine, as in humans).

ERROR: AUTOANTIBODIES

Antibodies against thyroid hormones have been reported in a small proportion of dogs, especially with hypothyroidism, and could interfere with the radioimmunoassay of thyroxine (and tri-iodothyronine). T_4 values may be falsely elevated or depressed depending upon the precise nature of these antibodies and the procedures used in the assay.

In the case of double antibody RIA procedures, where the autoantibody to T_4 does not cross-react with the second test antibody, the *apparent* plasma T_4 concentration will be elevated. This can result in the paradox of a clinical case of hypothyroidism seeming to possess a high level of T_4. (Similarly, autoantibodies to T_3 can produce falsely high T_3 values.) In such cases, the finding of a significant concentration of autoantibody (the measurement of which is now commercially available (Serono)) will clarify the diagnosis.

Note

Thyroxine levels may be comparatively higher in smaller canine breeds.

Causes of decreased plasma thyroxine (T₄) levels

Summary

- Hypothyroidism
- Hyperadrenocorticism
- Other illnesses ('euthyroid sick syndrome')
- Drug administration
- Thyroxine/tri-iodothyronine therapy
- Iodine deficiency [rare]

HYPOTHYROIDISM

Usually this is primary hypothyroidism, where the defect is in the thyroid gland itself. It is not an uncommon condition in dogs (due mainly to lymphocytic thyroiditis or idiopathic atrophy – occasionally to neoplasia), but it is rare, or at least rarely recognized clinically, in the cat (see Panel 8.1, p. 396).

Secondary and tertiary hypothyroidism could occur due to defects arising in the pituitary gland and hypothalamus respectively. Secondary hypothyroidism is present in less than 5% of hypothyroid dogs but tertiary hypothyroidism has *not* been reported. Neither condition has been recognized in the cat.

The different types of hypothyroidism are best distinguished from each other, and from other disorders which cause low thyroxine levels, by performing a TSH stimulation test (and/or a TRH stimulation test) (see p. 399).

CHECK   for increases in cholesterol and in CPK activity, and for a non-regenerative normocytic/normochromic anaemia.

HYPERADRENOCORTICISM (CUSHING'S SYNDROME)

Glucocorticoids decrease basal T_4 levels by a number of possible mechanisms including interference with the synthesis of T_4, decreased binding of it to proteins and cells, and/or increased clearance, *and* the inhibition of TSH and TRH secretion.

Over half of all hyperadrenocorticism cases show an abnormally low total T_4 level.

OTHER ILLNESSES (SO-CALLED 'EUTHYROID SICK SYNDROME')

Acute and chronic illnesses in dogs that possess *normal* thyroid function (i.e. are euthyroid, *not* hypothyroid) may result in abnormally low total T_4 levels. It is believed that this is largely attributable to either a decrease in plasma protein levels (due to decreased synthesis or increased loss) or the reduced affinity of the proteins for thyroxine.

Free (i.e. active) thyroxine levels remain normal but the protein binding of thyroxine is reduced, creating a fall in the total thyroxine level.

This situation can occur in association with diabetes mellitus (worsening with the development of ketoacidosis), chronic renal failure, cirrhosis (liver failure) and chronic active hepatitis, congestive heart failure, infections – including canine distemper, bacterial bronchopneumonia and sepsis – cardiomyopathies, polyneuropathies, intervertebral disc lesions, megaoesophagus, nephrotic syndrome, malabsorption and protein-losing enteropathies, starvation, systemic lupus erythematosus, autoimmune haemolytic anaemia, dermatological disorders (e.g. generalized demodicosis and generalized bacterial furunculosis), lymphosarcoma and terminal illnesses.

This euthyroid sick syndrome can be distinguished from primary hypothyroidism by the performance of a TSH (or TRH) stimulation test (see p. 399).

DRUG ADMINISTRATION

A number of drugs may result in reduced total T_4 concentrations including anticonvulsants (primidone, phenytoin and phenobarbitone), mitotane, phenylbutazone, penicillin, diazepam, iodide, propylthiouracil, salicylates, sulphonylureas (e.g. chlorpropamide), androgens and, in particular, glucocorticoids. The mechanisms responsible are (as above) either a decrease in plasma proteins or their reduced affinity for thyroxine.

Again a distinction from primary hypothyroidism can be made on the basis of the TSH (or TRH) stimulation test (see p. 399).

THYROXINE/TRI-IODOTHYRONINE THERAPY

Recent, or concurrent, therapy with T_4 or T_3 is likely to produce low thyroxine values due to the (temporary) suppression of TSH secretion. Therapy is best discontinued for 1–2 months before estimating the T_4 level.

IODINE DEFICIENCY [RARE]

There are more than adequate amounts of iodine in the diet of almost all small animals in developed countries (in canned foods, in fish and fish products, e.g. cod liver oil, and from the use of iodized salt). Even where a diet is *iodine deficient* (e.g. a solely meat and rice diet), it takes an extremely long time for any sign of the deficiency to appear.

Note

- Thyroxine levels may be lower in certain breeds (i.e. around the lower limit of the normal range), in particular in the Labrador Retriever, German Shepherd Dog, Boxer, Cocker Spaniel, Beagle, Greyhound, Alaskan Malamute, Siberian Husky and other large and giant breeds.
- Antibodies against thyroid hormones have been reported in a small proportion of dogs, and these could interfere with the radioimmunoassay of T_4 (and T_3). T_4 values may be falsely depressed or elevated depending upon the precise nature of these antibodies and the procedures used (e.g. for hormone separation) in the assay. Falsely *elevated* values are those most commonly found.

Cortisol

Cortisol is also known (chiefly in pharmacology) as hydrocortisone.

SI units of measurement are generally nanomoles per litre (nmol/l), although micromoles per litre (μmol/l) have also been adopted. Other units used previously have been μg/dl and ng/ml.

CONVERSION FACTORS

To make the necessary conversion multiply by the appropriate figure given below.

To convert to	From nmol/l	From μmol/l	From μg/dl	From ng/ml
nmol/l	–	1000	27.6	2.76
μmol/l	0.001	–	0.0276	0.00276
μg/dl	0.0362	36.2	–	0.1
ng/ml	0.362	362	10	–

NORMAL REFERENCE RANGE FOR BASAL CORTISOL LEVELS

Dog

- By radio-immunoassay (RIA) 20–250 nmol/l (0.7–9 μg/dl), although many laboratories quote an upper limit which is lower, e.g. frequently 170 nmol/l (= 6 μg/dl) and even 110 nmol/l (= 4 μg/dl).
- By fluorimetric method 55–330 nmol/l (2–12 μg/dl).

Cat

The reported range by each method appears similar to that in the dog, although the upper limit may be lower in each case.

Cortisol levels estimated by fluorimetric methods are much higher than those by radio-immunoassay because corticosterone is also measured (its concentration is about 25% that of cortisol but its fluorescence is four times greater). Levels estimated by competitive protein binding are approximately 15% higher than by RIA (again due to corticosterone); by an enzyme-linked immunosorbent assay (ELISA) they are esssentially the same; by high performance liquid chromatography (HPLC) they are about half those derived by RIA.

The precise range will vary depending upon the method employed by a particular laboratory, and the laboratory concerned should be consulted about its normal reference range.

However, the 'normal' range is of little practical value in the diagnosis of hyperadrenocorticism and hypoadrenocorticism because a high proportion of such cases show values which are *not* outside it.

ACCURACY

Falsely elevated values

These can be due to:

- Fluorescence of other substances, especially spironolactone (and also non-specific fluorescence and that due to unclean glassware) with the fluorimetric method.
- Therapeutic doses of prednisolone (or prednisone) with RIA.

Falsely low values

These are possible in samples kept for more than 5 days at room temperature.

SOURCE

Cortisol is the major glucocorticoid secreted by the adrenal cortex and its production is stimulated and regulated by adrenocorticotrophic hormone (ACTH = corticotrophin) synthesized in the adenohypophysis (anterior pituitary gland). ACTH production is, in turn, regulated by corticotrophin-releasing hormone (CRH = corticotrophin-releasing factor (CRF)) originating from the hypothalamus.

Cortisol has diverse effects in the body, among them promoting gluconeogenesis and diuresis, stimulating RBC and neutrophil production by the bone marrow (but inhibiting lymphocyte and eosinophil output), interrupting cell division elsewhere and causing immunosuppression. It is transported in the blood bound to an α-globulin (transcortin) and (weakly) to albumin, with 5–10% being free.

High levels are due to hyperadrenocorticism (Cushing's syndrome) and low levels to hypoadrenocorticism (see Panel 8.2, p. 401).

Causes of increased plasma cortisol levels

Summary

- Naturally occurring hyperadrenocortism (Cushing's syndrome)
- Prior to parturition [unusual]

Error: drug therapy

NATURALLY OCCURRING (SPONTANEOUS) HYPERADRENOCORTISM (CUSHING'S SYNDROME)

This is due to an increase in cortisol output from the adrenal cortex, *either* under the stimulus of excessive ACTH produced in the adenohypophysis (anterior pituitary gland) *or* from an autonomously secreting adrenal tumour (adenoma or carcinoma). (See Panel 8.2, p. 401).

PRIOR TO PARTURITION [UNUSUAL]

One to four days before parturition in the bitch (and probably also in the queen) cortisol levels rise.

ERROR: DRUG THERAPY

Falsely elevated values can be due to:

- Drugs, especially spironolactone, causing fluorescence (or non-specific fluorescence) with the fluorimetric method of estimation.
- Prednisolone or prednisone (giving relatively slight increases) with the RIA method.
- Anticonvulsant drugs (primidone, phenytoin and phenobarbitone) and oestrogens and progestogens, which *may* cause an increase in cortisol levels.

Causes of decreased plasma cortisol levels

> **Summary**
> - Hypoadrenocorticism – spontaneous or iatrogenic
> - Iatrogenic Cushing's syndrome
> - Mitotane therapy

HYPOADRENOCORTICISM

This may be one of the following types.

Spontaneous primary

This is where there is atrophy or destruction of the adrenal cortices (primary adrenal failure) resulting in a deficiency of both glucocorticoids and mineralocorticoids (Addison's disease, or Addison-like disease) – rare in the cat.

Iatrogenic primary

This is due to:

- Excessive dosage with mitotane (see below) – usually only the production of glucocorticoids is affected.
- Adrenalectomy – reducing all corticoid levels.

Spontaneous secondary [rare]

This is where there is damage to the hypothalamus or anterior pituitary gland reducing the output of ACTH and thus of glucocorticoids.

Iatrogenic secondary

This arises following the withdrawal of long-term systemic glucocorticoid therapy (including depot preparations) that has resulted in adrenocortical atrophy. There may be concurrent signs of (iatrogenic) Cushing's syndrome attributable to this therapy. In the cat this condition has arisen during therapy with megestrol acetate.

IATROGENIC CUSHING'S SYNDROME

Glucocorticoid administration, especially long term and/or in high dosage, suppresses ACTH production by the normal feed-back mechanism thereby provoking bilateral adrenocortical atrophy and reduced cortisol production.

Where the glucocorticoids concerned are synthetic, i.e. are *not* cortisol itself, the estimated cortisol level will usually be low because they are not measured by the method. In addition these administered glucocorticoids can produce the signs of Cushing's syndrome.

MITOTANE THERAPY

This drug is used for the treatment of spontaneous primary Cushing's syndrome. If the dose is excessive the therapy will destroy too great a proportion of the adrenal cortices resulting in low cortisol levels and signs of hypoadrenocorticism (see Panel 8.2, p. 401).

Insulin

SI units of measurement are picomoles per litre (pmol/l). Previous units were microunits per millilitre (µU/ml).

CONVERSION FACTORS

- To convert µU/ml to pmol/l multiply by 7.18.
- To convert pmol/l to µU/ml multiply by 0.14.

NORMAL REFERENCE RANGE FOR BASAL INSULIN LEVELS

Measurement is by RIA = immunoreactive insulin (IRI) assay.

Dog and cat: fasting levels = 36–180 pmol/l (= 5–25 µU/ml).

However, the precise range will vary slightly with each laboratory, depending upon the method used and, accordingly, each individual laboratory should be consulted about its normal reference range.

ACCURACY

- Samples collected following feeding will be misleading; insulin levels can increase up to five-fold.

- Falsely low values may result from haemolysis, or from allowing blood cells to remain in contact with the plasma (or serum) after collection, due to the action of insulinases.

Insulin levels are abnormally low in type I (insulin-dependent) diabetes mellitus, normal or slightly elevated in non-obese type II (insulin-resistant) diabetes mellitus, and significantly elevated in obese type II diabetes mellitus.

Causes of increased plasma insulin levels (hyperinsulinism)

HYPERINSULINISM DUE TO AN AUTONOMOUSLY SECRETING TUMOUR

This is a tumour of the beta cells of the islets of Langerhans in the pancreas.
Levels may be very high (>430 pmol/l, >60 μU/ml) but are variable.
Diagnosis is based on the level of insulin relative to the level of glucose in a fasting animal (see 'Amended insulin:glucose ratio', p. 286).

INSULIN-RESISTANT (TYPE II) DIABETES MELLITUS

Levels may be slightly elevated, or within the normal range, in non-obese type II diabetics, but are significantly elevated in those showing obesity.

POSTPRANDIAL INCREASE

Insulin levels can increase as much as five-fold after feeding, and remain high for several hours.

Causes of decreased plasma insulin levels (hypoinsulinism)

Summary

- Insulin-dependent (type I) diabetes mellitus
- Severe trauma
Error: insulinases

INSULIN-DEPENDENT (TYPE I) DIABETES MELLITUS

This results from the presence of insufficient functional beta cells to maintain an adequate insulin concentration. It may be the result of failure to correct the underlying cause of insulin-resistant (type II) diabetes mellitus before beta cell exhaustion has ensued.
Values are usually extremely low, e.g. 7–15 pmol/l (1–2 μU/ml).

SEVERE TRAUMA

The release of noradrenaline (norepinephrine) following trauma suppresses insulin secretion and, if severe, results in hypoinsulinaemia. (This and other effects can cause a three to four times increase in plasma glucose levels.) Reduced insulin secretion may persist for up to 3 days, in part due to the anti-insulin effect of corticosteroids.

ERROR: INSULINASES

These enzymes from the RBCs *may* lower the insulin level if:

- Cells are allowed to remain in prolonged contact with the plasma (or serum).
- There is extensive haemolysis.

Panel 8.1 Thyroid disorders

Hypothyroidism

This results from a deficiency of the metabolic hormones thyroxine (T_4) and tri-iodothyronine (T_3). The condition is one of the most common endocrine disorders of the dog and occurs from middle age onwards (although from as young as 2 years old in giant breeds). It is, however, rarely diagnosed in the cat.

PRIMARY HYPOTHYROIDISM

Dog

In the dog over 95% of cases of hypothyroidism are primary (i.e. the lesion is in the thyroid gland itself). For clinical signs to appear three-quarters or more of the follicles must have disappeared and/or have been replaced by other types of tissue. About half the canine primary cases are due to atrophy of the follicles (idiopathic atrophy) and their replacement by adipose tissue. An equal number of cases are due to an autoimmune thyroiditis (lymphocytic thyroiditis) causing follicular destruction, which terminates in the widespread deposition of fibrous tissue. Very occasionally there is bilateral malignancy and neoplastic tissue replaces the functional follicles in both thyroid lobes.

Cretinism (congenital hypothyroidism), characterized by disproportionate dwarfism, is an extremely rare disorder.

Cat

In the cat primary hypothyroidism has been associated with a number of pathological changes in the thyroid gland, but it most often follows bilateral thyroidectomy or (uncommonly) excessive dosage with anti-thyroid drugs or radioactive iodine as therapy for hyperthyroidism.

SECONDARY HYPOTHYROIDISM

This arises where the lesion is in the adenohypophysis (anterior pituitary gland), reducing the secretion and release of thyroid-stimulating hormone (TSH) and thus the stimulus for the thyroid to secrete thyroxine. This type of hypothyroidism accounts for less than 5% of canine cases, and is not recorded in the cat.

TERTIARY HYPOTHYROIDISM

This is caused by a lesion in the hypothalamus, thereby limiting its output of thyroid-releasing hormone (TRH = thyroid-releasing factor (TRF)) which is necessary to provoke the release of TSH (Figure 8.1). It has not yet been recorded in either the dog or the cat.

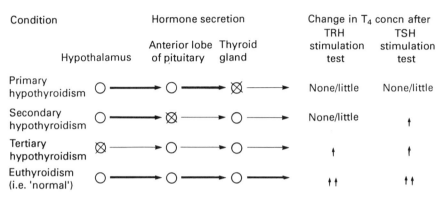

Condition	Hormone secretion			Change in T_4 concn after	
				TRH stimulation test	TSH stimulation test
	Hypothalamus	Anterior lobe of pituitary	Thyroid gland		
Primary hypothyroidism	○ ⟶	○ ⟶	⊗ ⟶	None/little	None/little
Secondary hypothyroidism	○ ⟶	⊗ ⟶	○ ⟶	None/little	↑
Tertiary hypothyroidism	⊗ ⟶	○ ⟶	○ ⟶	↑	↑
Euthyroidism (i.e. 'normal')	○ ⟶	○ ⟶	○ ⟶	↑↑	↑↑

T_4 = thyroxine, TRH = thyrotrophin-stimulating hormone, TSH = thyroid-stimulating hormone

⊗ = site of defect ⟶ = normal secretion ⟶ = reduced secretion

↑ = increased T_4 concentration, provided the thyroid gland is not markedly atrophic

↑↑ = greater increase in T_4 concentration

Figure 8.1 Results of TSH and TRH stimulation tests. In Cushing's syndrome, the 'euthyroid sick syndrome' or following administration of certain drugs, including glucocorticoids, the TSH stimulation test produces *an increase in T_4 output* similar to that seen in cases of secondary or tertiary hypothyroidism

All three types should present with identical clinical signs, although in the dog the diversity of the signs, and the fact that they may be present in any combination, complicates the diagnosis. Hypothyroidism mimics many other diseases. In the cat the prime features are lethargy, obesity and a dry coat with excessive shedding of hair and skin changes (e.g. bilaterally symmetrical alopecia and skin thickening). These are also the classic manifestations in the dog, although they need *not necessarily* be present. Other features recorded in dogs include muscle weakness, bradycardia, skin oedema (giving puffy folds over the neck and forehead, and consequently a worried expression), peripheral neuropathies (leading to paralysis), ocular lesions, constipation, diarrhoea and/or vomiting, a lack of libido and of oestrous cycles, and infertility.

NON-SPECIFIC LABORATORY FINDINGS

Changes seen in *non-specific laboratory tests* in hypothyroidism include the following.

In both species

- A mild, non-regenerative, normocytic/normochromic anaemia (PCV: dog <0.37 l/l, <37%; cat <0.30 l/l, <30%).

- An elevated plasma cholesterol level (in two-thirds to three-quarters of dogs). It is believed that the higher the cholesterol level the more likely it is that hypothyroidism is the cause.

In the dog

In the dog, where the disorder is much more common, other frequent changes are:

- Lipaemia, due to an increase in triglycerides.
- An increase in creatinine kinase (CK) activity.
- Mild to moderate increases in the activity of the enzymes ALT, AST, ALP and LD, due to secondary liver damage.

Other possible findings in the dog are:

- A macrocytic anaemia (increased MCV) due to impaired folate metabolism.
- An increased total WBC count due to infection.
- Proteinuria in association with lymphocytic thyroiditis and glomerulonephritis.

SPECIFIC TESTS

These tests of hypothyroidism involve the radio-immunoassay of T_4 (and T_3), *but*:

- T_3 levels add little to the information provided by the T_4 levels and can be less accurate in indicating true thyroid status.
- The output of T_3 in response to TSH varies more than that of T_4 and can complicate the interpretation of a TSH stimulation test.

For these reasons T_4 measurements are preferred, being thought more reliable than those of T_3.

Note

1. Measurements of T_4 (and T_3) should *not* be performed while animals are on treatment with thyroid hormones or shortly afterwards, because TSH secretion by the pituitary gland is suppressed and will cause secondary hypothyroidism even in a euthyroid animal. Treatment should preferably be discontinued for 1–2 months before carrying out any of the tests below.
2. Improbably high levels of T_4 (and/or T_3) justify the performance of tests to detect and measure autoantibodies, which may be responsible for hypothyroidism (see p. 389).

Basal (i.e. resting) total T_4 level

- Values within the normal range imply that an animal is *not* hypothyroid, especially when well above the lower limit.
- Values below the normal range suggest hypothyroidism (especially if very low), *but* other illnesses and/or drug administration will *also* result in low values (see 'Causes of decreased plasma thyroxine', p. 389).

TSH stimulation test

This is an essential diagnostic test and is used chiefly to distinguish dogs with primary hypothyroidism from those that are euthyroid (i.e. are producing adequate free thyroxine), but have low total T_4 levels due to illness or drug usage. It will also distinguish primary from secondary or tertiary hypothyroidism (see Figure 8.1.)

Method

T_4 levels (in the dog) are estimated in plasma (or serum) samples collected *before* and *6 hours after* the intravenous administration of 0.1 iu bovine TSH/kg body weight; in the cat 1 iu TSH/kg is recommended.

- Dogs suffering from primary hypothyroidism show little or no increase in their low basal T_4 levels.
- Euthyroid dogs whose basal T_4 levels are low due to illness or drugs, and also dogs suffering from secondary or tertiary hypothyroidism, significantly increase their T_4 levels, i.e. usually to above 26 nmol/l (= 2 µg/dl = 20 ng/ml). Some dogs, e.g. a number with Cushing's syndrome, *will* show a rise in T_4 values but may not reach this level. Where the thyroid is severely atrophic due to secondary hypothyroidism the test may need repeating on 3 consecutive days (i.e. the thyroid needs additional stimulation with TSH) before this response is seen. (CARE – repeated intravenous injections of bovine TSH can be the cause of an anaphylactic reaction.)
- Euthyroid dogs generally have higher basal T_4 levels (usually above 17 nmol/l, >1.3 µg/dl, >13 ng/ml) and show a greater increase after 6 hours, i.e. to above 52 nmol/l (>4 µg/dl, >40 ng/ml).
- Among *cats*, euthyroid animals would normally be expected to show a doubling of T_4 values, *but* this response may occasionally be shown by hypothyroid animals and occasionally not be shown by euthyroid cats, i.e. the test is not entirely satisfactory.

TRH stimulation test

This is *not* usually required if the TSH test is available.
This test is used:

- To confirm cases of secondary hypothyroidism detected by the TSH stimulation test, i.e. by identifying any case of tertiary hypothyroidism (rare).
- More importantly, when commercial TSH is not available to clinicians, to distinguish euthyroid animals (especially those with low basal T_4 values due to illness or drugs) from those with primary or secondary hypothyroidism.

Method

T_4 values are estimated in plasma (or serum) samples collected *before* and *6 hours after* the intravenous injection of 0.1 mg TRH/kg body weight (in the dog *or* cat), *or* (in the dog) *before* and *4 hours after* the intravenous administration of 0.2 mg TRH per dog (total dose).

- Dogs with primary or secondary hypothyroidism show little or no increase in their low basal T_4 levels.
- Euthyroid dogs show at least a 50% increase in the T_4 value 6 hours after receiving 0.1 mg/kg intravenously *or* an increase of at least 13 nmol/l (= 1 µg/dl = 10 ng/ml) 4 hours after 0.2 mg per dog intravenously.
- In euthyroid *cats*, the T_4 concentration should double 6 hours after giving 0.1 mg/kg intravenously.

Hyperthyroidism

This is due to the excessive secretion of the metabolic hormones thyroxine and tri-iodothyronine. It arises in cats and dogs in, or beyond, middle age.

It is the most common endocrine disorder of the older cat but an uncommon condition in dogs. In each case there is autonomous hypersecretion of thyroxine and tri-iodothyronine by thyroid neoplasms, unregulated by TSH. In the cat the vast majority of these tumours are benign, i.e. adenomas, whereas in the dog they are invariably malignant (carcinomas). Benign thyroid tumours in the dog appear either to be non-functional or to function normally (i.e. they do not hyperfunction).

The clinical signs are identical in both species, in particular weight loss, polyphagia, poor hair coat (unkempt, hair loss), polyuria and polydipsia, diarrhoea, vomiting, restlessness and panting. Paradoxically, in some cats inappetance/anorexia may follow or alternate with polyphagia.

A goitre (thyroid gland enlargement) is present; it is invariably prominent in the dog and may cause difficulty in swallowing, breathing and barking. In the cat, affected glands are freely mobile and may be intrathoracic.

LABORATORY FINDINGS IN CATS

These include:

- Increased activity of the liver enzymes, ALT, AST and ALP (and LD) – in almost all cases, due to secondary hepatic changes, e.g. localized hypoxia.
- Increased urea and creatinine levels in 40% of cases, probably associated with increased protein breakdown and reduced renal perfusion.
- An elevated inorganic phosphate level (in half of cases) and hypocalcaemia (in 20% of cases).
- Mild increases in the PCV, RBC count and haemoglobin concentration are features in half of cats with hyperthyroidism, due to increased RBC production following the stimulation of erythropoiesis and an increase in oxygen requirements. Macrocytosis (shown by an increased MCV) is seen in 50% of cases.
- A steroidal blood picture is seen, due to long-term stress, possibly associated with adrenocortical hyperplasia, i.e. a slight increase in total WBC count, neutrophilia (with a shift-to-the-left), eosinopenia and lymphopenia. (Because the stress is long term (i.e. not short lived) glucose levels are usually *not* raised, although a small proportion of cases shows concurrent diabetes mellitus.)
- Hepatic changes cause an elevated plasma bilirubin level in 20% of cases and marginal reductions in cholesterol and triglyceride levels occasionally.
- Increased faecal fat content in many cases, attributed to a decrease in pancreatic enzyme secretions.
- The urinary specific gravity can cover a wide range (1.005–1.065) – a feature which can be valuable in distinguishing polyuria/polydipsia due to renal failure (where there is a narrow range of specific gravity – isosthenuria).

LABORATORY FINDINGS IN DOGS

These are less consistent than in cats but *may* include a mild increase in PCV, an increase in the plasma calcium level (associated with thyroid carcinomas) and a marginal fall in the plasma cholesterol level.

(Dogs with *non-functional* thyroid tumours show increases in ALT and ALP activities in 40% of cases, a mild increase in plasma urea in less than 25%, hypercalcaemia (with carcinomas) and a mild regenerative anaemia of malignancy in 10%.)

The *specific diagnostic test* in both the dog and cat is the finding of elevated T_4 (and T_3) levels. Usually a single (basal) T_4 value is diagnostic. However, occasionally a value from a hyperthyroid cat will fall just below the upper limit of the normal range. In such cases, performance of the T_3 suppression test (see Appendix I, p. 474) will clearly distinguish hyperthyroid individuals.

The TSH stimulation test (although often suggested) has *not* proved valuable in clearly diagnosing hyperthyroidism.

In cases where basal T_4 values are equivocal it is better to concentrate on interpreting the other diagnostic features and to repeat the T_4 estimation after 1–2 months.

Panel 8.2 Adrenal disorders

Hyperadrenocorticism (Cushing's syndrome)

This term denotes the presence of an excess of glucocorticoids, which provokes a wide variety of clinical signs.

SPONTANEOUS (i.e. NATURALLY OCCURRING) HYPERADRENOCORTICISM

Dog

In the dog this is a relatively common endocrine disorder arising from middle age onwards (i.e. 4 years of age and older). Eighty-five to 90% of cases are the result of excessive ACTH production by the anterior pituitary lobe causing bilateral adrenocortical hyperplasia; such cases are termed 'pituitary-dependent hyperadrenocorticism'. It seems likely that in the majority of these cases pituitary tumours (usually adenomas) autonomously secrete ACTH which stimulates the excessive synthesis of cortisol; in the remainder the over-secretion of ACTH is stimulated by an excessive output of CRH (corticotrophin-releasing hormone) from the hypothalamus.

Ten to 15% of cases are due to an autonomously secreting *adrenocortical tumour*, which is equally likely to be an adenoma or carcinoma.

Cat

In the cat the disorder is rare but again it is seen from middle age onwards.

In the limited number of cases known, the proportion of pituitary-mediated cases and those due to adrenocortical tumours appears similar to that in the dog.

IATROGENIC HYPERADRENOCORTICISM

Glucocorticoid administration (e.g. for 1–2 weeks) will produce some signs of Cushing's syndrome in the dog; other signs require long-term/high dose therapy before appearing. Cats, on the other hand, seldom develop iatrogenic Cushing's syndrome.

The incidence of *clinical signs* is similar in both dog and cat, with polyuria/polydipsia, polyphagia, abdominal enlargement and changes in the skin and haircoat (including bilaterally symmetrical alopecia) occurring in the vast majority of cases. Muscular atrophy and weakness, depression, apparent obesity, hepatomegaly and panting at rest are also commonplace.

Ten per cent of dogs show calcinosis cutis and ectopic calcification may involve internal organs, including the adrenal gland itself.

At times englargement of a pituitary neoplasm compresses adjacent areas of the brain producing CNS disturbances, including blindness, head pressing and circling.

The onset of clinical signs is usually slow and progressive, although with adrenal carcinomas it may be so rapid that skin changes fail to develop.

NON-SPECIFIC LABORATORY TESTS

Changes in *non-specific laboratory tests* vary in the dog and cat.

Typical steroid-induced haematological changes

These are more prominent in dogs, particularly the pattern of WBCs – i.e. eosinopenia (often 0% on differential WBC count), lymphopenia (often <15% on differential WBC count), neutrophilia and monocytosis (the latter seldom seen in cats).

There may also be an increase in the total WBC count and sometimes in the PCV.

In the dog (although *not* the cat) other features include the following.

Increased ALP activity

In most dogs this is due to induction of a specific isoenzyme in the liver.

A mild increase in ALT activity

This is due to secondary liver damage in 50% of cases.

A fall in urea and/or creatinine levels

In some cases this is due to excessive water losses, i.e. with polyuria.

Reduced plasma inorganic phosphate

This occurs in a third of affected dogs.

A mild increase in plasma sodium

This, together with a similar fall in plasma potassium levels, can arise in up to half of the canine cases.

In both dogs and cats the following changes occur.

Elevated plasma cholesterol

This arises in at least three-quarters of dogs and cats and is frequently associated with lipaemia.

Increased plasma glucose

This occurs in all cats and approximately half of dogs.

Glycosuria

Glycosuria denoting overt diabetes mellitus is shown by three-quarters of cats but only 10% of dogs.

Changes in urinary specific gravity

In more than three-quarters of dogs the specific gravity is extremely low (if drinking is not inhibited by hospitalization); but this is *not* seen in cats, probably related to the concurrent glycosuria.

Increased lipase and amylase

Dogs with hyperadrenocorticism appear more likely to develop acute pancreatitis and therefore may show increased activities of plasma lipase and amylase.

SPECIFIC TESTS

These usually involve the measurement of plasma (or serum) cortisol levels. (The measurement of urinary corticosteroids has been advocated but collection of 24-hour urine samples can be difficult to arrange.)

Basal (i.e. resting) cortisol level

This is usually of little value in diagnosis since as few as 10% of primary cases in dogs show an elevated cortisol concentration. Nevertheless, an elevated value would indicate hyperadrenocorticism, and the higher the value the more confidence there would be in the diagnosis.

Consequently, the ACTH stimulation test and/or the low dose dexamethasone suppression (screening) test are usually needed to confirm the existence of primary Cushing's syndrome, and the high dose dexamethasone suppression test is employed to distinguish between cases due to pituitary dysfunction and those due to adrenal neoplasia.

These tests are chiefly employed in the dog but also function satisfactorily in cats.

The use of combined dexamethasone suppression and ACTH stimulation tests (e.g. Eiler and Oliver, 1980) is *not* recommended.

ACTH stimulation test

Administering ACTH results in the release of sizable *reserves* of stored cortisol from both hyperplastic and neoplastic adrenal glands (i.e. there is an exaggerated response to ACTH).

Method

Cortisol levels are assayed in plasma (or serum) samples collected:

- In the dog, before and 2 hours after the intramuscular (or intravenous) injection of 0.25 mg tetracosactrin (synthetic ACTH, e.g. Synacthen) for any size of dog.
- In the cat, before and half an hour after the intrasmuscular (or intravenous) injection of 0.125 mg tetracosactrin per cat.

Note

The pre-ACTH sample is useful primarily to identify iatrogenic cases (producing extremely low values) when the basal cortisol level has not already been determined. Otherwise it is *not* essential.

Post-ACTH values in the dog
- Post-ACTH values of more than 550 nmol/l (>20 µg/dl) usually indicate hyperadrenocorticism (using either fluorimetric methods or RIA – although refer to the individual laboratory).

Note

- Anticonvulsant therapy (primidone, phenytoin or phenobarbitone) can lead to an erroneous diagnosis because it may cause an elevated post-ACTH cortisol value as well as increased liver enzyme activities and several clinical signs (e.g. polyuria/polydipsia and polyphagia) that are consistent with Cushing's syndrome.
- Failure of cortisol values to double or treble during the period of the test should be *disregarded* – it is not essential to the diagnosis.

- Slightly lower post-ACTH values (e.g. 470–550 nmol/l, 17–20 µg/dl) are equivocal.
- Lower values than 470 nmol/l (=17 µg/dl) *suggest* normal adrenocortical function, *but* 15% of the pituitary-mediated cases of Cushing's syndrome and *almost a half* of those due to adrenal neoplasia do not show any significant elevation.

Note

Failure of the cortisol level to increase significantly in a dog showing clinical and non-specific laboratory features of Cushing's syndrome does not eliminate that diagnosis.

Post-ACTH values in the cat
- Values of more than 420 nmol/l (>15 µg/dl) indicate hyperadrenocorticism.
- Values between 360 and 420 nmol/l (13–15 µg/dl) are equivocal.
- Values of less than 360 nmol/l (<13 µg/dl) suggest normality.

Low dose dexamethasone suppression (screening) test

In both the dog and cat cortisol levels are estimated in plasma (or serum) samples collected *8 hours after* the intravenous injection of 0.01 mg dexamethasone/kg body weight.

- In normal animals the dexamethasone will suppress ACTH secretion and reduce cortisol production.
- Post-dexamethasone cortisol levels will be: in the dog <40 nmol/l (<1.5 µg/dl), and in the cat <30 nmol/l (<1 µg/dl).
- Dogs and cats with Cushing's syndrome do not show such a high degree of suppression and therefore the cortisol values are higher.

Note

- Apparent failure to suppress in dogs that do not have Cushing's syndrome can be due to previous therapy with anticonvulsants or with glucocorticoids (the latter *may* be measured, along with cortisol, in the assay).
- Suppression occurs in a very small number (5%) of early pituitary-mediated cases in dogs; repeating the test at least 2 months later usually demonstrates a lack of suppression.
- Suppression can occur with *intermittently* secreting adrenal tumours.

High dose dexamethasone suppression test

This test has not been evaluated in the cat. Cortisol levels are estimated in plasma (or serum) samples collected *before* and *3 and 8 hours after* the intravenous injection of 0.1 mg dexamethasone/kg body weight, i.e. a higher dose of dexamethasone than used in the screening test (see above).

The expectation is that:

- In normal dogs *both* of the post-dexamethasone values are less than 50% of the baseline value.
- In pituitary-dependent Cushing's syndrome usually at least one of the post-dexamethasone values is less than 50% of the baseline value.
- With adrenal neoplasia both values are more than 50% of the baseline value due to poor, or no, suppression. However, about 15% of pituitary-dependent cases are also poorly suppressed and therefore will give this result too; the ultimate differentiation is based on inspection of the adrenal glands following exploratory laparotomy.

ACTH assay

Reliable ACTH assays would be the preferred method of distinguishing pituitary-mediated and adrenal neoplastic types of Cushing's syndrome – the former giving high/high–normal values (generally >40 pg/ml) and the latter generally producing low values. Regrettably such assays are not yet routinely available.

Hypoadrenocorticism

This denotes deficient production of *either* both gluco- and mineralocorticoids (in spontaneous primary cases or following adrenalectomy) *or* of glucocorticoids alone.

It is a relatively uncommon condition in the dog and extremely rare in the cat.

The majority of cases (in dogs and cats) have a primary cause, i.e. are due to damage to the adrenal cortex.

SPONTANEOUS PRIMARY HYPOADRENOCORTICISM (ADDISON'S DISEASE)

In 90% of canine cases this is due to immune-mediated bilateral adrenocortical atrophy. Less commonly the cortical cells are destroyed by neoplastic metastases, amyloidosis, chronic granulomatous diseases (e.g. histoplasmosis, blastomycosis, tuberculosis), fibrosis or infarction. (Rarely thrombosis of the adrenal blood vessels may be responsible.)

A deficiency of both gluco- and mineralocorticoids results.

IATROGENIC PRIMARY HYPOADRENOCORTICISM

This can (exceptionally) be due to adrenalectomy, initially affecting production of all steroids although subsequently mineralocorticoid production usually recovers.

However, more frequently this condition is due to overdosage with the adrenal suppressant drug mitotane (= o,p'-DDD) in the treatment of hyperadrenocorticism. Normally this reduces glucocorticoid secretion only, but occasionally complete adrenocortical failure is a sequel.

SECONDARY CASES OF HYPOADRENOCORTICISM

These can develop where there is a deficiency of ACTH secretion giving rise to a deficiency of glucocorticoids alone.

These may again be either *spontaneous*, the result of damage to the hypothalamus or the anterior lobe of the pituitary (principally by trauma, inflammation or neoplasia) or *iatrogenic*, attributable to the withdrawal of long-term systemic glucocorticoid treatment after it has produced adrenocortical atrophy (and in cats following therapy with progestogens especially megestrol acetate).

Iatrogenic cases are the more frequent, although clinical signs often do not result.

Clinical signs of hypoadrenocorticism may be sudden in onset (addisonian crisis, with shock and acute renal failure), but more usually develop progressively. Such chronic cases most often show anorexia, vomiting and depression (in three-quarters, two-thirds and a half of affected dogs respectively) and muscular weakness of fluctuating severity; all of these signs are a consequence of the lack of glucocorticoids.

Diarrhoea, weight loss and abdominal discomfort may also arise. Where there is a deficiency of mineralocorticoids as well, the previous signs are intensified with trembling, polyuria and polydipsia, resulting from an excessive loss of sodium.

These signs may only be apparent during episodes of stress, causing them to 'wax and wane'.

Radiography often reveals a smaller heart (microcardia), and typical ECG changes follow the increase in plasma potassium levels (peaked T waves, shortened Q–T intervals and flattened or absent P waves).

IMPORTANT BUT NON-SPECIFIC LABORATORY FINDINGS

These consist of:

- A non-regenerative anaemia (normocytic/normochromic) – although commonly it is masked by concurrent dehydration.
- An absolute or relative eosinophilia *or* a normal eosinophil count where a reduction would have been expected due to stress, plus lymphocytosis and neutropenia.

- An increased (although not grossly elevated) plasma urea level – slightly more common in primary cases (this is due to poor renal perfusion (prerenal ARF) and, consequently, plasma creatinine levels do not usually rise correspondingly).
- A decrease in the plasma sodium level (accompanied by decreases in chloride and total carbon dioxide content) and an increase in the plasma potassium level – often, although not invariably, this produces a sodium:potassium ratio in dogs of less than 27:1, which is diagnostically significant.
- A fall in the plasma glucose level in a third of primary canine cases and two-thirds of secondary cases, although occasionally primary cases may show hyperglycaemia.
- An increased plasma calcium level in approximately 50% of dogs, most often in those that are severely ill; it arises less often in cats.
- An elevated inorganic phosphate level in the majority of cats.
- A urinary specific gravity of less than 1.030 in 80% of dogs and cats.
- Occasionally hypocholesterolaemia is seen.

SPECIFIC LABORATORY TESTS

Basal cortisol level

This is of limited usefulness because the value is below the normal range in only a third to a half of cases of hypoadrenocorticism.

ACTH stimulation test

Cortisol levels are measured in plasma (or serum) samples collected:

- In the dog before and 1 hour after the intramuscular (or intravenous) injection of 0.25 mg tetracosactrin (synthetic ACTH, e.g. 'Synacthen') for any size of animal.
- In the cat before and half an hour after the intramuscular (or intravenous) injection of 0.125 mg tetracosactrin.

Pre-ACTH values are either below, or in the lower part of, the normal range, and the post-ACTH values fail to reach 170 nmol/l (6 µg/dl) by RIA or 330 nmol/l (12 µg/dl) by the fluorimetric method, whereas these values would be exceeded in normal dogs. Generally the increase in cortisol concentration is slight in animals with hypoadrenocorticism, and it may even fall during the test.

Note

This test will not distinguish between primary and secondary cases of hypoadrenocorticism; a single injection of ACTH does not sufficiently stimulate the adrenal cortex. To make this distinction would require measurement of the ACTH levels.

ACTH assay

Reliable ACTH assays will distinguish primary causes of hypoadrenocorticism (high cortisol values) from secondary cases (low cortisol values), but unfortunately these assays are not yet routinely available.

Panel 8.3 Endocrine pancreatic disorders

Diabetes mellitus

This is a disorder of carbohydrate, fat and protein metabolism caused by the inability to produce or to utilize adequate amounts of insulin.

TYPE I (INSULIN-DEPENDENT) DIABETES MELLITUS

This has been presumed to be the *most common* type in small animals. There is hypoinsulinism resulting from a lack of functional beta cells. It appears likely that, particularly in genetically susceptible individuals, environmental factors, such as drugs or infectious agents (especially viruses), trigger the development of an immunity to the beta cells which is principally cell mediated. Due to this autoimmunity beta cells are progressively destroyed until insufficient remain to produce adequate levels of insulin in response to hyperglycaemia. Destruction of beta cells may also be the end result of chronic relapsing pancreatitis, neoplasia or trauma.

The secretion of insulin is also inhibited by:

- Catecholamines, i.e. adrenaline and noradrenaline (epinephrine and norepinephrine), that are produced in excess by functional phaeochromocytomas (tumours of the adrenal medulla).
- (Reversibly) by the drugs xylazine, diazoxide and clonidine.

Insulin levels are extremely low ($7-15$ pmol/l $= 1-2 \mu$U/ml) and 50% of cases are ketotic when first presented.

TYPE II (INSULIN-RESISTANT) DIABETES MELLITUS

Current opinion is that this may be the most common form of diabetes mellitus in mature dogs.

It can be a consequence of:

- Overeating, causing obesity and hyperinsulinism which reduces the number of receptor sites (it seems possible that obesity occurs in 50% of type II cases in dogs).
- Excess growth hormone, stimulated by high levels of progesterone (in canine dioestrus) or by progestogens (in oestrous control).
- Excess glucocorticoids (as therapy or in Cushing's syndrome).
- Excess thyroxine (in hyperthyroidism in the cat).

In all of these situations decreased cellular sensitivity to insulin develops, i.e. insulin resistance.

Insulin resistance or antagonism may also follow the excessive secretion of oestrogens, androgens or glucagon (e.g. by tumours), renal failure and/or acidosis, and the development of antibodies against insulin or the insulin receptors.

As a result the beta cells increase their output of insulin to compensate for its diminishing effect. Insulin levels are either within normal limits or higher than usual, being significantly elevated in obese animals. If the primary cause remains untreated, the beta cells can ultimately become exhausted in their attempt to produce more insulin, culminating in a fall in insulin levels, and then type I diabetes mellitus supervenes.

SO-CALLED TYPE III DIABETES MELLITUS

Type III (covert or chemical) diabetes refers to a state of glucose intolerance (as demonstrated by an abnormal glucose tolerance test result) *without* clinical signs. Such cases may represent mild and reversible drug-induced diabetes, but might include early cases of other forms of type I or type II diabetes.

Clinical signs of diabetes mellitus are of polyuria, polydipsia, polyphagia (until ketosis develops) and weight loss, i.e. muscle wasting. Cataracts and hepatomegaly are frequent features.

Roughly half of the dogs in both groups (types I and II) are ketotic when initially diagnosed and this ketoacidosis results in inappetance, hyperpnoea, vomiting, dehydration and depression, leading ultimately to coma and death.

NON-SPECIFIC LABORATORY FINDINGS

In the *early stage* these are:

- Hyperglycaemia (the principal finding) due to the lack of insulin or its effect.
- Glycosuria (when the renal threshold is exceeded, i.e. >10 mmol/l in the dog and >16 mmol/l in the cat), which many believe encourages and facilitates urinary tract infections.
- Increased ALT and ALP activities (commonly) resulting from the development of a fatty liver.
- Possibly a prolonged BSP clearance or an increased level of bile acids.
- Frequently an increased triglyceride level due to its decreased storage, giving rise to lipaemia.
- Often an increased plasma cholesterol level.
- An increase in plasma bilirubin in 10–20% of cats.
- Possibly an elevated PCV due to *dehydration*, which can also cause decreased renal perfusion with a rise in the level of *plasma urea* (without a proportionate rise in the plasma creatinine level) and (especially in cats) a rise in the levels of total protein and albumin in plasma.

In the ketotic stage, as well as even higher plasma glucose levels, there are almost invariable elevations of ALP, ALT and AST activity, evidence of dehydration (increases in PCV, urea and proteins) and (commonly) increases in triglycerides and cholesterol.

Other features may appear, namely:

- A fall in the total carbon dioxide level, indicating acidosis.
- A fall in the plasma levels of both sodium and potassium, due to polyuria (less commonly there may be increases).
- An increased total WBC count with toxic changes in the neutrophils (see p. 180).
- Increased activities of plasma lipase and amylase, in association with acute pancreatitis.
- Ketonuria, in addition to the glycosuria.

In the treatment of ketoacidotic diabetes mellitus, *hypophosphataemia* may develop, as in humans (Feldman and Nelson, 1987).

Note

In the infrequent cases of hyperosmolar non-ketotic diabetes mellitus, the plasma level of glucose is very high (even up to 135 mmol/l = 2400 mg/dl), with the signs of dehydration being intensified (i.e. high values for PCV and plasma urea) and the osmolality of the plasma (or serum) often exceeds 350 mosmol/kg.

SPECIFIC TESTS

The measurement of insulin concentration is usually not essential in diabetes mellitus but it will aid the distinction of type I (with very low levels) from type II (in which levels are normal or elevated (see p. 395)).

Performance of glucose tolerance tests may aid the diagnosis of some cases where there is uncertainty, but generally they are not recommended because they are influenced by factors such as fear and excitement, and may even precipitate ketoacidosis (see p. 284).

Hyperinsulinism

In dogs, usually above 6 years of age, neoplasms of the beta cells of the pancreas may develop which secrete excessive amounts of insulin (or pro-insulin) independently of normal control mechanisms. (This disorder rarely occurs in cats.) These tumours (insulinomas) can respond to glucagon and so are not entirely autonomous. The majority of them, if not all, appear to be malignant (i.e. carcinomas) or to have malignant potential.

The resultant clinical signs are those of hypoglycaemia, ranging from restlessness and ataxia to weakness, depression, collapse and a variety of neurological signs, including uncontrolled barking, twitching and convulsions (seizures). Such signs are intermittent and usually short-lived. Generally they arise following fasting, exercise or excitement, or 2–6 hours after feeding. Perhaps surprisingly, weight gain is a feature of 20% and polyuria/polydipsia of 10% of canine cases.

The *main laboratory finding* is that of hypoglycaemia, although occasionally 'normal' plasma glucose values are obtained. Often increases in the activities of ALP and ALT, and a decrease in the level of plasma albumin, are also noted.

The usual method of confirming the diagnosis is to determine the amended insulin:glucose ratio, in a fasted animal, as described on p. 286.

Part 3 Urinalysis

Introduction

The four main components of urinalysis are:

1. Physical examination.
2. Chemical examination.
3. Examination of the sediment.
4. Bacterial culture, preferably also establishing that there are a *significant number* of bacteria.

These aspects are dealt with in Chapters 9–12.

All four components could be investigated by a commercial laboratory, but because the physical and chemical examinations are relatively easy to perform, these tests are often carried out in the veterinary practice – and possibly the examination of the sediment as well. The advantage of performing tests in the practice is that changes in the urine occurring after collection will be minimized. However, the recognition of the various elements in urinary sediment may prove difficult. The bacterial culture is best performed by a specialized laboratory because the expertise and facilities within a practice are usually inadequate, and the identification of organisms and the performance of sensitivity tests can present problems. It is, however, most desirable that the laboratory establishes the concentration of organisms in the urine, rather than simply that 'some' bacteria are present, which would always be expected with free flow specimens.

Methods of urine collection

FREE FLOW

This avoids any interference, although the main problem is avoiding contamination if bacterial culture is required.

Dogs

Either:

- Urine is collected into a metal or ceramic dish (preferably sterilized, e.g. in an autoclave or domestic oven, or alternatively boiled for 10 minutes and allowed to dry without wiping) and transferred to a Universal container.
- Urine is collected *directly* into a Universal container (disposable gloves should be worn because this can prove messy).

Ideally, a mid-stream urine (MSU) is collected and the hair is disturbed as little as possible.

Cats

- The animal is restrained and gentle pressure applied to a full bladder to cause urination (although care is essential), collecting the urine in a Universal container as above.
- Urine is collected in a litter tray (containing no litter or other material and previously scalded with boiling water) and transferred to a Universal container.
- A special urine collection device is used consisting of two plastic trays, one above the other, the upper one having small holes and containing large, inert granules (e.g. washed aquarium gravel or polystyrene chips). Urine collecting in the bottom tray is again transferred to a Universal container.

Urine can also be collected in a metabolism cage (with either species) although samples are usually contaminated, i.e. unsuitable for bacterial culture, and other tests should be performed as soon as possible after collection.

CATHETERIZATION

This is convenient, although occasionally difficult, and in a proportion of cases it will cause a urinary tract infection (UTI). Lubricants, which are often unsterile and give rise to fat droplets in the specimen, should be avoided.

CYSTOCENTESIS

This requires the insertion of a 22 gauge needle with syringe attached, through the ventral abdominal wall at a 45° angle, backwards into a full bladder near to its junction with the urethra. The skin should be cleaned and disinfected beforehand and the bladder immobilized with the fingers, although not squeezed. The technique can cause trauma and haemorrhage, both to the abdominal wall and the internal organs, and could lead to urine leakage from the bladder. If sterility is poor it could result in a UTI, or even peritonitis. However, it is the preferred method of many clinicians.

General points regarding collection

- As much urine as possible should be collected (up to 25–30 ml usually, but much more if a urinometer is to be used).
- Sterile containers should be used, preferably Universal containers (even if the sample is not required for culture, bacterial contamination speeds up decomposition).
- Potentially chemically unclean containers, e.g. jam jars, should be thoroughly cleaned, rinsed and dried before use.
- Most preservatives (e.g. toluene, formalin) kill bacteria, preventing bacterial culture and interfering with some of the chemical tests. The exception is boric acid, which preserves bacteria in urine, although even this is unnecessary unless a long delay is likely between collection and examination without the possibility of refrigeration. The concentration must not be excessive as this will prevent the growth of bacteria on culture. It is used chiefly for postal samples intended for bacterial culture.
- Samples are best refrigerated between collection and examination, but should not be tested while cold. They need to be warmed to room temperature.
- Freezing is suitable if urine is intended for physical and chemical tests, but will damage sediment and adversely affect bacteria.

If information about possible bacterial infection is required, *either* carry out a bacterial screening method first, i.e. before dipping test strips, pipettes, urinometer etc. into the sample) *or* split the sample and keep back an uncontaminated portion for bacterial culture later.

Chapter 9

Physical examination of urine

Conventionally, physical examination includes the measurement of urinary volume, a record of the urine's appearance (colour, transparency and odour) and the determination of its specific gravity.

Urinary volume (quantity)

It is pointless to measure the volume of a random urine sample; measurement is only valuable when *all* the urine formed over a known period is collected, ideally at least 24 hours. This is seldom possible without using a 'metabolism cage'. Any such measurement would therefore be made in the practice, rather than by an outside laboratory.

NORMAL REFERENCE RANGE (ADULTS)

Dog: 20–40 ml/kg per day.
Cat: 18–25 ml/kg per day.

Water output correlates better with body surface area than body weight, and so values are relatively higher for smaller animals and lower for larger animals.

AGE

Young animals produce slightly more urine than adults of a comparable weight.

DIET

Urinary output increases with:

- Increased food intake.
- Diets high in protein and salt because of the need to excrete more urea, sodium and potassium.
- The increased intake of well-liked drinks ('flavoured water'), e.g. milk, soup, tea etc., because of the need to excrete surplus water (O'Connor and Potts, 1988).

Production of an abnormally increased volume of urine (>50–70 ml/kg per day) is termed 'polyuria'. Production of an abnormally decreased volume of urine (<7 ml/kg per day) is termed 'oliguria'.

Complete cessation of urinary output (anuria – in fact <2 ml/kg per day) is rare and usually associated with complete urinary obstruction.

Causes of polyuria

Polyuria (excessive urine production) is not an unusual disorder and has several possible causes that can be classified under the three headings: polyuria associated with impaired secretion or action of ADH, polyuria due to excess of solute, and polyuria due to other diuretic effects.

Polyuria associated with impaired secretion or action of antidiuretic hormone

Impaired secretion of ADH
- Hypothalamic–hypophyseal diabetes insipidus – very high urine volume.
- Phaeochromocytoma (uncommon).
- Hyperinsulinism (pancreatic islet cell tumour) (uncommon).
- Drugs (atropine, phenytoin, clonidine, adrenaline).
- Psychogenic polydipsia – very high urine volume (uncommon?).
- Overhydration with intravenous fluids.

Impaired action of ADH
- Nephrogenic diabetes insipidus (uncommon).
- Hyperadrenocorticism (Cushing's syndrome).
- Pyometra (and other toxaemia).
- Hypercalcaemia, e.g. due to malignant tumours causing pseudohyperparathyroidism, which in turn impairs the action of ADH and may lead to nephrocalcinosis and chronic renal failure.
- Hypokalaemia (uncommon).
- Hyperthyroidism.
- Liver disorders – these disorders may cause polyuria by a number of mechanisms, not only impaired action of ADH.
- Drugs (methoxyflurane, amphotericin B, demeclocycline and, in excess, glucocorticoids and prostaglandin E_2).

Polyuria due to excess solute

- Increased salt or protein intake.
- Osmotic diuretics, e.g. hypertonic dextrose or mannitol solutions.
- Diabetes mellitus.
- Acromegaly (uncommon).
- Primary renal glycosuria (uncommon).
- Fanconi's syndrome (uncommon).
- Primary glomerular diseases and nephrotic syndrome (uncommon).
- Hyperviscosity syndrome (uncommon).
- Chronic renal failure (many causes).
- Acute renal failure (including urinary tract obstruction, e.g. feline urological syndrome).

Polyuria due to other diuretic effects

Diuretics that diminish active reabsorption
- Carbonic anhydrase inhibitors (e.g. acetazolamide).
- Benzothiadiazine (thiazide) derivatives (e.g. hydrochlorothiazide).
- Loop diuretics (e.g. frusemide (furosemide), ethacrynic acid).
- Aldosterone antagonists (e.g. spironolactone).

Reduced medullary tonicity

- Hypoadrenocorticism.
- Liver disorders – these disorders may cause polyuria by a number of mechanisms.
- Low protein diet (uncommon)
- Pyelonephritis (uncommon).

Uncertain aetiology

- Hypocalcaemia (uncommon).
- Lymphocytic thyroiditis (uncommon).

Polyuria exists when the urine volume exceeds 50 ml/kg per day (Allen and Wilke, 1988) and is quite definitely present beyond 70 ml/kg per day (Bush, 1988).

In the markedly polyuric/polydipsic (pu/pd) disorders, i.e. diabetes insipidus and pyschogenic polydipsia, urine production (and thirst) is usually over five times normal and may reach ten times normal or higher.

Polyuria and polydipsia are generally recognized by owners when there has been a 50% increase in urinary volume and/or water consumption.

The volume, appearance and specific gravity of urine are often related, i.e. as the volume progressively increases:

- Urine appears progressively paler (less yellow).
- The specific gravity progressively falls.

Note

- Colour may be affected by abnormal excretion of pigments, either yellow (bilirubin, nitrofurantoin) or otherwise (e.g. blood).
- Specific gravity may *not* fall if solute excretion increases in line with that of water – see 'Polyuria due to excess solute', p. 415 and 'Changes in specific gravity', p. 421.

Polyuria due to osmotic diuresis is generally less severe than that due to impaired secretion or activity of antidiuretic hormone.

Also polyuria is primary, i.e. comes first, and polydipsia is secondary, i.e. follows later, except in psychogenic polydipsia, increased salt intake and overhydration with intravenous fluids (in the last condition there is *no* polydipsia).

Causes of oliguria

Oliguria is present when the production of urine is less than 7 ml/kg body weight per day. (Anuria is defined as less than 2 ml/kg body weight per day.)

CHECK   that there is no urethral or bladder obstruction by passing a catheter.

Usually the urine will appear deeper yellow (due to increased concentration of normal pigments) but the specific gravity does not necessarily increase; that depends on the disorder.

ACUTE RENAL FAILURE (INITIAL STAGE)

Prerenal acute renal failure

Oliguria occurs in prerenal ARF (poor perfusion) due to severe dehydration, shock, haemorrhage, hypoadrenocorticism, myocardial dysfunction (e.g. congestive heart failure and arrhythmias) and hypoalbuminuria (in glomerulonephritis). The specific gravity is more than 1.030 in the dog and more than 1.035–1.040 in the cat.

Renal acute renal failure (intrarenal acute renal failure)

Oliguria occurs in intrarenal ARF due to acute interstitial nephritis, i.e. acute leptospirosis or acute tubular necrosis due to nephrotoxins or ischaemia (see 'Causes of increased plasma urea levels', p. 227). The specific gravity of the urine is less than 1.030 in the dog, and less than 1.035 in the cat.

Postrenal acute renal failure and postrenal azotaemia

With postrenal ARF (urinary tract obstruction, e.g. feline urological syndrome) or bladder rupture, the specific gravity of the urine is variable.

CHRONIC RENAL FAILURE (TERMINAL STAGE)

In the rare oliguric terminal stage of chronic renal failure, urinary specific gravity is less than 1.030 in the dog and less than 1.035 in the cat.

Note

In many cases of chronic and acute renal failure the specific gravity lies between 1.008 and 1.018, but with a marked loss of functional nephrons (>75% in the dog, even more in the cat) it falls to isosthenuric values: 1.008–1.012.

Appearance of urine

This is divided into colour, transparency and odour. These features are best recorded as soon as a sample is collected. They may not be reported on by a commercial laboratory.

COLOUR

Normal urine appears yellow due to the presence of urochrome (a combination of urobilin and urobilinogen with a peptide), with smaller amounts of uncombined urobilin and uroerythrin. Urochrome excretion is relatively constant and therefore its concentration reflects urine production:

- Dark amber indicates a high concentration in the urine (as in oliguria).
- Very pale, almost colourless, urine indicates that it is dilute (as in polyuria).

Abnormal colours

These may arise as follows.

Red/pink
This is the most common colour change. It may be due to:

- Haematuria (intact RBCs in the urine).
- Haemoglobinuria (haemoglobin free in the urine).

These are the two most common causes of a red colour, i.e. haemoglobin inside or released from RBCs, and both can be detected by chemical strip tests as described under 'Causes of haematuria', p. 450 and 'Causes of haemoglobinuria', p. 453.

- Myoglobin, in freshly passed urine (which darkens later); it is also detected by the chemical strip tests for blood (see below).
- Porphyrins, in domestic short-haired and Siamese cats with inherited porphyria; teeth and urine appear brownish to pink and fluoresce in ultraviolet light (rare disorder).
- Bromsulphthalein (BSP, Bromsulphalein = sulfobromonphthalein), used as a test of liver function or phenolsulphonphthalein (PSP), used as a test of renal function in *alkaline* urine.
- Phenytoin (anticonvulsant) – at times.

Red-brown/brown-black
This can be due to:

- Myoglobin (i.e. causing myoglobinuria), particularly with exertional rhabdomyolysis (wrongly termed 'azoturia') in Greyhounds that are unfit or raced over a longer distance than usual. (Occasionally myoglobin will give a red or green colour, depending on whether the urine is examined very soon, or a long time, after being released.) It is detected by chemical tests for blood (see p. 454).
- Methaemoglobin formed from haemoglobin in stale urine samples or where bladder emptying is delayed. It is also detected by the chemical test for blood.

Yellow/yellow-orange
This is due to:

- Concentrated urine, usually resulting from dehydration.
- Bilirubin, e.g. with hepatocellular or obstructive jaundice. This can be detected by chemical strip tests (see 'Causes of bilirubinuria', p. 441).
- Drugs, e.g. nitrofurantoin, sulphasalazine (salicylazosulfapyridine) – may appear brownish.
- Riboflavin in large dosages.
- Phenolsulphonphthalein (PSP) in *acid* urine.

Blue
This can be due to methylene blue used as a urinary antiseptic – not advised, especially in the cat, because it can cause haemolytic anaemia.

Green
This can be due to:

- Biliverdin resulting from the oxidation of bilirubin in an old sample; it will *not* be detected by chemical strip tests for bilirubin.
- A mixture of methylene blue or acriflavine with urochrome.
- Myoglobin occasionally (see above), and detected by chemical tests for blood.
- *Pseudomonas aeruginosa* infection of the urine – rarely. Bacteria should be evident on urinary culture, or even in the sediment.

Other causes of colour changes described in humans rarely occur in animals.

TRANSPARENCY

Dog and cat urine is normally transparent (i.e. clear). Turbidity may be due to the following.

Crystalluria

This occurs quite commonly. Salts in solution precipitate out as the urine cools, particularly if refrigerated. Commonly these salts are amorphous phosphates (giving a white precipitate) or urates (giving a buff colour).

Excessive numbers of cells

The turbidity results from excessive cells (and sometimes casts), e.g. WBCs (pus cells), RBCs and epithelial cells alone or (often) in combination. Flocculent particles which settle on standing are usually clumps of WBCs or epithelial cells.

Micro-organisms

Turbidity is caused by bacteria or yeasts in large numbers.

Natural secretions

Turbidity can be caused by increased amounts of secretions, i.e. strands of mucus and semen (especially prostatic fluid and sperms).

However, cloudiness alone is very non-specific and examination of the urinary sediment is needed to establish the cause.

ODOUR

Natural odours

These are due to:

- Pheromones, especially obvious in male cats.
- Metabolites of food, e.g. fish, meat etc., especially the volatile fatty acids.

Abnormal odours

Ammonia
This is the most common abnormal odour. In freshly passed urine it indicates a urinary tract infection with urease-producing bacteria, splitting urea to ammonia (especially *Proteus* spp.). Otherwise it suggests that the sample is *stale*, which is the most common cause.

Acetone
This gives the sweetish 'solvent' smell of ketonuria – almost the only cause of which is the ketoacidotic stage of diabetes mellitus.

Putrefaction
This is associated with bacterial breakdown of urinary proteins or, less often, marked epithelial necrosis in the urinary tract.

Drugs or drug metabolites
For example penicillins.

Specific gravity (SG = relative density or RD)

By definition the specific gravity of water is 1.000. (There are no units because specific gravity is a ratio.)

$$\text{Specific gravity} = \frac{\text{weight of any volume of a substance (e.g. water or urine)}}{\text{weight of the same volume of pure water}}$$

MAXIMUM RANGE POSSIBLE

Dog: 1.001–1.065.
Cat: 1.001–1.080.

NORMAL REFERENCE RANGE

Dog: 1.015–1.045.
Cat: 1.035–1.060.

Glomerular filtrate (produced by a physical process) has a specific gravity of 1.008–1.012 (290–300 mosmol/kg), i.e. its specific gravity and osmolality are the same as that of plasma.

From this filtrate kidneys that function normally can produce urine which is either more, or less, concentrated depending upon the total amount of water and solutes in the body.

In general most of the non-nitrogenous solutes will be reabsorbed (to conserve them) resulting in a urinary specific gravity of between 1.015 and 1.045 in the dog and 1.035 and 1.060 in the cat. *However*:

- If there is excess water to be eliminated the specific gravity can be as low as 1.001 in both species.
- If there is a deficiency of water the urine can be concentrated to as high as 1.065 in the dog or 1.080 in the cat.

In real life situations short periods of dehydration are more likely to occur than overhydration, due to the combination of intermittent access to water and increased losses by evaporation (from the mouth and respiratory tract) caused by exercise and barking.

METHODS COMMONLY USED TO MEASURE SPECIFIC GRAVITY

Urinometer

This is a modified hydrometer, where the scale reading represents the second and third decimal places of the specific gravity (i.e. a reading of 34 represents a specific gravity of 1.034). But a large volume of urine is needed (45 ml); even miniature urinometers usually need at least 15 ml. However, the urine can be diluted and a correction made (i.e. with one part urine and one part water multiply the scale reading by 2; with one part urine and two parts water multiply the scale reading by 3; greater dilutions are too inaccurate).

Refractometer

Actually this instrument measures the refractive index (shown on the right-hand side of the scale) that has been correlated with the specific gravity (measured by more accurate methods) of typical *human* urine. The left-hand side of the scale shows the specific gravity reading. Measurement requires only 1–2 drops of urine.

Accuracy

The accuracy of both instruments can be checked with distilled water at the recommended temperature (both should read 1.000). Accuracy is better with refractometers using *new* scales (see below); urinometers are difficult to read (the stem leans to one side, urine may froth) and if the paper scale in the glass stem should move there is a considerable error.

Note

- The older Atago 'Uricon' refractometers (which have a pink background to the scale) give specific gravity readings 15–20% higher than those obtained using a urinometer, but later models (with a blue background to the scale) have a revised scale (which is marked *Int* on the bottom left-hand side of the scale). This new scale provides much better correlation. A conversion of old to new scales is given in Figure 9.1.
- **CHECK** the temperature at which the urinometer or refractometer was calibrated; results require temperature correction if the sample used is at a significantly different temperature (i.e. if refrigerated). In practice this is much more important with urinometers; the small amount of urine used in refractometers quickly reaches room temperature.
- Some multiple-band test strips carry a specific gravity band. (Principle: urinary specific gravity is related to the concentration of ions in the sample, and increasing the ionic concentration causes progressive dissociation of a polyelectrolyte and a local change in pH, producing a colour change in an indicator in the band.)

  Unfortunately in the dog and the cat, readings of this band do *not* correlate with refractometer and urinometer readings, i.e. the band is *not reliable* and *should be ignored*.

- Specific gravity can also be estimated using a specific gravity bottle, density gradient column or mixed solvent titration, all of which are extremely time consuming to set up.
- As an alternative to specific gravity a laboratory can use an osmometer to measure *osmolality*; this is a measure of the number of particles of solute in the solution (working on the principle of depression of freezing point or depression of vapour pressure).

  The units are milliosmoles per kilogram (mosmol/kg). There is not a linear relationship between osmolality and specific gravity; osmolality is related only to the number of particles, specific gravity also depends on the molecular weight of the particles (most of the osmotic pressure of urine is due to sodium chloride and urea). Therefore they are not directly comparable (it is possible for urines of the same specific gravity to have different osmolalities and vice versa) but *approximately*: osmolality (mosmol/kg) = the last two digits of specific gravity × 30; *and* specific gravity = last two digits of osmolality (mosmol/kg) × 0.033.

- An estimation of the total *protein* content (in g/l) of a *plasma* or *serum* sample can be obtained from a *refractive index* reading, using the formula, $\dfrac{\text{Refractive index} - 1.3365}{0.000175}$

Changes in specific gravity (or osmolality)

Four main abnormalities can occur.

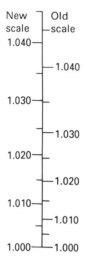

Figure 9.1 Conversion of refractometer scale. The scale used in the older model of the Atago 'Uricon' refractometer (right-hand side) is compared with the revised scale used in the newer model (left-hand side)

AN INCREASED LOSS OF WATER WITHOUT AN INCREASED LOSS OF SOLUTE

This gives a low or low–normal specific gravity. The causes are summarized in 'Causes of polyuria' (p. 415) under the headings 'Polyuria associated with impaired secretion or action of antidiuretic hormone' and 'Polyuria due to other diuretic effects'. The specific gravity can be in the lower part of the usual range or below it, depending upon the severity of the disorder; the greater the polyuria the lower the specific gravity. Those disorders (hypothalamic–hypophyseal diabetes insipidus and pyschogenic polydipsia) which can result in the greatest polyuria invariably have a specific gravity of less than 1.007 and it frequently falls even lower.

Eighty-five per cent of dogs with *Cushing's syndrome* have specific gravity values of less than 1.007 in their own familiar environment; hospitalization inhibits drinking somewhat but the specific gravity is invariably still less than 1.015. (In contrast cats with *Cushing's syndrome* have a specific gravity of more than 1.020 in three-quarters of cases, probably related to glycosuria which is a more frequent feature than in the dog.)

In *canine pyometra* cases specific gravity values are commonly less than 1.015 in the later stages and may be less than 1.008 (although initially they can be more than 1.030). Cats with hyperthyroidism can (rarely) have a urinary specific gravity of 1.006, although it is very variable (1.006–1.060).

Seventy per cent of dogs with hypercalcaemia have a specific gravity of less than 1.015, and it is less than 1.030 in 80–90% of dogs and cats with hypoadrenocorticism.

AN INCREASED LOSS OF WATER ACCOMPANIED BY, AND DUE TO, AN INCREASED LOSS OF SOLUTE

This gives a 'normal' or slightly raised specific gravity. The causes are summarized in 'Causes of polyuria' (p. 415) under the heading 'Polyuria due to excess of solute'. *With the important exceptions* of chronic renal failure and acute renal failure (dealt with below), the specific gravity is generally within the usual range or slightly above it.

> **Note**
>
> The contribution made by excess solutes is not as great as might be expected.
> Specific gravity increases by 0.001 for each additional 14 mmol/l (= one-quarter per cent) of glucose or 3–5 g/l (= 300–500 mg/dl) of albumin. Protein losses seldom exceed 10 g/l, which would add only an extra 0.003 to the specific gravity, and even in poorly controlled diabetes mellitus, the urinary glucose level is not usually above 220 mmol/l (= 4%), which would add 0.016 to the specific gravity.

A DECREASED LOSS OF WATER WITHOUT A CORRESPONDING DECREASE IN THE LOSS OF SOLUTES

This gives a raised specific gravity. With poor renal perfusion the urinary specific gravity in the dog is invariably 1.030 and in the cat above 1.035–1.040. It can result from severe dehydration or haemorrhage, reduced cardiac output in heart failure, severe shock, obstruction of the renal blood vessels (with infarcts or thrombi) etc.

CHECK for elevated PCV and total protein values indicating dehydration, and examine the urea and creatinine levels. An increase in the urea value, which is proportionately much greater than the increase in the creatinine value, indicates poor renal perfusion (see p. 228).

A REDUCED ABILITY TO CONCENTRATE OR DILUTE THE GLOMERULAR FILTRATE

This gives a 'fixed' specific gravity. In chronic renal failure (CRF) and acute renal failure (ARF), the intrarenal and postrenal loss of functional nephrons reduces the kidney's ability to concentrate or dilute the glomerular filtrate. A loss of two-thirds of the normal number of functional nephrons results in inability to produce urine outside the specific gravity range of:

- 1.007–1.029 in the dog.
- 1.007–1.034 in the cat.

Repeat urine samples that are consistently in this range *suggest* the development of chronic renal failure, especially if the daily water input and output begins to increase.

CHECK for increased plasma urea and creatinine levels, but *note* that in the cat (and in early primary glomerular disease in both dog and cat) azotaemia (an increase in urea and creatinine values) may occur *before* the inability to concentrate the urine.

Urine of this specific gravity can also be a feature of both the oliguric and polyuric phases of intrarenal acute renal failure and postrenal (obstructive) acute renal failure.

A loss of three-quarters of the normal number of functional nephrons results (in the dog) in inability to produce urine any more concentrated or dilute than the glomerular filtrate (termed 'isosthenuria'), i.e. classically in the range 1.008–1.012 (its specific gravity/osmolality is identical with that of plasma), although a slightly wider range (1.007–1.015) is often found. In the *cat* though, urine *may* still be concentrated up to and beyond a specific gravity of 1.025, but with even further nephron loss it will, similarly, remain roughly fixed between 1.008 and 1.012 (Ross and Finco, 1980). This is seen especially in polyuric chronic renal failure as well as acute renal failure.

The polyuria of these disorders is related to the need to remove a normal (in CRF) or accumulated (post-ARF) solute load via fewer functional nephrons.

Following the polyuric phase of intrarenal ARF or postrenal (obstructive) ARF the ability to produce urine of specific gravity 1.025 or greater indicates the restoration of renal function and is a good prognostic sign. With postrenal ARF (urinary tract obstruction, e.g. feline urological syndrome, or bladder rupture) the specific gravity is variable.

> **Note**
>
> Finding a specific gravity within the ranges mentioned above does not of itself establish a diagnosis of renal failure – other findings, especially increases in urea and creatinine levels, are necessary. In many polyuric disorders an equally low specific gravity is common, and isosthenuric values (between 1.008 and 1.012) are frequent in pyometra.

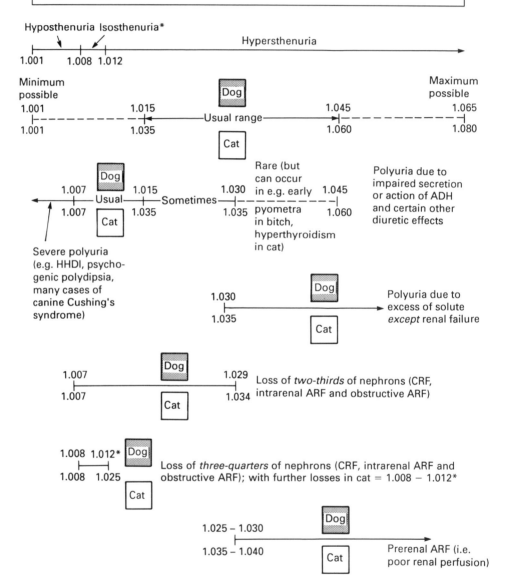

Figure 9.2 Urinary specific gravity in health and disease. Canine values above each line; feline values below. HHDI = hypothalamic–hypophyseal diabetes insipidus; CRF = chronic renal failure; ARF = acute renal failure; ADH = antidiuretic hormone. *Isosthenuric range is generally accepted to be 1.008–1.012, but is probably wider, i.e. 1.007–1.015

Chapter 10

Chemical examination of urine

Substances filtered by the *normal* kidney generally have a molecular weight of less than 68000, e.g. water, urea, glucose, electrolytes etc. Two on the borderline are haemoglobin (molecular weight 64500 although this is usually excreted as a dimer (two subunits) with a molecular weight of 32000) and albumin (molecular weight 66000). Other proteins (globulins and fibrinogen) have a higher molecular weight (160000–900000). The negative charge on proteins also restricts filtration because the glomerular walls have a negative charge as well. Most filtered substances that are useful to the body are completely reabsorbed (e.g. amino acids, glucose and vitamins) unless the renal threshold for that substance is exceeded. Others (allantoin and creatinine) are not reabsorbed. The levels of still others, e.g. electrolytes and water, are regulated according to the body's needs.

Urinary pH and the level of chemical constituents of the urine can be most conveniently measured using commercial strip tests and almost certainly these will be used by commercial laboratories.

These strips are designed to be used with human urine; no special veterinary strips are made. Consequently, the sensitivity of the different test areas is adjusted to detect what would be regarded as abnormal levels of those substances in human urine. These human sensitivities are not necessarily applicable to dogs and cats and the fact that a 'higher' reading is obtained on a test area does not necessarily imply an abnormality. For example, a protein reading of 0.5 g/l (50 mg/dl, or +), or four times that amount if the specific gravity is high, is quite normal in the dog, as can be bilirubin readings of one plus (+).

Some test areas are not reliable in small animals, particularly the specific gravity band, but also those for urobilinogen (giving a large number of false positives and false negatives) and nitrite (with a large number of false negatives).

It is possible for a laboratory to 'read' urine test strips with a reflectance photometer, e.g. Urotron RL9 system (BCL), but this will not alter the inherent reliability of the test areas.

Different commercial strips employ different chemical reactions; consequently they vary in:

- Their sensitivity to the substance being tested for.
- The substances which will interfere with the test (i.e. giving false negative and/or false positive reactions).

It is important to read the manufacturers' instructions because these products are frequently misused; in general:

- They should be stored in a cool dry place, i.e. away from direct sunlight and heat, with their caps firmly in place, *but* not in a refrigerator because condensation will cause rapid deterioration. (Desiccant packets inside containers should not be removed.)
- The test band areas should not be handled.
- The urine should be at room temperature when tested (i.e. if refrigerated it should be allowed to return to room temperature).
- Ideally all preservatives should be absent and the urine should not be centrifuged or filtered before use.
- Strips should be dipped into sufficient urine to cover *all* the test areas, but not allowed to remain a long time in the urine which will leach out reagents.
- Readings should be made at exactly the times stated and, in the case of plastic strips, the correct *side* of the strip must be read.
- The strips must be within their expiry date. (Outdated strips can often be recognized by darkening of the test areas.)

Urinary pH

pH indicates the acidity or alkalinity of the urine (= $-\log_{10}$ of the hydrogen ion concentration). The total pH range is 0–14 (strong acid–strong alkali) with neutrality at pH 7, but pH values for dog and cat urine can only range between the extremes of 4.5 and 8.5. Values outside this range are virtually impossible.

There are no units of measurement.

NORMAL REFERENCE RANGE

Dog and cat: 5.5–7, and usually 6–7 (most frequently 6.5 in dog and 6–6.5 in cat).

Urinary pH is largely related to diet. Animals fed large amounts of protein foods (carnivores) have an acid urine. With an increasing proportion of plant-derived foods (high in organic potassium salts), the urine becomes progressively less acid, even slightly alkaline.

The pH can alter throughout the day, e.g. becoming less acid after eating a meal – the 'alkaline tide'.

MEASUREMENT OF pH

pH *can* be measured with a pH meter, universal indicator (as a liquid or as test papers) or 'narrow range' pH papers, but in general it will be estimated using the pH band of a urine test strip.

Error

The cause of an unexpected result can be *not* dipping the pH band into the urine when using a multiple test strip.

Causes of increased urinary acidity, i.e. pH<5.5

Summary

- Respiratory acidosis
- Hypoxaemia (oxygen debt)
- Shock (circulatory collapse)
- *Severe* vomiting (paradoxical aciduria)
- Ketoacidosis (in diabetes mellitus)
- Severe diarrhoea
- Severe azotaemia
- Increased protein breakdown
- Acidifying drugs
- Acidifying diets
- Ethylene glycol or metaldehyde poisoning

RESPIRATORY ACIDOSIS

This is due to decreased excretion of carbon dioxide with:

- Diseases resulting in decreased pulmonary ventilation, usually severe lung diseases (pneumonia, pulmonary oedema) and obstructions of the airway, but also heart failure etc.
- Drugs (e.g. anaesthetics) causing respiratory depression and trauma to the respiratory centre.

HYPOXAEMIA (OXYGEN DEBT)

This is closely associated with respiratory acidosis (above). A decrease in oxygen usually becomes apparent before an increase in carbon dioxide levels. Metabolic acidosis results from the accumulation of organic acids (in particular lactic acid) following an increase in anaerobic glycolysis. Causes include:

- Inadequate ventilation/perfusion due to airway obstruction (tracheal damage, bronchospasm or laryngospasm).
- Impaired oxygen diffusion.
- Right-to-left cardiac shunts.
- General or regional hypoventilation due to, for example, chronic respiratory disease or severely abnormal filling of the pleural cavity (hydrothorax, pneumothorax or diaphragmatic hernia).

SHOCK (CIRCULATORY COLLAPSE)

This causes reduced tissue perfusion which leads to an accumulation of acidic metabolites.

SEVERE VOMITING

In the dog, severe vomiting (paradoxical aciduria of vomiting) follows dehydration and lactic acidosis, loss of alkaline duodenal contents and increased hydrogen and chloride ion reabsorption.

KETOACIDOSIS

This is seen as a feature of diabetes mellitus, commonly in the dog and occasionally in the cat. Metabolic acidosis (lactic acidosis) is also seen in the much rarer disorder of hyperosmolar non-ketotic diabetes mellitus.

(Starvation usually does not cause significant ketonaemia in dogs (de Bruijne, 1979, 1982) or in cats, unlike humans. However, starvation of diabetic dogs and cats may induce ketoacidosis.)

SEVERE DIARRHOEA

This is due to loss of non-reabsorbed bicarbonate ions in the digestive juices.

SEVERE AZOTAEMIA

The acidosis of chronic or acute renal failure is due to the retention of organic acids from protein breakdown.

INCREASED PROTEIN CATABOLISM

This is due to:

- Very high protein diets (exogenous protein).
- Glucocorticoids or long-term pyrexia (giving rapid breakdown).

ACIDIFYING DRUGS

These include phosphates (e.g. sodium acid phosphate), methionine, ammonium chloride, frusemide (furosemide) and even sodium chloride.

ACIDIFYING DIETS

These include commercially produced diets, e.g. s/d and c/d diets.

ETHYLENE GLYCOL OR METALDEHYDE POISONING

These poisons produce acid metabolites.

Causes of alkaline urine, i.e. pH>7

Summary

- Low protein, high vegetable diets
- Respiratory alkalosis
- Vomiting
- Renal tubular acidosis [rare]
- Alkalizing drugs
- Urinary tract infection with urease-producing bacteria
- Stale urine [most common]
- Urinary retention
- Postprandial alkaline tide

Error: contamination (ammonia or detergent)

LOW PROTEIN, HIGH VEGETABLE DIETS

These usually give a pH around 7.2–7.5.

RESPIRATORY ALKALOSIS

This arises due to hyperventilation (as with *mild/moderate* respiratory disorders, such as pneumonia, pulmonary oedema and pneumothorax etc., fever, anxiety and the use of mechanical ventilators) with increased losses of carbon dioxide as a consequence.

VOMITING

Alkalosis is due to the loss of hydrogen ions. The finding of an alkaline urine, in association with vomition, is indicative of frequent repeated vomiting or pyloric obstruction.

RENAL TUBULAR ACIDOSIS [RARE]

Both proximal and distal types of renal tubular acidosis can result in an alkaline urinary pH.

ALKALIZING DRUGS

For example sodium bicarbonate (given in excess in the the treatment of acidosis or urolithiasis), sodium lactate, potassium citrate, acetazolamide and chlorothiazide.

URINARY TRACT INFECTION WITH UREASE-PRODUCING BACTERIA

Particularly infection with *Proteus* spp. or staphylococci (often producing urine of pH 8 or 8.5). This is the second most common cause of a high urinary pH, and will not be 'corrected' with urinary acidifiers.

STALE URINE [MOST COMMON]

This is the most common cause due to loss of carbon dioxide (especially in open vessels) and the bacterial decomposition of urea.

URINARY RETENTION

This occurs because of obstruction in the urinary tract and an alkaline urine develops as a result of the last two causes mentioned above.

POSTPRANDIAL ALKALINE TIDE

Following feeding this occurs as a response to gastric acid secretion, and produces a *transiently* alkaline urine.

ERROR: CONTAMINATION OF COLLECTING VESSELS

This may occur, for example, with ammonia or detergent.

Urinary protein

Significant levels are often due to renal damage (especially primary glomerular diseases) and urinary tract infections.

Testing will usually be with commercial strips.

SI units of measurement are grams per litre (g/l). If multiplied by 100, values in g/l are converted to the older units of mg/dl (= mg/100 ml), i.e. 2 g/l = 200 mg/dl.

Commercial strip tests are *more sensitive* to albumin (which is mainly of renal origin) than to other proteins (globulin, haemoglobin, myoglobin, Bence-Jones protein and mucoprotein).

Twenty per cent sulphosalicylic acid (salicylsulphonic acid) is more sensitive to these other proteins (as well as being sensitive to albumin), although it can give a *false positive result* with the presence of radiographic contrast media, high levels of penicillins, tolbutamide, contamination with thymol (as a urine preservative), cephalosporins or sulphafurazole (sulfisoxazole). Turbidity, related to the amount of protein present, is produced on bringing together one drop of acid with one drop of urine on a slide or adding six drops of urine to half an inch (1 cm) of acid in a test tube.

Sulphosalicylic acid gives a *false negative result* with highly buffered alkaline urine; therefore avoid testing stale urine.

NORMAL REFERENCE RANGE

In normal *dogs* protein concentrations up to 0.5 g/l (50 mg/dl) are of little significance. Even double this amount may be present. About half of this urinary protein is albumin from the kidney. (Of the small quantity of filtered albumin more than 90% is reabsorbed in the proximal tubule.) The other half of the protein comes from the distal tubules and collecting ducts, the lower urinary tract and the genital tract, i.e. Tamm–Horsfall mucoprotein plus some immunoglobulins against infection.

Therefore a trace or 0.3 g/l (= + or 30 mg/dl) reading has no significance.

However, protein concentration depends on the volume of water being excreted as well as the amount of protein, i.e. with more concentrated urine higher concentrations of protein can be normal. For example at specific gravities above 1.020, 1 g/l (100 mg/dl), and with specific gravities above 1.030, 2 g/l (200 mg/dl) can be normal. The best guide is to measure the protein loss over 24 hours.

To determine the 24-hour protein loss it was necessary to collect all the urine (e.g. in a metabolism cage), assess the protein level in an aliquot and calculate the total loss in relation to body weight. Protein loss in mg/kg body weight/day =

$$\frac{\text{No. of litres of urine/24 hours} \times \text{Protein concn (g/l)} \times 1000}{\text{Body weight (in kg)}}$$

The alternative is to use the fact that creatinine excretion per 24 hours is fairly constant to calculate protein excretion, by measuring the levels of both protein and creatinine in a random urine sample (Barsanti and Finco, 1979).

Normal protein losses in urine average 15 mg/kg body weight per day (ranging from 0 to 30 mg/kg body weight per day) in both males and females.

Protein levels are best interpreted in association with the urinary sediment, e.g. the finding of casts implies proteinuria is of renal origin, whereas a large number of WBCs suggests inflammation — which if present is usually in the lower urinary tract.

ACCURACY

Commercial strip tests work on the 'protein error of pH indicators' principle, i.e. the ability of the amino acids of proteins to bind with and alter the colour of some acid–base indicator.

False positive results may be obtained:

- With highly buffered alkaline urines.
- With contamination with quaternary ammonium compounds (e.g. cetrimide and benzalkonium chloride) or chlorhexidine.
- During and after infusion of polyvinyl pyrrolidone as a blood substitute.
- By soaking the strip in the urine (instead of briefly dipping it) which leaches out the citrate buffer.

Commercial tests for blood are more sensitive than those for protein and therefore a negative result for protein does not necessarily indicate the absence of blood.

Haemoglobin and myoglobin will be detected by tests for blood (see p. 448).

Bence-Jones protein (light chain polypeptides of immunoglobulins) may be released in some cases of plasma cell myeloma (multiple myeloma), macroglobulin-aemia of lyphoproliferative disorders and, being readily filtered, appears in the urine (see Panel 5.1, p. 295). It is not detected by commercial strip tests but can be detected using 20% sulphosalicylic acid. It is best identified in the urine by electrophoresis, producing a characteristic band in the globulin region of the trace. This is more reliable than thermal tests (Bence-Jones protein precipitates out at 40–60°C and re-dissolves again around 85–100°C).

Amino acids may be excreted in the urine in high concentrations in certain genetic disorders of the dog due to defective tubular reabsorption, i.e. without there being abnormally high concentrations in the blood. For instance:

- Cystinuria, where the main, or only, amino acid in the urine is cystine. This is best detected by the cyanide–nitroprusside test (Lewis, 1932), although cystine crystals may be evident in the urinary sediment.
- Fanconi's syndrome, especially in Basenjis, where a number of amino acids including cystine are excreted, together with glucose, phosphate and sometimes electrolytes. There is also an associated proteinuria.

(Generalized aminoaciduria is best detected by paper chromatography.)

Causes of proteinuria

Summary

Renal origin
- Mild–moderate – many renal disorders, especially chronic renal failure
- Severe – primary glomerular disorders

Other sources
- Inflammation in rest of urinary (or genital) tract
- Haematuria
- Haemoglobinaemia
- Myoglobinaemia
- Hyperproteinaemia
- Natural secretions
- Waxy and granular casts in the urine

Error: effects of buffers, disinfectants and drugs

RENAL ORIGIN

The protein is chiefly albumin because of its smaller molecule.

Mild–moderate proteinuria

Protein levels are less than 10 g/l (<1 g/dl) and are not necessarily present in every case of the following disorders.

Chronic renal failure

This results in values usually below 3 g/l (300 mg/dl) and frequently below 1 g/l (100 mg/dl) because the associated polyuria results in dilution of the protein. Causes are:

- Hydronephrosis.
- Pyonephrosis.
- Nephrolithiasis.

With these three causes (above) there may be *no* urine flow from the affected kidney but the disorder will contribute to the 75% (or more) loss of nephrons.

- Pyelonephritis.
- Neoplasia.
- Polycystic kidney.
- Disorders producing an *end-stage kidney*: chronic interstitial nephritis, chronic amyloidosis, chronic (exudative) glomerulonephritis (see Note 1, p. 434), chronic pyelonephritis and familial renal diseases.

Acute renal failure

This is caused by acute interstitial nephritis and acute tubular necrosis (due to ischaemia or nephrotoxins).

Early renal amyloidosis

Proliferative, and early membranous, glomerulonephritis

See Note 1, p. 434. Usually the protein concentration exceeds 2.5 g/l (250 mg/dl).

Glomerulosclerosis

This occurs in long-standing (2 years plus) diabetes mellitus (unusual).

Physiological causes

These may sometimes be responsible – strenuous exercise, extreme heat or cold, stress.

Fanconi's syndrome

The proteinuria is due to renal tubular dysfunction.

Chronic passive congestion

This is associated with heart or liver disease or the presence of abdominal masses.

Fever

Infectious diseases

Proteinuria may be noted in leptospirosis, infectious canine hepatitis, feline infectious peritonitis, FeLV infection, and (although not in the UK) ehrlichiosis, coccidioidomycosis and Rocky Mountain spotted fever, in association with glomerulonephritis or other renal damage.

Primary renal glycosuria and other familial renal disorders
These conditions, e.g. in Cocker Spaniels and Norwegian Elkhounds, may be accompanied by proteinuria.

Severe proteinuria

The protein levels are more than $10\,g/l$ ($>1\,g/dl$). Causes are:

- Membranous glomerulonephritis (advanced) (see Note 1, p. 434).
- Renal amyloidosis (advanced).

Both these disorders result in the nephrotic syndrome (see Note 2, p. 434). As renal damage progresses proportionately more globulins appear in the urine.

Note

Proteinuria may itself cause tubular damage, which may be recognized by the appearance in the urine of the enzyme γ-glutamyltransferase (GGT).

OTHER (NON-RENAL) SOURCES OF PROTEIN

Proteinuria is usually mild.

Inflammation elsewhere in the urinary or genital tracts

Especially cystitis due to urinary tract infection (including discharges and pus, e.g. in prostatitis and pyometra).

Haematuria

This may arise anywhere in the urinary or genital tracts, and causes a protein reaction since blood contains plasma proteins.

Haemoglobinaemia

This is the result of intravascular haemolysis – see Note 3 (p. 434) and see also Panel 2.3 (p. 95).

Myoglobinaemia

This follows rhabdomyolysis – see Note 3 (p. 434) and see also 'Causes of myoglobinuria' (p. 454).

Hyperproteinaemia

This can follow:

- The parenteral administration of plasma (the renal threshold for plasma proteins is approximately $100\,g/l$ ($= 10\,g/dl$)).
- An abnormal increase in the production of immunoglobulins, e.g. with multiple myeloma (see Note 3, p. 434).

Natural secretions

These include semen, prostatic fluid and oestral discharges – see Note 3 below.

Waxy and granular casts in the urine

Error: falsely elevated levels of urinary protein

These may occur:

- With commercial strip tests – due to highly buffered alkaline urine (avoid testing stale urine), contamination with quaternary ammonium compounds (cetrimide and benzalkonium chloride) and chlorhexidine, the presence of polyvinyl pyrrolidone, and as a result of 'soaking' the test strip.
- With 20% sulphosalicylic acid due to the presence of sulphafurazole (sulfisoxazole), cephalosporins, penicillins in high dosage, radiographic contrast media (intravenous or retrograde) or tolbutamide, or contamination with thymol.

Notes

1. Immune-complex glomerulonephritis may be part of systemic lupus erythematosus (see Panel 2.7, p. 125) or associated with canine scabies or lymphocytic thyroiditis (ultimately resulting in hypothyroidism). In the cat glomerulonephritis is often associated with FeLV infection; protein losses are seldom marked.
2. All the features of the nephrotic syndrome, except oedema, may occur with moderate proteinuria due to glomerulonephritis or amyloidosis.
3. Proteins other than albumin are best (or only) detected using 20% sulphosalicylic acid.

Urinary glucose

Commercial quantitative strip tests specific for glucose have largely replaced earlier tests for reducing sugars (e.g. copper reduction methods such as Clinitest) which are *not* recommended.

SI units of measurement are millimoles per litre (mmol/l). Previously levels were expressed in mg/dl (= mg/100 ml) or as a percentage (1 g/dl, i.e. 1000 mg/dl = 1%).

Table 10.1 details the conversions between different units.

CONVERSION FACTORS

Some commercial strips will measure glucose levels up to 111 mmol/l (2%), others to 280 mmol/l (5%).

In the main glucose will be present due to diabetes mellitus, *although glycosuria may* at times be induced by other disorders, e.g. Cushing's syndrome, hyperthyroidism, acromegaly, phaeochromocytoma and, particularly, by the administration of glucorticoids or progestogens (e.g. megestrol acetate).

Table 10.1 Glucose conversions

mmol/l	% (g/dl)	g/l	mg/dl (mg/100 ml)
2.8	0.05 (1/20)	0.5	50
5.6	0.1 (1/10)	1	100
14	0.25 (1/4)	2.5	250
17	0.3 (1/3)	3	300
28	0.5 (1/2)	5	500
56	1	10	1000
111	2	20	2000
167	3	30	3000
223	4	40	4000
280	5	50	5000

Conversion factors

To convert mmol/l to mg/dl multiply by 18
To convert mmol/l to % multiply by 0.018
To convert mg/dl to mmol/l multiply by 0.056
To convert % to mmol/l multiply by 56

ACCURACY

Bacteria

In urine samples bacteria can utilize the glucose causing a progressive decrease in its concentration; therefore tests should be on freshly voided (or, failing that, refrigerated) urine samples.

But some tests are affected by low temperatures – therefore let urine samples regain room temperature before testing.

Modern commercial tests

These are based on the glucose oxidase/peroxidase reaction and *false positive* results can be obtained if there is contamination with hydrogen peroxide, hypochlorite or chlorine. Formalin, generated by hexamine in acid urine, gives *false negative* results.

Ascorbic acid

The levels of urinary ascorbic acid can reach 0.9 g/l in the dog and 0.5 g/l in the cat. Such high levels can slightly depress glucose readings, as may high levels of ketones or bilirubin.

Older tests

With older tests for reducing sugars (e.g. Clinitest), which react with many reducing substances, *false positive* results can be obtained with formalin (derived from hexamine in acid urine), nalidixic acid, chloral hydrate, high doses of salicylates, high ascorbic acid levels and, of course, other reducing sugars (lactose, galactose, pentose, fructose, maltose etc.). Cephalosporins may cause a black colour to develop.

Error

In non-hyperglycaemic cats with urethral obstruction and haematuria, a positive glucose reaction has been obtained and attributed to an unknown oxidizing substance reacting with the indicator in the glucose test strip to give a *false positive* reaction (pseudoglycosuria).

Note

- There is normally a minute amount of glucose in urine (much less than detected by conventional test methods) which forms the basis of the hypoglycosuria screening test for significant bacteriuria.
- In dogs and cats on normal diets, it is not usual for the blood glucose level to rise above the upper limit of normal after a meal (postprandial hyperglycaemia) and therefore glycosuria following a meal is *not* usual. If it did occur it would suggest hypoinsulinism.

Causes of glycosuria

Summary

With hyperglycaemia
- Diabetes mellitus
- Disorders inducing diabetes mellitus
- Drugs inducing diabetes mellitus
- Acute pancreatitis
- Removal of insulinoma
- Severe stress
- Injection of dextrose (or other carbohydrate)
- Convulsions
- Chronic liver disease [rare]
- Drug therapy for hyperinsulinism
- Serious insulin overdosage – Somogyi effect [rare]
- Xylazine (sedative) [rare]
- Feline urological syndrome

Without hyperglycaemia
- Primary renal glycosuria
- Fanconi's syndrome
- Other familial renal disorders
- Acute renal failure (intrarenal or postrenal)
- Lead or cholinesterase poisoning
- Chronic renal failure [rare]
- Phloridzin [rare]

Error: False reaction in feline urological syndrome

These causes of glycosuria are divided into those associated with hyperglycaemia and those that are not.

GLYCOSURIA ASSOCIATED WITH HYPERGLYCAEMIA

Glycosuria results when the renal threshold is exceeded (in the dog = 10 mmol/l (180 mg/dl), in the cat = 16 mmol/l (290 mg/dl), although there is an indication that in *diabetic* cats the threshold may be lower, i.e. 11 mmol/l (200 mg/dl)).

Diabetes mellitus

Glycosuria is a feature of all types, i.e. hypoinsulinism, insulin-resistant, ketoacidotic and (rare) hyperosmolar non-ketotic.

Disorders which may induce diabetes mellitus

These include:

- Hyperadrenocorticism (glycosuria in <10% of dogs but three-quarters of cats).
- Acromegaly in bitches (in dioestrus or on progestogen therapy) causes glycosuria in one-third.
- Hyperthyroidism in cats (glycosuria in <10%).
- Phaeochromocytoma (a tumour usually found in the adrenal medulla) producing adrenaline and noradrenaline (epinephrine and norepinephrine).

Drugs which may induce diabetes mellitus

Drugs include glucocorticoids, ACTH and progestogens (e.g. megestrol acetate and medroxyprogesterone acetate).

Acute pancreatitis

Usually any glycosuria is transient although the disorder can give rise to diabetes mellitus.

Following pancreatic surgery to remove an insulinoma

Severe stress

Glycosuria is due to the transient release of adrenaline (epinephrine), *especially in cats* where the resultant blood glucose level can reach 22–28 mmol/l (400–500 mg/dl).

Parenteral administration of dextrose or other carbohydrates

The most common cause is the administration of dextrose by intravenous drip.

Convulsions

These may be due to hypocalcaemia or primary central nervous system disorders.

Chronic liver disease [rare]

Drug therapy for hyperinsulinism

Treatment with streptozotocin or alloxan has been performed in order to destroy the beta cells in cases of hyperinsulinism.

Serious insulin overdosage [rare]

This can result in a *transient* hyperglycaemia (Somogyi effect).

Xylazine

This sedative (like clonidine) inhibits insulin secretion and can produce up to a 500% increase in plasma glucose level in cats (Feldberg and Symonds, 1980).

Feline urological syndrome (FUS)

The blood glucose level may be high due to stress or possibly insulin inhibition by uraemic toxins.

GLYCOSURIA OCCURRING WITHOUT HYPERGLYCAEMIA [RARE]

Primary renal glycosuria and Fanconi's syndrome

In both of the above inherited defects the renal threshold for glucose is abnormally low.

Acute renal failure

With significant tubular damage (intrarenal ARF, e.g. due to nephrotoxins such as gentamicin) and ARF due to obstruction (e.g. FUS), filtered glucose is incompletely reabsorbed leaving small quantities. (This is generally a useful feature for distinguishing between acute and chronic renal failure.)

Poisoning with lead or anticholinesterases

For example, poisoning with organophosphates.

Chronic renal failure [very rare]

Some other familial renal disorders

Glycosuria occurs at times – i.e. it is a variable feature, e.g. in Norwegian Elkhounds and Cocker Spaniels.

Phloridzin [rare]

Glycosuria occurs following administration of the drug phloridzin.

ERROR: FELINE UROLOGICAL SYNDROME

A false positive reaction has been obtained in cases of urethral obstruction in cats, attributed to an unknown oxidizing substance in the urine reacting with the indicator in the test strip.

Urinary ketones

These can be measured by commercial strip or tablet tests.

The concentration can be expressed in SI units (in mmol/l) but is often recorded as trace, small, moderate or large amounts (trace, +, ++ or +++) corresponding to concentrations ranging from 0.5 mmol/l to 8–10 mmol/l or above.

Ketones are inevitably present in *ketoacidotic diabetes mellitus*.

SOURCE

Ketones should be absent from the urine.

Any significant shift in energy production from carbohydrates to fats results in the increased oxidation of fatty acids, and the production of intermediate metabolites (acetone, acetoacetic acid and β-hydroxybutyric acid) increases faster than they can be oxidized by the tissues. Two of these ketones are acids giving a keto*acid*osis. Acetone (and to a lesser extent acetoacetic acid) gives the sweet, solvent smell of ketones in the urine.

ACCURACY

- Strip tests react solely or mainly with acetoacetic acid and only to a slight extent with acetone. Tablet tests react with both.
- Acetone is soluble in toluene; therefore if toluene is used as a urine preservative (improbable nowadays), it will decrease the acetone levels.
- Bacteria in urine may decrease the acetoacetic acid concentration (although this is only a marginal effect).
- Bromsulphthalein (BSP) used as a test of liver function, phenolphthalein (used as a purgative) and high levels of cysteine can give a similar, although rather reddish, colour with commercial tests.
- Out-of-date test strips may fail to react with ketones, even when these are present in high concentrations, giving a negative reading.

Causes of ketonuria

> **Summary**
> - Diabetes mellitus
> - Low carbohydrate/high fat diets [rare]
> - Hypoglycaemic syndromes [rare]
> - Severe trauma

DIABETES MELLITUS

Ketonuria is almost invariably due to diabetes mellitus, and is inevitably present in ketoacidotic diabetes mellitus. It is found in half the dogs, but only occasionally in cats, at the time of the initial diagnosis of diabetes.

Therefore when insulin doses are being regulated using urinary glucose levels, it helps to include a ketone band on the test strip.

Ketones add to the osmotic diuresis of diabetes mellitus and therefore increase the polyuria.

LOW CARBOHYDRATE–HIGH FAT DIETS [RARE]

HYPOGLYCAEMIC SYNDROMES [RARE]

For example, hyperglycinaemia due to insulinomas. Ketonaemia has also been recorded in association with hypoglycaemia in a pregnant bitch.

Starvation usually does *not* cause significant ketonaemia in dogs or in cats, unlike humans (de Bruijne, 1979, 1982), although the starvation of diabetic dogs and cats may induce ketoacidosis.

SEVERE TRAUMA

Following trauma, lipolysis is increased and ketones produced in large quantities; these may be eliminated in the urine.

Urinary bilirubin

Testing is usually with commercial strip tests, which are two to four times *less* sensitive to bilirubin than the tablet test Ictotest. This is an advantage because the renal threshold for bilirubin in dogs is low, and so using a strip bilirubin is less readily found in the urine of normal dogs.

Strip tests can detect as little as 3–7 µmol/l (0.2–0.4 mg/dl).

Detectable concentrations are usually recorded as small, moderate or large (=+,++ and +++).

CONVERSION FACTORS

- To convert mg/dl to µmol/l multiply by 17.1.
- To convert µ/l to mg/dl multiply by 0.059.

NORMAL REFERENCE RANGE

Dog

At least 20% of normal dogs (i.e. not having bilirubinaemia) will eliminate sufficient bilirubin in their urine to produce a one plus (+) reading. When canine urine is within its usual specific gravity range (1.015–1.045) *only ++ or +++ readings are significant.*

Cat

Generally, bilirubinuria is not found in normal cats (the renal threshold for bilirubin is nine times higher than in the dog) and therefore *any reading is significant.*

SOURCE

Bilirubin (unconjugated bilirubin=free bilirubin), derived from degradation of the haemoglobin of aged RBCs by the mononuclear phagocyte system, is transported to the liver, conjugated with glucuronic acid and secreted in the bile. Unconjugated bilirubin, bound to albumin and insoluble in water, cannot be excreted by the kidney, but conjugated bilirubin (not protein bound and water soluble) can be. Therefore the bilirubin found in urine (i.e. in bilirubinuria when the renal threshold for bilirubin is exceeded) is always conjugated bilirubin.

The highest urinary levels of bilirubin are associated with obstruction to bile flow, especially extrahepatic, and with liver disease involving damage to the liver cells. A variable degree of bilirubinuria is associated with severe acute intravascular haemolysis, occurring about 3 days afterwards. *But* urinary bilirubin levels alone provide very limited information, revealing little about liver function, and in addition false positive and negative readings can occur.

CHECK any abnormal readings by reference to the total and direct-reading bilirubin levels in the plasma (see p. 254) and obtain further evidence of liver disorders by performing additional tests on plasma (see Panel 6.1, p. 333).

ACCURACY AND SENSITIVITY

- Large quantities of chlorpromazine metabolites can give a false positive reaction.
- Oxidation of bilirubin to biliverdin, which will not react with commercial tests, occurs rapidly, especially at room temperature and on exposure to light, so a fresh sample (or refrigerated sample) of urine should be tested.
- The sensitivity of the test is reduced by high levels of ascorbic acid, or nitrite in cases of urinary tract infections.

Causes of bilirubinuria

Summary

Loss of liver function
- Toxic substances
- Infectious diseases
- Chronic active hepatitis
- Feline liver disorders
- Myeloproliferative disorders
- Endocrine disorders (cat)

Bile flow obstruction
- Intrahepatic
- Extrahepatic
- Inflammation of biliary tree
- Congestive cardiopathy
- Congenital cystic disease (dog) [rare]
- Chronic infectious diseases

Rupture of biliary tree
Severe acute haemolysis
Breakdown of large haematoma or massive internal haemorrhage [unusual]
Salicylate poisoning (?haemolysis)
Fever/starvation
Error: chlorpromazine metabolites

At times bilirubinuria may *precede* hyperbilirubinaemia and clinical jaundice (e.g. in leptospirosis and infectious canine hepatitis); for additional information see 'Plasma bilirubin' (p. 254).

LOSS OF LIVER FUNCTION

This is consequent upon hepatocellular disease. Inevitably, such a disorder is intimately bound up with intrahepatic cholestasis (i.e. obstruction to bile drainage in the liver).

It is chiefly due to toxic and infectious agents. Causes include the following.

Toxic substances

For example, chlorinated hydrocarbons, phenolic compounds (disinfectants, creosote), aflatoxin B_1, paraquat and thallium (see Table 6.2).

Infectious agents

This includes especially canine adenovirus-1 (causing infectious canine hepatitis), leptospirae (chiefly *Leptospira icterohaemorrhagiae*) and possibly the coronavirus responsible for feline infectious peritonitis.

Chronic active hepatitis

This may be due to:

- Excessive copper storage (e.g. in Bedlington Terriers and West Highland White Terriers).
- Leptospiral or canine adenovirus-1 infections.
- Drug therapy, e.g. primidone.
- Idiopathic causes.

Feline liver disorders

These include cholangiohepatitis, hepatic lipidosis (the most common feline liver disorder in the USA, though currently thought to seldom occur in the UK) and lymphocytic cholangitis – all essentially of unknown origin.

Myeloproliferative disorders

Endocrine disorders in cats

The incidence of bilirubinuria occurs in:

- Diabetes mellitus (10–20% of cases).
- Hyperthyroidism (20% of cases).

OBSTRUCTION TO THE FLOW OF BILE (CHOLESTASIS)

This may be either intrahepatic or extrahepatic.

Intrahepatic

The drainage of bile can be impeded by:

- Acute inflammatory swelling of the liver cells (hepatitis) and the bile canals (cholangitis) that may be due to toxic materials or infectious agents.
- Diffuse neoplasia, amyloidosis or fibrosis (in cases of chronic active hepatitis).

There is clearly some overlap with loss of liver function arising from hepatocellular disease as a cause of the bilirubinuria.

Extrahepatic

Obstruction can be due to:

- Compression of part of the bile system by neoplasms, or abscesses in the biliary tract, or close to it.
- Blockage of the bile duct or gall bladder by calculi (i.e. gall stones).

Biliary tract inflammation (cholangitis)

This can be intra- or extrahepatic and is attributable to:

- Bacterial infection, ascending or haematogenously spread.
- Bile retention.
- Acute pancreatitis.

Congestive cardiopathy

This condition results in right-sided heart failure and liver swelling.

Congenital cystic disease of the biliary tree in the dog [rare]

Chronic infectious diseases

These may cause problems following their dissemination to the liver, e.g. histoplasmosis, coccidioidomycosis or blastomycosis (although not in the UK).

RUPTURE OF THE BILIARY TREE

This leads to bile peritonitis and usually occurs in the dog as a result of trauma.

SEVERE ACUTE (INTRAVASCULAR) HAEMOLYSIS

The onset of bilirubinuria is variable.

Provided conjugation proceeds normally, significant bilirubinuria would be expected 3–4 days after the haemolytic crisis.

CHECK – the absence of bile salts in the urine, and the presence of anaemia, are useful diagnostic features.

There is also evidence that, in the dog, the renal tubular cells can produce bilirubin from haemoglobin and can convert unconjugated to conjugated bilirubin resulting in bilirubinuria – so that a small amount of bilirubin may appear in the urine even in the early stages of haemolysis.

BREAKDOWN OF LARGE HAEMATOMA OR HAEMORRHAGE [UNUSUAL]

Bilirubinuria occurs as a result of phagocytosis of RBCs from an exceptionally large haematoma or a massive internal haemorrhage.

SALICYLATE (ASPIRIN) POISONING IN THE CAT

Bilirubinuria is presumed to be the result of increased haemolysis (Aliakbari, 1975).

FEVER AND STARVATION

Because of the low renal threshold in the dog, mild bilirubinuria can be found in cases of fever and in starvation.

ERROR: CHLORPROMAZINE METABOLITES

In large amounts these can give a false positive reaction, for bilirubin.

Urinary bile salts

These would be expected where bilirubinuria is due to obstruction of bile flow, or to hepatocellular damage, but not where there is haemolysis.

Foam test

The foam test, i.e. shaking producing a foam (and one that is yellow–orange if bilirubin is present) is unreliable; foaming can also occur with high protein levels.

Hay's test

This is preferred; bile salts reduce the surface tension and this causes the rapid descent of any fine powder sprinkled on the surface, e.g. flowers of sulphur. This test is unnecessary if the level of bile salts in the plasma is estimated.

Both of the above tests can give false positive results if detergent is present.

Urinary urobilinogen

This is *not* a reliable test in the dog and cat because there are too many complicating factors.

It would be expected that the normal small amount of urobilinogen in the urine would increase in cases of haemolytic jaundice and liver damage but not in cases of obstructive jaundice where obstruction is complete.

The SI units for urobilinogen are micromoles per litre (μmol/l). Previously results were expressed in mg/dl which are equivalent to Ehrlich units/dl.

CONVERSION FACTORS

- To convert from mg/dl (= Ehrlich units/dl) to μmol/l multiply by 16.9.
- To convert from μmol/l to mg/dl (= Ehrlich units/dl) multiply by 0.06.

NORMAL REFERENCE RANGE

Usually there is a low level in normal dogs and cats (8–17 μmol/l) *but see the warning* at the start of this section.

Higher than normal urinary levels would be expected with haemolytic jaundice (following severe intravascular haemolysis) and with most cases of damage to the liver cells (i.e. those insufficient to provoke jaundice), and *lower* levels than usual would be xpected with obstruction to bile flow, i.e. obstructive jaundice, and with *severe* liver lamage (responsible for hepatocellular jaundice).

However, there are many causes of false readings (see 'Causes of increased levels of arinary urobilinogen', p. 446 and 'Causes of decreased levels of urinary urobilinogen', . 447), and it is not possible to establish the complete absence of urobilinogen with :ommercial tests. Consequently, in the dog and cat the results of this test obtained with multiple test strips should either be *ignored* or interpreted in relation to other indings (see Panel 6.1, p. 333).

SOURCE

Conjugated bilirubin is transported to the duodenum in the bile (see 'Plasma bilirubin', p. 254) where it is converted into colourless urobilinogen (faecal urobilinogen=stercobilinogen). A small proportion (10–15%) is reabsorbed and passes in the portal vein to the liver (see Figure 5.3). The majority is re-excreted into the bile but some (approximately 20% of that reabsorbed) is excreted in the urine.

ACCURACY

Commercial strip tests

These:

- Cannot establish the complete absence of urobilinogen.
- May produce a greyish-green colour if there is a large amount of bilirubin present (due to its conversion to biliverdin).

Long-term oral antibacterial therapy

This can destroy the normal intestinal flora resulting in failure to reduce conjugated bilirubin to urobilinogen.

Anaerobic bacteria

The presence of anaerobic bacteria in the liver of normal dogs means that they are capable of producing urobilinogen in the liver even when the bile duct is completely blocked.

The Ehrlich reaction

This reaction (used by Ames) can:

- Give false positive reactions in the presence of a number of drugs, including sulphonamides.
- Give false negative results if large amounts of nitrite are present in cases of urinary tract infection.

Fresh urine samples

Fresh samples are required otherwise urobilinogen will be oxidized to urobilin which does not react in the test.

Causes of increased levels of urinary urobilinogen

Summary
- Severe acute intravascular haemorrhage
- Moderate loss of liver function
- Increased bacterial fermentation
- Alkaline urine

Error: drugs/out-of-date strips/sulphonamides

An increased level would be *expected* if one of the following was present.

SEVERE ACUTE INTRAVASCULAR HAEMOLYSIS

Increased urinary urobilinogen in association with haemolytic anaemia, because eventually there is increased production of conjugated bilirubin.

A MODERATE LOSS OF LIVER FUNCTION

The degree of damage due to hepatocellular disease, e.g. toxic or infectious hepatitis, needs to be sufficiently severe to reduce the re-excretion of urobilinogen in the bile, but not so severe that it appreciably reduces the conjugation of bilirubin.

However, the test is thought to be unreliable in the dog and the cat because increased levels can also be present if one of the following conditions *also* pertains.

INCREASED BACTERIAL FERMENTATION IN THE GUT AND INCREASED ABSORPTION OF UROBILINOGEN

The cause may be severe constipation, bacterial overgrowth in the gut, intestinal obstruction or bacterial enteritis.

AN ALKALINE URINE

This causes increased urinary excretion of urobilinogen.

ERROR: FALSELY HIGH LEVELS OF UROBILINOGEN IN URINE

These *can* be due to:

- Drugs which appear red in acid urine (e.g. phenazopyridine, although seldom used in small animals).
- Out-of-date strips.
- The presence of sulphonamides, especially sulphafurazole (= sulfisoxazole), which affects the Ehrlich reaction (used by Ames).

Causes of decreased levels of urinary urobilinogen

Summary
- Significant decrease in conjugated bilirubin formation
- Significant decrease in bile excretion
- Decreased bacterial activity in the intestine
- Polyuria
- Intestinal malabsorption
- Delayed urine testing
Error: formalin/nitrite

A decreased level would be *expected* if one of the following was present.

SIGNIFICANTLY INCREASED FORMATION OF CONJUGATED BILIRUBIN

This may occur due to severe loss of liver function following hepatocellular damage, and is usually accompanied by some intrahepatic obstruction to the excretion of conjugated bilirubin.

SIGNIFICANTLY DECREASED EXCRETION OF BILE

The bile carries the conjugated bilirubin and decreased excretion can be caused especially by extrahepatic obstruction, e.g. bile duct obstruction or compression.

However, the urobilinogen test is thought to be unreliable in the dog and cat because urinary concentrations can also be low if one of the following conditions also pertains.

DECREASED BACTERIAL ACTIVITY IN THE INTESTINE

The result is that conjugated bilirubin is not converted into urobilinogen, e.g. following suppression or elimination of the normal gut flora with *long-term antibiotic therapy*.

INCREASED URINE PRODUCTION (POLYURIA)

Polyuria dilutes the urobilinogen.

INTESTINAL MALABSORPTION

This can impair the absorption of urobilinogen.

DELAY IN URINE TESTING

Delay causes urobilinogen to be oxidized to (non-reacting) urobilin, especially at room temperature and with exposure to sunlight. *Fresh* urine samples are required.

ERROR: FALSE NEGATIVE RESULTS

These can arise:
- If formalin is present, e.g. as a urinary preservative or from the metabolism of a urinary antiseptic such as hexamine.
- If large amounts of nitrite are present, e.g. in cases of urinary tract infection, when the urobilinogen test uses the Ehrlich reaction.

Urinary blood pigment

Commercial strip tests are available which can distinguish:

- Haematuria, i.e. an abnormally large number of intact RBCs in the urine.
- Haemoglobinuria or myoglobinuria, i.e. haemoglobin or myoglobin which is free within the urine and *not* contained within cells.

With haematuria individual RBCs lyse on the test area giving individual spots of colour, i.e. a speckled appearance, whereas if there is free pigment the colour change is uniform throughout the area.

In cases of myoglobinuria, free pigment in the plasma has been filtered and excreted by the kidney. In cases of haemoglobinuria the same may be true, but some cases are due to the lysis of RBCs in the kidney or, more likely, in the urine, especially if testing is delayed (with despatched samples), i.e. the case is, in fact, one of haematuria.

The combination of both a uniform colour change on the test area plus speckling indicates partial haemolysis of RBCs in the urine.

NORMAL REFERENCE RANGE

This is not well established for the dog and cat; in humans up to $5\,\text{RBCs/}\mu\text{l}$ ($= 5 \times 10^3\,\text{RBCs/ml}$) can be normal, which is the lowest limit of the strip's sensitivity. The trace result on the strip corresponds to $5\text{--}15 \times 10^3\,\text{RBCs/ml}$.

The amount of blood pigment may be recorded as trace, small, medium or large (trace, $+$, $++$ or $+++$) and is related to the number of intact RBCs or the number of RBCs that have released haemoglobin; it is slightly less sensitive to free haemoglobin than to intact RBCs.

A positive test for blood with reagent strips, but a failure to find intact RBCs in the urinary sediment, can occur with haemoglobinuria, myoglobinuria or minute haematuria, i.e. very small numbers of RBCs.

The test will also respond to RBCs in RBC casts. The lowest limit of detection by the strip ($5\text{--}15 \times 10^3\,\text{RBCs/ml} = 5\text{--}15\,\text{RBCs/}\mu\text{l}$ urine) corresponds to less than 1 red blood cell per high power field when the urinary sediment (obtained by conventional techniques) is examined microscopically.

Usually when blood is present protein will also be found, but the test sensitivity for blood is 50 times greater than that for protein (the blood test area will detect a haemoglobin concentration of $0.001\,\text{g/l}$, whereas the protein test area will not react positively until the haemoglobin concentration reaches $0.05\,\text{g/l}$ (Jansen and Lumsden, 1985)). Consequently, a positive blood reaction may occur in the absence of a positive protein result.

ACCURACY

A false positive result

This may follow contamination with:

- Hydrogen peroxide.
- Hypochlorite bleaches.
- Bacterial peroxidases (unlikely).

A false negative result

This can be due to the presence of:

- Formalin.
- Very large amounts of ascorbic acid, which at times may be present in canine or feline urine (reducing sensitivity).

High levels of nitrite (associated with UTIs) may delay the reaction with haemoglobin or myoglobin and high levels of protein ($>5\,g/l$) may diminish it.

Other red colours in the urine can quickly be differentiated from blood pigment by this test (e.g. red colours due to phenolphthalein (a laxative) in acid urine, phenazopyridine or phenytoin).

Haematuria

Haematuria denotes an abnormally large number of intact RBCs in the urine, which are derived from either the urinary or genital tracts.

Gross haematuria (an obvious red colour in the urine) occurs when there are more than 2.5×10^6 RBCs/ml urine ($>2.5\times10^3/\mu l$ urine), which corresponds to a finding of 150 or more RBCs per high power field when urinary sediment is examined.

Below this concentration the presence of RBCs (or released haemoglobin) cannot be detected by the naked eye and is referred to as 'occult' (hidden) blood.

In theory haematuria and haemoglobinuria can be distinguished by centrifugation, but because RBCs may rapidly lyse examination of the urinary sediment alone may give a misleading impression of the *degree* of haematuria.

Causes of haematuria

Summary

From any part of the urinary tract
- Severe inflammation (bacteria, cyclophosphamide)
- Urinary calculi
- Neoplasia
- Trauma

From the kidney
- Acute leptospirosis
- Acute tubular necrosis
- Glomerulopathies
- Other nephropathies – infarcts, septicaemia etc.
- Crystalluria [rare]
- Renal parasites (not the UK)
- Idiopathic renal haemorrhage
- Radiation injury
- Renal cysts
- Telangiectasia – familial renal disease

From bladder/urethra
- Feline urological syndrome

From genital tract
- Prostatic disorders
- Disorders of penis and prepuce
- Disorders of uterus, vagina and vulva

Affecting other body systems also
- Defective haemostasis
- Severe liver dysfunction
- Severe septicaemia, toxaemia, viraemia
- Chronic passive congestion

Error: bacterial growth

ORIGINATING IN ANY PART OF THE URINARY TRACT

Severe inflammation

This is usually due to bacterial infection (urinary tract infections – UTIs).

Haematuria is most obvious with bladder infections (to CHECK culture the urine); it may not be marked if (rarely) the kidney alone is affected (e.g. pyonephrosis with partial obstruction or acute pyelonephritis).

Urinary tract infection localized in the bladder is the most *common* cause.

Note

Cystitis with haematuria can follow cancer treatment with cyclophosphamide.

Urinary calculi

CHECK – there may be signs of obstruction; catheterization and radiography are valuable in diagnosis.

Neoplasia

This includes benign (polyps) or, more often, malignant (transitional cell carcinoma) neoplasia, and tumours may be either large or small.

CHECK   – contrast radiography.

Trauma

For example a road accident or kick, *alternatively* (affecting the kidney and bladder) vigorous palpation, (bladder and urethra) catheterization, or (bladder) cystocentesis or *Capillaria plica* infection – very rarely.

ORIGINATING IN THE KIDNEY

Acute leptospirosis

This is caused by *L. canicola*

CHECK   – finding leptospires in the urine is conclusive evidence of their presence.

Acute tubular necrosis (ATN)

This is due to nephrotoxins or ischaemia (i.e. intrarenal acute renal failure).

CHECK   – in both acute leptospirosis and ATN, early oliguria is an important sign.

Glomerulopathies

These include proliferative glomerulonephritis (as with systemic lupus erythematosus) and renal amyloidosis.

Other nephropathies

For example renal infarcts, and as a sequel to septicaemia, cardiomyopathy or endocarditis.

Crystalluria

This was chiefly caused by the less-soluble sulphonamides in acid urine (improbable nowadays).

Renal parasites

Dioctophyma renale (giant kidney worm) and microfilaria of the heartworm *Dirofilaria immitis* (neither occur in the UK).

Idiopathic renal haemorrhage

CHECK   – diagnosis depends on ureteral catheterization at laparotomy plus, ideally, renal angiography.

Unilateral cases involve the left kidney. It is probably due to rupture of anomalous intrarenal blood vessels (Holt et al., 1987).

Radiation injury

Renal cysts

Telangiectasia in Pembroke Welsh Corgis

This is a familial disease with multiple organ involvement.

ORIGINATING IN THE BLADDER/URETHRA

Feline urological syndrome (FUS)

This is characterized by struvite crystal formation, cystitis and, in the male, urethral blockage.

ORIGINATING IN THE GENITAL TRACT

Prostate gland disorders

These include trauma, inflammation (prostatitis), neoplasia (usually adenocarcinomas), cysts and hyperplasia/hypertrophy (variable in degree but *common*).

Penis and prepuce

Causes include inflammation, neoplasia (transmissible venereal tumour) and trauma (e.g. mating, masturbation, licking, bite wounds, preputial foreign bodies).

Uterus, vagina and vulva

Causes include inflammation (metritis, chronic subinvolution of placental sites, vaginitis), neoplasia, trauma (mating, spaying, parturition, dystocia, foreign body) and, in the bitch, pro-oestral discharge.

GENERALIZED

This encompasses causes affecting other body systems also.

Defective haemostasis

For example warfarin poisoning and thrombocytopenia.

Severe liver dysfunction

Haematuria occurs with impaired prothrombin synthesis resulting in defective haemostasis.

Severe septicaemia, toxaemia or viraemia

Chronic passive congestion

ERROR: BACTERIAL GROWTH

This may result in a *false positive* result due to a reaction of the test strip with the peroxidases produced.

Note

- Haemorrhage also occurs with prolapse of the male urethra or female bladder, but the lesion is very rare and obvious.
- Haematuria may result from urine collection, especially catheterization, or squeezing the bladder to facilitate urine collection.

Haemoglobinuria

Free haemoglobin in the urine is derived from RBCs that have been lysed:

- Either intravascularly (or occasionally in the kidney) so that the haemoglobin is excreted via the kidney.
- Or in the urine, i.e. as a sequel to haematuria. The longer the RBCs remain in the urine, especially at extremes of pH or urinary concentration, the more likely it is that they will lyse.

Free haemoglobin in the urine appears pink or red (when there is >0.3–0.5 g/l in a transparent, pale-coloured urine), but with oxidation to methaemoglobin and dissociation of the haem group it progressively darkens to a brown-black colour.

Causes of haemoglobinuria

Summary

- Urinary lysis of RBCs
- Intravascular lysis of RBCs [rare]

URINARY LYSIS OF RBCs

The causes are therefore those of haematuria.

INTRAVASCULAR LYSIS OF RBCs [UNCOMMON]

The causes are essentially those responsible for acute haemolytic anaemia. The amount of haemoglobin suddenly liberated exceeds the capacity of haptoglobin to bind it and haemoglobin dimers are excreted by the kidney. It arises with:

- Certain cases of autoimmune haemolytic anaemia (see Panel 2.7, p. 125).
- Disseminated intravascular coagulation (DIC) (see Panel 4.2, p. 216), and with splenic torsion.
- Certain types of toxin, e.g. oxidant drugs (causing Heinz body anaemia), such as chlorate, nitrate, paracetamol (acetaminophen), benzocaine and propylthiouracil, and also dimethyl sulphoxide (DMSO), and snake venom.
- Physical lysis, due to intravenous injection of hypotonic solutions, severe burns and radiation.

- Incompatible blood transfusion.
- Haemolytic disease of the newborn.
- Feline haemobartonellosis (rarely).

Myoglobinuria

This condition is sometimes wrongly termed 'azoturia'. Myoglobin is the pigment responsible for oxygen transport in muscle and, following muscle injury, large amounts can appear in the blood (myoglobinaemia). When the plasma concentration exceeds 9–12 μmol/l (15–20 mg/dl), the surplus myoglobin is excreted in the urine, and a useful diagnostic feature is that at this concentration the plasma *does not* appear pigmented.

Urine containing myoglobin usually appears brown but it may range from red-brown to black and even, exceptionally, green. It deteriorates quickly unless the urine is refrigerated, and preferably made neutral (i.e. buffered to pH 7).

Myoglobin can be distinguished from free haemoglobin in the urine by examining a *blood* sample from the same patient that has been centrifuged immediately following collection, to avoid any haemolysis. If the plasma is *clear* (i.e. not pink or red) it denotes that the pigment in the urine is myoglobin; if the plasma *is* pink/red it indicates that the pigment in the urine is haemoglobin.

An alternative method is to see if the pigment can be precipitated from the urine by alkalinizing it (to pH 7.5–8 using sodium hydroxide solution) and then adding sodium sulphate (2.8 g/5 ml urine) to produce a precipitate. If after centrifugation the liquid part is free from pigment (all the pigment now being in the precipitate which has formed), the pigment is haemoglobin; if the liquid *remains* pigmented, it is myoglobin. Of course, exceptionally *both* pigments may be present.

Commercial strip tests will *not* distinguish between free haemoglobin and myoglobin, and usually commercial laboratories make no attempt to distinguish them by using the tests described above. As a result myoglobinuria is seldom diagnosed, except in racing Greyhounds where it is a well-recognized consequence of racing an animal over a longer distance than it is accustomed to ('tying up').

It seems probable that in the past cases of myoglobinuria following vigorous muscular exertion (exertional rhabdomyolysis) were wrongly diagnosed as haemoglobinuria.

Causes of myoglobinuria

Myoglobinuria is a sequel to rhabdomyolysis (the disintegration or dissolution of muscle tissue causing the release of myoglobin) which is due to ischaemia, trauma or toxaemia. The major causes are listed below.

SEVERE OR PROLONGED EXERCISE

This occurs especially in animals that are not adequately prepared, resulting in hypoxia of the muscles, e.g. 'canine hypoxic rhabdomyolysis' in racing Greyhounds (Pemberton, 1983). Otherwise this condition is termed 'exertional rhabdomyolysis', and popularly known as 'tying up' or, in a milder form, 'cramping'.

Other causes of myoglobinuria include:

- Heatstroke.
- Crush injuries.
- Snake bite.
- Electric shock.
- Severe burns, involving muscle tissue.
- Acute inflammation (myositis).
- Prolonged seizures, i.e. status epilepticus.

Urinary nitrite (Griess's test)

This is included on many commercial test strips as a screening test for *significant bacteriuria* (i.e. a significant number of bacteria in the urine), including Microstix where it is combined with two culture areas.

It is unfortunately an unreliable test with canine and feline urine.

SOURCE

Nitrate, absorbed from food and excreted in the urine, is reduced by bacteria in the urine to nitrite, which can be detected on the test area. This reduction occurs *provided that* the urine has been in the bladder long enough for the conversion to take place. Consequently an overnight urine sample is preferred.

NORMAL REFERENCE RANGE

In animals without a urinary tract infection there should be a negative result. Any pink colour suggests a significant bacterial infection.

ACCURACY

False negative results

The test is unreliable in dogs and cats because it detects a significant UTI in less than 50% of cases, i.e. there are many *false negative* results.

This is primarily because:

- High levels of ascorbic acid, which often occur in dog and cat urine, will inhibit the reaction.
- The urine may not contain sufficient quantities of reducible nitrate (derived in the main from vegetables in the diet).
- Some strains of streptococci, staphylococci and *Pseudomonas* spp. found in urine do not form nitrite from nitrate.

In addition *false negative results* can occur because:

- Antibacterial therapy has been given within the previous few days, inhibiting the growth and metabolism of bacteria, although not necessarily eliminating them (the presence of an antibacterial drug can be established using the strip test Micur-BT (BCL)).
- The urine has not been in the bladder long enough, i.e. in polyuric conditions where urine is being passed frequently.

- The animal has not eaten recently, i.e. it is anorexic or has been starved or fed intravenously.
- There are extremely large numbers of bacteria in the specimen examined 4 hours or more after being passed; these can reduce the nitrite even further, i.e. to nitrogen, which will *not* react (however, see 'False positive results', below).
- There is a high urinary specific gravity, which reduces the sensitivity of the test.

False positive results

These can occur:

- If stale urine is tested (passed more than 3–4 hours previously) because normal contaminants from the urethra can multiply and bring about the conversion to nitrite.
- If the animal is receiving a drug which masks or mimics the colour change, e.g. phenazopyridine or phenytoin.

Urinary leucocytes

This *chemical* test for WBCs detects esterases in neutrophils, which initiate a colour reaction.

NORMAL REFERENCE RANGE

The few WBCs *normally* present in urine would *not* be detected by this test.
The lowest test reading corresponds to approximately 15×10^3 WBCs/ml of urine (15 WBCs/µl). The test strip will also respond to WBCs in WBC casts.

SOURCE AND INTERPRETATION

An increased number of neutrophils indicates inflammation (usually acute) in the urinary tract and is commonly associated with cystitis due to a urinary tract infection. It is also found with pyelonephritis, infected renal cysts, renal abscesses, renal tubular damage due to nephrotoxins (e.g. gentamicin), urethritis, urinary calculi, pyometra, metritis, prostatitis and prostatic abscesses.
The presence of WBCs can indicate a UTI when recent antibacterial therapy has considerably reduced the number of bacteria in the urine and inhibited their growth on culture media, although not totally eliminating the infection.

ACCURACY

Depending on which commercial product has been employed, a test result *lower* than would otherwise have been obtained (reduced responsiveness) may be due to the presence of one or more of the following:

- Gross albuminuria.
- High levels of ascorbic acid.
- Ketones.
- Urinary preservatives.
- Cephalexin.

- High levels of glucose.
- Oxalic acid.
- Tetracycline
- High urinary specific gravity.
- Strong colours, e.g. due to bilirubin or nitrofurantoin, which can affect readings.

One manufacturer's leucocyte test may not be effective in the cat (Canfield, 1986).

Chapter 11

Urinary sediment

Examination of the urinary sediment is a valuable part of urinalysis but one which is often omitted.

A fresh or refrigerated sample is required; with time there is increasing alkalinity causing progressive lysis of blood cells and casts and, at times, changes in crystals.

Usually centrifugation is used to concentrate the sediment into approximately 10% of the urinary volume. The number of RBCs and WBCs in the sediment (after examining a number of high power fields – usually 10) is reported as the number per high power field (HPF).

'Normal urine' contains less than five RBCs and less than five WBCs per HPF, a few epithelial cells (squamous, transitional or renal tubular), a few hyaline or granular casts, some crystals, possibly some sperms and possibly fat droplets.

Abnormal urine may contain more RBCs, WBCs and casts (especially cellular casts), hyperplastic or neoplastic epithelial cells, bacteria, yeasts (or fungal hyphae), parasitic eggs and/or cystine, tyrosine or leucine crystals.

Leptospirae are preserved longest in alkaline urine (therefore it is advisable to give alkalinizing drugs for 24 hours before urine collection), and are best seen when the sediment is examined by dark-ground illumination.

Features of urinary sediment

RED BLOOD CELLS

Even a single RBC per HPF may be significant, certainly more than five per HPF indicates haematuria, equivalent to $80\,RBCs/\mu l$ of the original urine ($= 80 \times 10^3\,RBCs/ml$ urine). (For the significance of haematuria refer to 'Haematuria', p. 449.)

Note

- Haematuria may arise following catheterization or squeezing the bladder to induce urination, and also occurs in pro-oestrus in bitches.
- Highly concentrated urine may cause crenation of the RBCs, but very dilute urine (specific gravity <1.008) produces RBC lysis, although the RBCs may still be faintly visible as swollen 'ghost cells'.

WHITE BLOOD CELLS (PUS CELLS)

Certainly more than five WBCs per HPF indicates inflammation, and large numbers indicate acute inflammation in the urinary tract; the causes are as for the chemical leucocyte test (see p. 456). Often, although not necessarily, WBCs in the urine are associated with bacteria and RBCs, e.g. as in prostatitis.

Note

It may be difficult to distinguish the various types of WBC (usually they are neutrophils) and to differentiate them from renal tubular epithelial cells of similar size.

WBCs lyse in alkaline or hypotonic urine.

EPITHELIAL CELLS

Renal tubular cells

These are small, round cells which may show trailing cytoplasm, giving a comma shape.

They are difficult to distinguish from the smaller transitional cells and WBCs and are, therefore, of dubious significance unless they are present in casts.

Transitional cells

These are derived from the renal pelves, ureters, bladder or proximal urethra; their size depends on their position in the epithelium. Often they are found in clumps or sheets. Small, tapered transitional cells (tapered cells) derive from the renal pelvis.

These cells have a variable shape and granular cytoplasm. Large numbers suggest inflammation (e.g. due to infection, or mechanical or chemical irritation) or neoplasia. The cells may show hyperplasia.

Squamous cells

These are shed from the distal urethra, vagina or prepuce. They are very large, thin cells with an irregular outline and they may be folded. They can be present as sheets of cells. There are increased numbers in the urine at the time of oestrus.

Neoplastic epithelial cells of any of the above types may be recognized, appearing as larger cells with relatively larger nuclei and increased staining (e.g. cells shed from transitional cell carcinomas or rhabdomyosarcomas; rarely from renal carcinomas).

CASTS

These are cylindrical structures moulded into the shape of the tubules; they may have ends that are rounded, tapered or broken.

The basis of all types of cast is mucoprotein (Tamm–Horsfall protein) which is secreted in the nephron in the loop of Henle, the distal tubule and the collecting duct (where urine reaches its maximum concentration and acidity).

'Broad casts' originate from the collecting ducts and, in large numbers, usually indicate severe disease (e.g. chronic renal failure), although they are also found during recovery from acute renal failure.

On the basis of their composition, casts are classified as:

- Hyaline casts – consisting of a mucoprotein gel alone (these dissolve rapidly in dilute or alkaline urine).

- Cellular casts – which incorporate cells, i.e. RBCs (following renal haemorrhage and occasionally in acute glomerulonephritis), WBCs (due to renal inflammation, e.g. acute pyelonephritis) or tubular epithelial cells (as a result of degeneration and necrosis, especially in acute renal failure and pyelonephritis).

Subsequently cellular casts degenerate to give:

- Granular casts (first coarse, then, as degeneration continues, fine).
- Finally, waxy casts (commonly associated with chronic renal failure or renal amyloidosis).

Whether cellular, granular or waxy casts are found depends on the time elapsing before the cast is shed from the tubule and time of transit through the urinary tract, i.e. it reflects the duration of the degenerative process.

- Fatty casts (more commonly found in cats) as a result of degeneration of the tubular epithelial cells which contain considerable lipid. Frequently these occur in the nephrotic syndrome.

Up to two hyaline casts or one granular cast per low power field can be present in 'normal' urine.

Large numbers of casts indicate active, generalized renal disease, usually acute (e.g. ARF); fewer casts are encountered in chronic disorders (e.g. CRF).

Hyaline casts are the most common; granular casts are those most often found in renal disease. Haemoglobin may form casts following acute intravascular haemolysis and haemoglobinuria (consequently they have a red colour). Any casts may be stained yellow with bilirubin if there is also bilirubinuria.

Increased numbers of casts occur in aflatoxicosis, leptospirosis and nephrotoxicosis.

IMPORTANT NOTE

The absence of casts *does not* rule out any renal disease.

Casts will be dissolved and subsequently disappear in alkaline urine, and will be disrupted by high speed centrifugation.

BACTERIA

It is thought that more than 3×10^4/ml must be present before bacteria are detectable in urinary sediment.

Large numbers *suggest* a urinary tract infection but this needs confirmation by bacterial culture methods, i.e. the apparent presence or absence of bacteria in urinary sediment is not an effective substitute for bacterial culture/screening.

Bacteria may multiply en route to the laboratory, although this can be prevented by using boric acid as a urinary preservative. They can be stained (e.g. using Gram's method) for identification.

YEASTS AND FUNGI

Yeasts (ovoid and budding organisms) and fungi (producing segmented hyphae) are almost invariably contaminants in the urine.

PARASITES

These include:

- Eggs of *Capillaria plica* or *Dioctophyma renale*.
- Microfilariae of *Dirofilaria immitis*.

Only *Capillaria plica* occurs in the UK.

SPERMS

These are a normal finding in uncastrated male animals, and occasionally in the urine of females.

LIPID DROPLETS

Finding lipid droplets is not related to lipaemia (high lipid levels in the blood). A small number of droplets is normal in cats, but they can indicate degenerative changes in the renal tubular cells *or* contamination of the urine with lubricants.

MUCUS

This is produced in long ribbon-like strands by the mucous glands. A certain amount is normal in genital secretions, especially at oestrus. Otherwise large amounts suggest inflammation and irritation.

Error

Cells and granules can stick to mucous strands and resemble casts (although in general, mucous strands are far too long to be confused with casts).

CRYSTALS

Many crystals precipitate out as the urine cools from body temperature. The number of crystals depends upon the concentration of the urine, its pH, the solubility of salts etc. Oxalate and cystine crystals are less common in alkaline (e.g. stale) urine.

Some crystals always have significance:

- Cystine crystals are associated with congenital cystinuria and possibly cystine calculi.
- Tyrosine crystals.
- Leucine crystals.

Both tyrosine and leucine crystals (rare) can indicate severe liver disease.

Some crystals occur in normal dogs but *also* in dogs with urinary calculi and other diseases:

- Calcium oxalate and struvite crystals are more likely in cases of hyperparathyroidism.
- Calcium oxalate crystals, primarily monohydrate, are a feature of ethylene glycol poisoning. (Crystals resembling those of hippuric acid have also been described, but are in fact a form of calcium oxalate monohydrate.) Both calcium oxalate

dihyrate (weddellite) and monohydrate (whewellite) crystals may occur in the urine or apparently normal dogs and cats.

- Ammonium urate (ammonium biurate) crystals commonly occur in Dalmatians that have reduced activity of hepatic uricase and hyperuricosuria as inherited defects, and in dogs with hepatic disorders where there are high blood ammonia levels (portosystemic shunts and liver failure). Infrequently they develop in normal dogs and cats.
- Phosphate crystals – chiefly of struvite (magnesium ammonium phosphate) – may appear in some normal dogs and cats, especially in alkaline urine; often these are associated with some apatite (calcium phosphate) crystals in dogs; in combination they are known as triple phosphate.
- In the dog there is a frequent association between the presence of phosphate calculi and staphylococcal infection of the urine.
- In the cat the presence of struvite crystals is associated with the feline urological syndrome.

Note

At times urates and phosphates precipitate in the sediment in an amorphous form. (Amorphous urates, but not amorphous phosphates, will dissolve in sodium hydroxide solution. Amorphous phosphates, but not amorphous urates, are soluble in acetic acid; urates *may* form uric acid crystals.)

Other crystals are very rare:

- Carbonate – although described in old dogs these probably never appear.
- Cholesterol, in apparently normal dogs.
- Bilirubin – in concentrated urine from normal dogs or where there is abnormal bilirubin metabolism.
- Sulphonamides – although modern sulphonamides are much more soluble in acid urine.
- Other drugs, e.g. xanthine in dogs or cats dosed with excessive amounts of allopurinol.
- Uric acid (very rare in normal animals but readily formed by adding 10% acetic acid to urine containing urate crystals or amorphous urates).

Crystals of salts may appear as a wet preparation of the sediment dries out.

ARTEFACTS

Contaminants are occasionally present which are confused with true sediment, e.g. hairs, pollen grains, starch granules, cotton fibres, granules of unfiltered or dried stain, air bubbles (distinguished by having thick walls and varying in size) and also chips or scratches on the microscope slide or coverslip.

Chapter 12

Urinary culture and bacteriological screening methods

Where a urinary tract infection (UTI) is suspected it is important for the urine to be cultured. *But*:

- Urine samples must be collected with 'sterile' precautions to avoid contamination, 'preservatives' (except possibly boric acid) should not be added, and refrigeration is necessary if there is delay between collection and testing or despatch.
- Previous treatment with an antibacterial drug (for whatever reason) which is excreted via the kidneys can prevent the growth of bacteria (i.e. bacteria may not be killed but their growth on culture media will be inhibited). Ideally a week should be allowed between the last dose of drug and urine collection. (The presence of antibacterials can be detected with Micur-BT (BCL)).
- The sample should not be contaminated by dipping test strips, urinometers etc. into it *before* culture, and ideally the sample should be split and a portion reserved solely for culturing.

Significant bacteriuria

It is important to establish the *concentration* of bacterial organisms in the urine, since some of the normal bacterial population of the uretha are washed out of the urethra each time an animal urinates; merely finding *these* organisms, which are present in low numbers, will be misleading because they are not responsible for a urinary tract infection.

Only a high number of bacteria (significant bacteriuria) indicates a UTI and in the dog a significant number is taken as 10^5 or more bacteria per ml of urine. In the cat a figure of 10^4 or more/ml has been recommended for voided specimens and 10^3 or more/ml for catheterised samples (Lees and Rogers, 1986).

Tests which allow accurate estimates of numbers to be made are marked * in the listing below. With many tests it is difficult to get accurate estimates of numbers.

Note

Tests should always be carried out on uncentrifuged urine; centrifuging will concentrate the organisms and give a false impression of their concentration in the urine.

SCREENING METHOD

Full plating-out techniques (using a minimum of two culture plates of different media to permit quantitative counts to be performed) are expensive and for that reason *screening tests* are frequently carried out because they are cheaper and often quicker.

However, some of these screening tests are better than others and the listing below is provided to help both check the validity of tests used by commercial laboratories and in case it is intended to perform some testing in the veterinary practice.

Indirect tests

These tests are unreliable and are *not* recommended.

Examination for proteinuria
This is very non-specific.

WBC count on uncentrifuged urine
This is also very unreliable.

Examination of a Gram-stained smear of uncentrifuged urine
This is very time-consuming (need to examine 50 oil immersion fields).

Chemical tests for bacteria

- Triphenyltetrazolium chloride (TTC) test involves the incubation of urine with TTC for 4–6 hours; a red precipitate is produced if there is a significant number of bacteria.
- Catalase test – catalase from bacteria causes the release of oxygen from hydrogen peroxide.
- Hypoglycosuria test – very sensitive test to detect the minute amount (0.3 mmol/l) of glucose in normal urine. This glucose is expected to be absent in cases of significant bacteriuria, having been utilized by the bacteria. However, the test will not work with *Pseudomonas* organisms or in cases of diabetes mellitus.
- Nitrite test (Griess's test) – found on many commercial chemical strips and as part of Microstix (see p. 465). It works on the principle that a large number of bacteria convert nitrate (in the urine) to nitrite, which is detected because it produces a pink colour.

The last three tests are not influenced by contamination during urine collection (provided the sample is examined within 3 hours), although it is important for the urine to have been present in the bladder long enough for bacterial metabolism to have produced the change which is being detected. Overall *less than 50% of UTIs* are detected by such tests.

Direct semi-quantitative culture methods using less urine and culture media

Culture of a standard loopful of uncentrifuged urine
It is difficult to distinguish contamination from a UTI.

*Dip-inoculum transport media
A plastic 'slide', previously coated on one or both sides with culture medium, is dipped into urine, placed inside a Universal container and incubated. It was developed originally for postal samples to avoid the rapid multiplication of contaminant bacteria; it permits both an assessment of significant bacteriuria and identification of the organisms.

Strip culture tests

Filter paper strip
A strip that has one end folded to provide a standard area is dipped into the urine and the end touched on the surface of a culture plate. The area required is so small that a number of urine samples can be tested (in duplicate) on the same culture plate. This plate is incubated and the resultant number of colonies counted. More than a predetermined number per area indicates significant bacteriuria.

Microstix (Ames)
As well as the rather unreliable nitrite band (for immediate reading), each strip bears two culture areas, one able to grow all bacteria and one able to grow only Gram-negative organisms. After being dipped into the urine the strip is placed into a polythene pouch and incubated for 12–18 hours. The number of (red) colonies on each area (estimated from a chart) indicates the number (and type) of bacteria present. *Pseudomonas* spp. may give unusual background colours, i.e. grey or green. The presence of marked haematuria can interfere with colony counting.

RESULT OF TESTING

In 90% of cases where there is significant bacteriuria, a single organism is isolated, but the percentage of mixed infections rises to 25% in cases where urinary calculi are present. In the majority of first-time infections the organism involved is *Escherichia coli*, the others (derived from the bowel or skin) include *Proteus* spp., *Klebsiella*, *Aerobacter*, *Staphylococcus* (*aureus*, *intermedius* and *epidermidis*), *Streptococcus* (*faecalis* and others) and *Pseudomonas aeruginosa*.

SENSITIVITY TESTING

Where a significant bacteriuria is established it is important to determine the sensitivity of the organisms to antibacterial drugs.

Often in commercial testing a variety of unsuitable drugs is tested, e.g. drugs which cannot be given orally and/or are toxic (such as the aminoglycoside group, including streptomycin and neomycin) or which do not attain adequate concentrations in the urine (e.g. chloramphenicol).

In general the best drugs for treatment are ampicillin, amoxycillin, amoxycillin augmented with clavulanic acid, cephalexin and trimethoprim synergized with a sulphonamide. There is frequently bacterial sensitivity to nitrofurantoin (although this drug often produces vomiting), and to nalidixic acid and cinoxacin (these also cause vomiting and possibly nervous signs). Gentamicin may be used for stubborn infections (although it requires to be injected) and tetracyclines may be useful although they are bacteriostatic and many organisms show resistance to them. Enrofloxacin and enoxacin (quinolone derivatives) have also proved to have excellent broad-spectrum activity in urine.

Pseudomonas needs treatment with specialized drugs: polymyxins, the anti-pseudomonal penicillins, gentamicin or tobramycin.

Techniques

The techniques described in this appendix are those which it would normally be necessary or more convenient to perform within a veterinary practice, because:

- Either irreversible changes will occur in the sample within a short time rendering it unsuitable for certain tests, so that these tests cannot be acurately performed on samples collected and despatched to an external laboratory in the usual way.
- Or the test procedure requires the administration of some substance to the patient prior to the collection of one or more samples for testing.

The only alternative to performing these tests within the practice would be for the patient to be taken to the laboratory (by prior arrangement) and the necessary procedures carried out there.

Recommendations about the *collection* of samples are given in the introduction to each of the major sections ('Haematology', 'Plasma biochemistry' and 'Urinalysis').

Information about the *type* of blood sample required for individual tests (e.g. heparinized, citrated etc.) is displayed in Appendix II.

Haematological techniques

BLEEDING TIME

1. With the animal suitably restrained make a moderately deep cut with a' scalpel blade, approximately 0.25 cm long in an area of skin with comparatively few hairs, e.g. the inside of the ear. The flank or skin near the umbilicus may also be used, but this usually requires hair being clipped from the area and, if necessary, careful washing and thorough drying. *Note the time* when the cut is made.
2. At 30-second intervals gently touch the blood on the wound in a fresh area with a piece of filter paper (e.g. Whatman No. 1). Take care not to actually touch the edge of the wound because this may dislodge the platelet plug.
3. Continue until no blood soaks into the filter paper when it is touched. *Note the time.* This is the bleeding time and, in the dog and cat, it should be less than 5 minutes.

CLOTTING TIME (WHOLE BLOOD CLOTTING TIME)

It is more sensitive to use the activated clotting time (ACT) described later.

1. Avoiding undue trauma during insertion of the needle, collect blood into a plain tube, i.e. without anticoagulant. Immediately three-quarters fill a 20 cm length of fine capillary tube, with a lumen of approximately 1 mm (this can be made by heating a length of glass tubing in a Bunsen burner flame and then drawing the two

ends apart). In an emergency two dry microhaematocrit tubes that *do not* contain anticoagulant can be used, but these are more difficult to break. The tubes should be pre-warmed to 37°C, not cold. Start the stopwatch as the tube(s) are filled.
2. Plug the unfilled end of the tube(s) with modelling clay, e.g. Plasticine, and place it, sealed end downwards, in a vacuum flask containing water (or for smaller tubes, a beaker of water) at 37°C.
3. At 30-second intervals break off a small length, e.g. 0.5 cm, from the top of the tube, and as this is done note whether the blood inside separates cleanly.
4. As soon as a strand of fibrin is seen to be drawn out between the two parts of the tube as they are separated, *record the time*. This is the clotting time.

An alternative method (Lee–White) is as follows:

1. Carefully withdraw around 4 ml of blood into a dry *plastic* syringe avoiding undue trauma. If there is any difficulty in obtaining blood the technique should be repeated using another vein.
2. Immediately remove the needle from the syringe and discharge 1 ml of blood into three clean, dry, unsiliconized, glass tubes (75 mm × 10 mm) which have been previously warmed to 37°C. Start the stopwatch. (It is important that the tubes have no irregularity of the internal surface, e.g. chips, cracks, scratches or dried residues, that might decrease the time normally taken for the blood to clot.)
3. Every 30 seconds, take the last tube to be filled and gently tilt it as if to pour out the blood. As soon as the blood has clotted, so that the tube can be tilted past the horizontal without blood being spilt, *record the time*.
4. Tilt the remaining tubes at 30-second intervals *noting the times* at which clotting occurs in them also.
5. The average of the times for all three tubes is accepted as the clotting time (whole blood coagulation time).

Using either the capillary or the tube method (Lee–White method), the clotting time is usually less than 5 minutes in both dog and cat, but can be prolonged to 13 minutes in the dog or 9 minutes in the cat.

ACTIVATED CLOTTING TIME (ACT)

1. Without undue trauma fill a special 2 ml Vacutainer tube containing silicaeous earth (catalogue No. 6522, Becton-Dickinson). The tube should be pre-warmed to 37°C. Start the stopwatch.
2. Gently but thoroughly mix the blood and place it in a heating block at 37°C (or a waterbath or beaker of water at 37°C) and, after 45 seconds, and every 10 seconds thereafter, gently tilt the tube and note when a blood clot first appears. *Record the time*. This is the activated clotting time.
3. The same sample in the tube can be used (see later) to assess clot retraction.
   (a) In the dog the ACT is less than 95 seconds at 37°C; if the test is performed at room temperature rather than at 37°C, the ACT in the dog is less than 130 seconds.
   (b) In the cat the ACT is less than 90 seconds at 37°C.

CLOT RETRACTION

1. Withdraw 2 ml of blood from the patient and place it (without any anticoagulant) into a clean glass tube. *Alternatively*, use the tube of blood used to determine the activated clotting time (above).

2. Place the tube into an incubator or waterbath at 37°C.
3. Examine the blood after 1 hour. Usually clot retraction will be in progress and visual inspection alone will show the presence of clear serum around a firm clot. If poured away the volume of serum will usually measure at least 0.5 ml.
4. If retraction is *not* evident, re-examine after 2 hours (and if possible 4 hours) and, if no retraction is evident, again after 24 hours. Note the appearance of the clot, i.e. whether firm, or soft and jelly-like, or whether a crumbly clot which liquefies (see p. 211).

Usually in both dog and cat retraction takes place within 1–2 hours.

FIXING BLOOD SMEARS FOR SUBSEQUENT STAINING

Blood smears made soon after blood collection for subsequent staining and examination, either in the practice or by another laboratory, can be fixed to avoid deterioration by covering, or immersing, in absolute methanol (acetone free) for 2–10 minutes before drying naturally without excessive heat.

This is appropriate when smears are to be examined for *Haemobartonella felis* because it preserves the organisms. They can subsequently be stained with Giemsa stain for 45 minutes *or* equal parts of May–Grünwald stain and phosphate buffer (pH 7.2) for 15 minutes, followed by 1 part of Giemsa stain and 9 parts of phosphate buffer (pH 7.2) for 30 minutes.

Blood smears fixed in this way can also be stained with a Romanowsky or supravital stain and used to obtain an assessment of the number of platelets when it is not possible to count them, electronically or manually, within 2 hours.

STAINING BLOOD SMEARS FOR *HAEMOBARTONELLA FELIS*

Of the three staining methods frequently recommended for demonstrating *H. felis* in blood smears, acridine orange has been shown to be the best but it requires ultraviolet microscopy to examine the smear. Almost as good is staining with May–Grünwald–Giemsa, a method which is 50% more likely to reveal the organisms than Giemsa staining alone (Bobade and Nash, 1987); both of these methods utilize an ordinary light microscope for examination. All three methods are better than Leishman's staining method.

Giemsa method

1. Fix the blood smear in absolute methanol for 2–3 minutes.
2. Cover, or immerse, in Giemsa stain for 30–90 minutes (45 minutes is a reasonable compromise).
3. Wash with distilled water.
4. Air dry and examine.

May–Grünwald–Giemsa method

1. Fix the blood smear in absolute methanol for 2–10 minutes.
2. Cover, or immerse, in a mixture of equal parts of May–Grünwald stain and phosphate buffer (pH 7.2) for 15 minutes.
3. Cover, or immerse, in a mixture of one part of Giemsa stain to nine parts of phosphate buffer (pH 7.2) for 30 minutes.

4. Rinse with phosphate buffer.
5. Air dry and examine.

Acridine orange method

1. Fix the blood smear in 10% formol saline for at least 24 hours.
2. Cover, or immerse, in a solution containing one part acridine orange in 1000 parts 0.1 N hydrochloric acid (having a pH of 2 or 3) for 15 *seconds*.
3. Wash in distilled water.
4. Air dry and examine with an ultraviolet microscope.

Chains and single organisms in affected RBCs appear brilliantly fluorescent.

ESTIMATING THE PLATELET COUNT USING A STAINED BLOOD SMEAR

Staining may be with Romanowsky or supravital stains.

Counting the number of platelets per oil immersion field

Six to seven platelets per oil immersion field are roughly equivalent to a count of $100 \times 10^9/l$.

Counting the numbers of platelets and RBCs over the same area of smear

This requires that the RBC count in $10^{12}/l$ is also known.

$$\text{Platelet count (in } 10^9/l) = \frac{\text{No. of platelets counted} \times \text{RBC count (in } 10^{12}/l) \times 10^3}{\text{No. of RBCs counted}}$$

One platelet per 70 RBCs is *roughly* equivalent to a count of $100 \times 10^9/l$.

Counting the number of platelets and WBCs over the same area of smear

This is the most accurate method and can be combined with performance of the differential WBC count.

$$\text{Platelet count (in } 10^9/l) = \frac{\text{No. of platelets counted} \times \text{WBC count (in } 10^9/l)}{\text{No. of WBCs counted}}$$

All three methods of estimation can have considerable errors due to the clumping of platelets and uneven platelet distribution within the smear.

SAMPLE REQUIREMENTS FOR TESTS OF AUTOIMMUNITY

Antinuclear antibody (ANA) test

This requires *serum* which can be posted satisfactorily.

Lupus erythematosus (LE) cell test

Ten millilitres of blood should be collected, allowed to clot and the clotted blood kept at room temperature for 2 hours before examination.

Therefore, ideally the laboratory should be close at hand after blood collection.

Platelet factor-3 (PF-3) test

Serum should be collected from clotted blood within 2 hours, heated at 56°C for 30 minutes and then either tested immediately (which requires the animal and the laboratory to be close together) or frozen to −30°C (and despatched to the laboratory frozen).

Lipaemic and haemolysed serum give inconsistent results, and plasma is *not* suitable.

QBC-V SYSTEM

The QBC-V system (quantitative buffy coat analysis – veterinary) allows rapid measurements to be made of the packed cell volume (PCV), total WBC count and platelet count. Counts (both percentage and absolute) can also be obtained for the combined granulocytes (neutrophils, eosinophils and (if they exist) basophils) and the combined non-granulocytes (lymphocytes and monocytes). A *separate* count for each individual type of WBC is not possible although in the dog the number of eosinophils can be determined (when they exceed $0.1 \times 10^9/1$) and so, by difference, the number of neutrophils can be found.

A special capillary tube is filled with blood (as soon as possible after its collection into EDTA), sealed, the precision-made plastic 'float' inserted and the tube centrifuged. The constituents of the blood separate according to their density and, because the float occupies most of the diameter of the tube, the buffy coat is spread out over a much longer length than usual. This allows the boundaries between its constituents (the platelets and the two groups of WBCs) to be easily distinguished when the tube is viewed through the special reading instrument. The operator positions a pointer on each boundary in turn and when all have been registered an instant digital display of the parameters is provided.

Sometimes it is not possible to determine precisely the boundary between the RBCs and WBCs due to 'streaming' which arises when there are large number of immature RBCs (usually reticulocytes) present, and this is usually an accompaniment of a regenerative anaemia. However, the effect can also occur with myeloproferative disorders.

Values appear to correlate with measurements made by conventional laboratory methods sufficiently well for clinical purposes, and a particular advantage is that it offers a quick and reliable method of estimating platelet numbers.

Biochemical techniques

GLUCOSE TOLERANCE TEST

Oral glucose tolerance test (OGTT)

- The dog is fasted for at least 12 hours.
- Two grams glucose per kg body weight are given by mouth as a 25% solution (i.e. the total volume administered should be 8 ml/kg body wt).
- A blood sample is collected just before giving the glucose and after 30 minutes, 1 hour, 2 hours (and possibly 3 hours), into sample bottles containing *fluoride–oxalate* (colour coded yellow), or alternatively into grey Vacutainers.

In normal dogs the peak value (usually below 8.9 ml/l = 160 mg/dl) is reached after ½–1 hour, and the level falls to near the resting level (certainly <7 mmol/l, <125 mg/dl) after 2 hours.

In diabetics the level at 1 hour is usually above 8.3 mmol/l (150 mg/dl) and does not fall rapidly.

The intravenous glucose tolerance test (IVGTT)

- The dog is fasted for at least 12 hours.
- Glucose 0.5 g/kg body weight given as a 50% sterile solution by slow intravenous injection (lasting 30 seconds). The total volume administered should be 1 ml/kg body weight.
- A blood sample is collected just before giving the glucose and 15 minutes, 30 minutes, 1 hour and 2 hours afterwards, into fluoride–oxalate containers, as indicated above.

In normal dogs there is an immediate rise in the blood glucose level (>16.6 mmol/l (>300 mg/dl) after 15 minutes) which returns to the fasting level in approximately 1 hour.

In diabetics a return to the fasting value takes 2–3 hours.

Note

The excitement and stress associated with collecting one or more blood samples can itself elevate the glucose level, confusing the results.

XYLOSE ABSORPTION TEST

This is used as an indicator of carbohydrate *absorption* in the small intestine.

- The dog is fasted for at least 12 hours.
- D-xylose 0.5 g/kg body weight is given orally (preferably by stomach tube) as a 5% solution (i.e. the total volume should be 10 ml/kg body weight). With a large dog the total volume can be considerable and halving the volume (i.e. using a 10% solution) is recommended. Hypertonic solutions (e.g. 25%) delay stomach emptying and can give confusing results.
- A blood sample is collected just before giving the xylose and every half an hour afterwards for 3 hours, into fluoride–oxalate sample containers (colour coded yellow or, alternatively, grey Vacutainers).

In normal dogs the peak value (usually > 2.5 mmol/l, >37.5 mg/dl) is reached after 1–1½ hours.

In cases of intestinal malabsorption there is slower absorption and the peak is achieved later and is often less than 2 mmol/l (<30 mg/dl).

In the cat the test is imprecise and not recommended.

Conversion factors for xylose

- To convert mg/dl to mmol/l multiply by 0.067.
- To convert mmol/l to mg/dl multiply by 15.

FAT (LONG CHAIN TRIGLYCERIDE) ABSORPTION TEST

This can be used as an indicator of the ability to digest and absorb long chain triglycerides (Simpson and Doxey, 1983) which, with modifications, can determine the presence of exocrine pancreatic insufficiency, (presumed) bile salts deficiency or a solely absorptive defect. It is a much more reliable test than the previously used turbidity test.

- The dog is fasted for at least 12 hours.
- Corn oil (e.g. Mazola), which contains long chain triglycerides, is given orally (usually consumed voluntarily) at the rate of 3 ml/kg body weight.
- Blood samples are collected just before giving the corn oil and 3 hours afterwards, which is the time of peak triglyceride levels in normal dogs. Either heparinized plasma or serum can be used.

In *normal dogs* the level of triglycerides after 3 hours is greater than the initial level (in most cases double).

In dogs with *digestive/absorptive disorders*, the initial value is lower than normal (usually <0.7 mmol/l, <60 mg/dl), and there is little if any rise after 3 hours.

- In those dogs which produce abnormal results, repeating the test, but administering pancreatic lipase (e.g. Pancrex powder, 0.4 g/kg body weight) *in addition* to the corn oil, enables cases of exocrine pancreatic insufficiency to be detected. In such cases, the level of triglyceride after 3 hours shows a considerable increase over the previous value at 3 hours. The use of an acid-blocking agent, e.g. cimetidine, prior to pancreatin dosage will presumably enhance the action of the enzyme.
- In those cases where *no* increase in triglyceride level follows the addition of pancreatic lipase, repeating the test yet again with the further addition of bile salts (e.g. the administration of both lipase and bile salts in the form of Panteric tablets together with the corn oil) enables cases of bile salts deficiency to be recognized. There is a marked increase in the triglyceride level at 3 hours compared with the 3 hour level on the two previous occasions.
- Continually low triglyceride levels, i.e. despite the addition of lipase and bile salts to the corn oil, may be presumed to indicate a defect in the absorption of long-chain triglycerides.

BROMSULPHTHALEIN (BSP) CLEARANCE TEST (SULFOBROMOPHTHALEIN EXCRETION TEST, BROMSULFALEIN RETENTION TEST)

Technique

1. The animal should be fasted; this is to avoid bile salt secretion which stimulates BSP excretion.
2. Five mg BSP/kg body weight (as a 5% solution) is injected intravenously (i.e. the total volume = 0.1 ml/kg body weight).
3. Blood samples are collected into heparin (for plasma) either:
    (a) after 30 minutes or, preferably,
    (b) after 10, 20 and 30 minutes. Collecting a number of samples allows the half-life of BSP clearance to be calculated.

A blood sample can be collected prior to injection of BSP as a check on the absence of any interfering substance but is not essential.

Care is needed:

1. To avoid any perivascular injection because:
    (a) this is irritant and may cause sloughing;
    (b) it can give results which may suggest poor liver function because the BSP is progressively absorbed from the perivascular site, thereby keeping the level in the plasma higher than it would be otherwise.
2. To collect sample(s) after injection from a different vein.
3. To have the analysis performed as soon as possible, preferably the same day, because BSP in plasma is labile.

In most normal dogs less than 5% of the injected dose will remain in the blood after 30 minutes and more than 10% remaining indicates abnormal liver function or a reduction in the hepatic blood flow.

If the half-life of BSP clearance is calculated in normal dogs it should be less than 7 minutes; a half-life greater than 9 minutes indicates deficient liver function or interference with hepatic perfusion.

In normal cats, the half-life of BSP clearance is less than 5.5 minutes. Also, in normal cats, usually less than 2% of the dose remains after 30 minutes.

TSH STIMULATION TEST

This is used chiefly to distinguish dogs with primary hypothyroidism from those that are euthyroid (i.e. are producing adequate free thyroxine) but which have low total T_4 levels due to illness or drug usage. It will also distinguish primary from secondary or tertiary hypothyroidism (see Figure 8.1, p. 397).

T_4 levels are estimated in plasma (or serum) samples collected *before* and *6 hours after* the intravenous administration of TSH. The dose advised in the *dog* is 0.1 i.u. bovine TSH/kg body weight; in the *cat* 1 i.u. TSH/kg is recommended.

- Dogs suffering from primary hypothyroidism show little or no increase in their low basal T_4 levels.
- Euthyroid dogs whose basal T_4 levels are low due to illness or drugs, and also dogs suffering from secondary or tertiary hypothyroidism, significantly increase their T_4 levels, i.e. usually to above 26 nmol/l ($= 2 \mu g/dl = 20 ng/ml$).

    Some dogs, e.g. a number with Cushing's syndrome, *will* show a rise in T_4 values but may not reach this level.

    Where the thyroid is severely atrophic due to secondary hypothyroidism, the test may need repeating on 3 consecutive days (i.e. the thyroid needs additional stimulation with TSH) before this response is seen. (Care — repeated intravenous injections of bovine TSH can be the cause of an anaphylactic reaction.)
- Euthyroid *dogs* generally have higher basal T_4 levels (usually above 17 nmol/l ($>1.3 \mu g/dl$, $>13 ng/ml$)) and show a greater increase after 6 hours, i.e. to above 52 nmol/l ($>4 \mu g/dl$, $>40 ng/ml$).
- Among *cats* euthyroid animals would normally be expected to show a doubling of T_4 values, *but* this response may *occasionally* be shown by hypothyroid animals and *occasionally* not be shown by euthyroid cats, i.e. the test is not entirely satisfactory.

TRH STIMULATION TEST

This is *not* usually required if the TSH test is available.

This test is used:

- To confirm cases of secondary hypothyroidism detected by the TSH stimulation test, i.e. by identifying any case of tertiary hypothyroidsm (rare).
- More importantly when commercial TSH is not available to clinicians, to distinguish euthyroid animals (especially those with low basal T_4 values due to illness or drugs) from those with primary or secondary hypothyroidism.

T_4 values are estimated in plasma (or serum) samples collected *before* and *6 hours after* the intravenous injection of 0.1 mg TRH/kg body weight (in the dog *or* cat), or (in the dog only) *before* and *4 hours after* the intravenous administration of 0.2 mg TRH (total dose) per dog.

- Dogs with primary or secondary hypothyroidism show little or no increase in their low basal T_4 levels.
- Euthyroid dogs show at least a 50% increase in the T_4 value 6 hours after receiving 0.1 mg/kg intravenously *or* an increase of at least 13 nmol/l (= 1 g/dl = 10 ng/ml) 4 hours after 0.2 mg/kg intravenously.
- In euthyroid *cats* the T_4 concentration should double 6 hours after giving 0.1 mg/kg intravenously.

T_3 SUPPRESSION TEST

This test can be used in the diagnosis of hyperthyroidism in cats but is *only* required in those few suspected cases in which the T_4 level is found to lie within the normal range (12–52 nmol/l); probably most instances are attributable to early diagnosis, i.e. the T_4 level has not yet risen above the upper limit of normal.

- Collect a blood sample for measurement of the plasma (or serum) level of thyroxine (T_4).
- Administer orally to the cat 20 µg (tablet size) of liothyronine (Tertroxin, Pitman–Moore) every 8 hours for 2 consecutive days and again (seventh dose) on the morning of the third day.
- Four hours after this last (seventh) dose, collect a further blood sample and again estimate the T_4 level.

Interpretation

- In *non-hyperthyroid cats* the post-treatment T_4 value is suppressed to less than 50% (often around 10%) of the pre-treatment value.
- In *hyperthyroid cats*, the post-treatment T_4 value is more than 50% of the pre-treatment value.

ACTH STIMULATION TEST TO DETECT CASES OF HYPERADRENOCORTICISM (CUSHING'S SYNDROME)

Administering ACTH results in the release of sizeable *reserves* of stored cortisol from both hyperplastic and neoplastic adrenal glands (i.e. there is an exaggerated response to ACTH).

Cortisol levels are assayed in plasma (or serum) samples collected:

- In the dog, *before* and *2 hours after* the intramuscular (or intravenous) injection of 0.25 mg tetracosactrin (synthetic ACTH, e.g. 'Synacthen') for any size of dog.
- In the cat, *before* and *half an hour after* the intramuscular (or intravenous) injection of 0.125 mg tetracosactrin per cat.

> **Note**
>
> The pre-ACTH sample is useful primarily to identify iatrogenic cases (producing extremely low values) when the basal cortisol level has not already been determined. Otherwise it is *not* essential.

In the dog
- Post-ACTH values of more than 550 nmol/l (>20 µg/dl) usually indicate hyperadrenocorticism (using either fluorometric methods or RIA – although refer to the individual laboratory).

> **Note**
>
> - Anticonvulsant therapy (primidone, phenytoin or phenobarbitone), can lead to an erroneous diagnosis because it may cause an elevated post-ACTH cortisol value as well as increased liver enzyme activities and several clinical signs (e.g. polyuria/polydipsia and polyphagia) that are consistent with Cushing's syndrome.
> - Failure of cortisol values to double or treble during the period of the test should be *disregarded* – it is not essential to the diagnosis.

- Slightly lower post-ACTH values (e.g. 470–550 nmol/l = 17–20 µg/dl) are equivocal.
- Lower values than 470 nmol/l (= 17 µg/dl) *suggest* normal adrenocortical function, *but* 15% of the pituitary-mediated cases of Cushing's syndrome and almost a half of those due to adrenal neoplasia do not show any significant elevation.

> **Note**
>
> Failure of the cortisol level to increase significantly in a dog showing clinical and laboratory features of Cushing's syndrome does not eliminate that diagnosis.

In the cat, post-ACTH values:

- More than 420 nmol/l (>15 µg/dl) indicate hyperadrenocorticism.
- Between 360 and 420 nmol/l (13–15 µg/dl) are equivocal.
- Less than 360 nmol/l (<13 µg/dl) suggest normality.

ACTH STIMULATION TEST TO DETECT CASES OF HYPOADRENOCORTICISM (ADDISON'S DISEASE)

Cortisol levels are assayed in plasma (or serum) samples collected:

- In the dog *before* and *1 hour after* the intramuscular (or intravenous) injection of 0.25 mg tetracosactrin (synthetic ACTH, e.g. Synacthen) for any size of animal.
- In the cat *before* and *half an hour after* the intramuscular (or intravenous) injection of 0.125 mg tetracosactrin.

Pre-ACTH values are either below, or in the lower part of, the normal range, and the post-ACTH values fail to reach 170 nmol/l (6 μg/dl) by RIA or 330 nmol/l (12 μg/dl) by the fluorometric method, whereas these values would be exceeded by normal dogs. Generally, the increase in cortisol concentration is slight in animals with hypoadrenocorticism, and it may even fall during the test.

Note

This test will not distinguish between primary and secondary cases of hypoadrenocorticism; a single injection of ACTH does not sufficiently stimulate the adrenal cortex. Measurement of the ACTH level is required to make this distinction.

LOW DOSE DEXAMETHASONE SUPPRESSION (SCREENING) TEST

This test may be used as an alternative to the ACTH stimulation test to detect cases of hyperadrenocorticism (i.e. Cushing's syndrome).

In both the dog and cat cortisol levels are estimated in plasma (or serum) samples collected *8 hours after* the intravenous injection of 0.01 mg dexamethasone/kg body weight.

- In *normal* animals the dexamethasone will suppress ACTH secretion and reduce cortisol production. Post-dexamethasone cortisol levels will be:
  (i) *in the dog* <40 nmol/l (<1.5 μg/dl);
  (ii) *in the cat* <30 nmol/l (<1 μg/dl).
- Dogs and cats with Cushing's syndrome do not show such a high degree of suppression and therefore the cortisol values are higher.

Note

- Apparent failure to suppress in dogs that do not have Cushing's syndrome can be due to previous therapy with anticonvulsants or with glucocorticoids (the latter *may* be measured, along with cortisol, in the assay).
- Suppression occurs in a very small number (5%) of early pituitary-mediated cases in dogs; repeating the test at least 2 months later usually demonstrates a lack of suppression.
- Suppression can occur with *intermittently* secreting adrenal tumours.

HIGH DOSE DEXAMETHASONE SUPPRESSION TEST

This test has not been evaluated in the cat. It is used in the dog to distinguish between cases of hyperadrenocorticism (Cushing's syndrome) that are pituitary mediated and those due to adrenal neoplasia.

Cortisol levels are estimated in plasma (or serum) samples collected *before* and *3 and 8 hours after* the intravenous injection of 0.1 mg dexamethasone/kg body weight, i.e. a higher dose of dexamethasone than used in the screening test (see above).

The expectation is that:

- In normal dogs both of the post-dexamethasone values are less than 50% of the baseline value.

- In pituitary-dependent Cushing's syndrome usually at least one of the post-dexamethasone values is less than 50% of the baseline value.
- With adrenal neoplasia both values are more than 50% of the baseline value due to poor, or no, suppression. However about 15% of pituitary-dependent cases are also poorly suppressed and therefore will give this result also, and the ultimate differentiation in such cases is based on inspection of the adrenal glands following exploratory laparotomy.

Appendix II

Normal reference ranges

Bear in mind:

1. Normal reference ranges for different laboratories may vary because of differences in the test methods; wherever possible check values against the ranges provided by the laboratory performing the estimations.
2. Enzyme activity is measured in international units per litre (iu/l), but the exact value will *vary* with the method of determination, i.e. it depends upon the substrate and the buffer which are used and upon the incubation temperature; consequently, for enzymes it is *impossible* to state 'normal' ranges that will apply to *all* methods.
3. One in 40 of all values from 'normal' animals will be above the normal reference range and a similar proportion will be below it.
4. Some values within the normal range, particularly near either end, will in fact be 'abnormal', i.e. will have changed due to disease but remain inside the range (see p. 4).

Type of sample	Parameter	Dog		Cat	
		SI units	Gravimetric units	SI units	Gravimetric units
E	Packed cell volume (PCV)	0.37–0.55 l/l*	37–55%*	0.30–0.45 l/l	30–45%
E	Haemoglobin concentration	12–18 g/dl (120–180 g/l) (7.5–11.5 mmol/l)	12–18 g/dl	8–15 g/dl (80–150 g/l) (5–9.5 mmol/l)	8–15 g/dl
H	Glycosylated haemoglobin	4–8% of total Hb		4–8% of total Hb	
H	Methaemoglobin	<2% of total Hb		<2% of total Hb	
E	Red blood cell count	$5.5–8.5 \times 10^{12}$/l	$5.5–8.5 \times 10^{6}$/μl	$5–10 \times 10^{12}$/l	$5–10 \times 10^{6}$/μl
E	Reticulocyte count	approx. 1% of total RBCs		1.5–11% of total RBCs	

Code		0–5 mm/1 hour		0–12 mm/1 hour	
E	Erythrocyte sedimentation rate (ESR)†	0–5 mm/1 hour		0–12 mm/1 hour	
E	Mean corpuscular volume (MCV)	60–77 fl	60–77 μm³	39–55 fl	39–55 μm³
E	Mean corpuscular haemoglobin concentration (MCHC)	32–36 g/dl	32–36 g/dl	30–36 g/dl	30–36 g/dl
E	Mean corpuscular haemoglobin (MCH)	19.5–24.5 pg	19.5–24.5 pg	12.5–17.5 pg	12.5–17.5 pg
E	Total white blood cell count	6–17 × 10⁹/l	6–17 × 10³/μl	5.5–19.5 × 10⁹/l	5.5–19.5 × 10³/μl
E	Differential WBC count				
	Absolute number of WBCs				
	Unlobulated neutrophils	0–0.3 × 10⁹/l	0–0.3 × 10³/μl	0–0.3 × 10⁹/l	0–0.3 × 10³/μl
	Adult neutrophils	3–11.5 × 10⁹/l	3–11.5 × 10³/μl	2.5–12.5 × 10⁹/l	2.5–12.5 × 10³/μl
	Eosinophils	0.1–1.25 × 10⁹/l	0.1–1.25 × 10³/μl	0.1–1.5 × 10⁹/l	0.1–1.5 × 10³/μl
	Basophils	0	0	0	0
	Lymphocytes	1–4.8 × 10⁹/l	1–4.8 × 10³/μl	1.5–7 × 10⁹/l	1.5–7 × 10³/μl
	Monocytes	0.15–1.35 × 10⁹/l	0.15–1.35 × 10³/μl	0.1–0.85 × 10⁹/l	0.1–0.85 × 10³/μl
	Percentage of WBCs				
	Unlobulated neutrophils	0–3%		0–3%	
	Adult neutrophils	60–80%		35–75%	
	Eosinophils	2–10%		2–12%	
	Basophils	0		0	
	Lymphocytes	10–34%		20–55%	
	Monocytes	1–11%		1–4%	
E/X	Platelet count	200–500 × 10⁹/l	200–500 × 10³/μl	300–700 × 10⁹/l	300–700 × 10³/μl
X	Bleeding time	<5 minutes		<5 minutes	
X	Clotting time	<13 minutes		<9 minutes	
X	Activated clotting time (ACT)	<95 seconds (37°C) or <130 seconds (room temp)		<90 seconds (37°C)	
X	Clot retraction time	1–2 hours		1–2 hours	
C	Activated partial thromboplastin time (APTT)	<11 seconds		<15 seconds	
C	Prothrombin time (PT) *or* one stage prothrombin time (OSPT)	7–10 seconds		7–12 seconds	
C	Thrombin time (TT) *or* thrombin clotting time (TCT)	<11 seconds		<20 seconds	
E	Fibrinogen	1–5 g/l	0.1–0.5 g/dl	0.5–3 g/l	0.05–0.3 g/dl
T	Fibrinogen degradation products (FDPs)	<10 mg/ml		<10 mg/ml	

Type of sample	Parameter		Dog		Cat	
			SI units	Gravimetric units	SI units	Gravimetric units
H	Urea		2.5–7 mmol/l	15–40 mg/dl	5–11 mmol/l	30–65 mg/dl
H	Creatinine		40–130 µmol/l	0.5–1.5 mg/dl	40–130 µmol/l	0.5–1.5 mg/dl
H	Total plasma protein		55–77 g/l*	5.7–7.7 g/dl*	58–80 g/l*	5.8–8 g/dl*
H	Albumin		25–40 g/l*	2.5–4 g/dl*	25–40 g/l*	2.5–4 g/dl*
H	Globulin		25–45 g/l*	2.5–4.5 g/dl*	28–55 g/l*	2.8–5.5 g/dl*
H	Globulin fractions					
	α_1		2–5 g/l	0.2–0.5 g/dl	2–11 g/l	0.2–1.1 g/dl
	α_2		3–11 g/l	0.3–1.1 g/dl	4–9 g/l	0.4–0.9 g/dl
	total α		5–13 g/l	0.5–1.3 g/dl	6–16 g/l	0.6–1.6 g/dl
	β_1		6–13 g/l	0.6–1.3 g/dl	3–9 g/l	0.3–0.9 g/dl
	β_2		6–14 g/l	0.6–1.4 g/dl	4–10 g/l	0.4–1 g/dl
	total β		12–22 g/l	1.2–2.2 g/dl	7–16 g/l	0.7–1.6 g/dl
	γ_1		4–13 g/l	0.4–1.3 g/dl	3–24 g/l	0.3–2.4 g/dl
	γ_2		4–9 g/l	0.4–0.9 g/dl	12–19 g/l	1.2–1.9 g/dl
	total γ		8–18 g/l	0.8–1.8 g/dl	15–35 g/l	1.5–3.5 g/dl
H	Albumin:globulin ratio (A:G ratio)		0.5–1.7		0.4–1.7	
H	Bilirubin (total)		1.7–10 µmol/l	0.1–0.6 mg/dl	2–5 µmol/l	0.12–0.3 mg/dl
H	Bile acids					
	RIA	Fasted	1–10 µmol/l	–	<2 µmol/l	–
		2 hours post-feeding	<16 µmol/l	–	<10 µmol/l	–
	Enzymatic assay	Fasted	<30 µmol/l	–	<25 µmol/l	–
		2 hours post-feeding	<50 µmol/l	–	<30 µmol/l	–
H	Triglycerides		0.6–1.2 mmol/l	50–100 mg/dl	0.6–1.2 mmol/l	50–100 mg/dl
H	Cholesterol (total)		2.5–8 mmol/l	100–300 mg/dl	2–6.5 mmol/l	75–250 mg/dl
F	Glucose		3.3–6 mmol/l*	60–100 mg/dl*	3.3–6 mmol/l	60–100 mg/dl
E	Ammonia		25–70 µmol/l	45–120 µg/dl	60–100 µmol/l	100–170 µg/dl
H	Bromsulphthalein (BSP) retention		<5% dose (30 min)		<2% dose (30 min)	
H	Bromsulphthalein (BSP) half-life		<7 min		<5.5 min	
H	Sodium		140–155 mmol/l	140–155 mEq/l (320–355 mg/dl)	145–157 mmol/l	145–157 mEq/l (335–360 mg/dl)

Potassium	H	3.6–5.8 mmol/l	3.6–5.8 mEq/l (14–22.5 mg/dl)	3.6–5.5 mmol/l	3.6–5.5 mEq/l (14–21.5 mg/dl)
Chloride	H	100–120 mmol/l	100–120 mEq/l (350–420 mg/dl)	115–130 mmol/l	115–130 mEq/l (405–455 mg/dl)
Total carbon dioxide content (bicarbonate)	H	17–24 mmol/l	17–24 mEq/l	17–24 mmol/l	17–24 mEq/l
Calcium	H	2–3 mmol/l	4–6 mEq/l (8–12 mg/dl)	1.8–3 mmol/l	3.6–6 mEq/l (7.2–12 mg/dl)
Inorganic phosphate	H	0.8–1.6 mmol/l*	1.4–2.9 mEq/l* (2.5–5 mg/dl)	1.3–2.6 mmol/l	2.3–4.7 mEq/l (4–8 mg/dl)
Iron	H	15–42 µmol/l	84–233 µg/dl	12–38 µmol/l	68–215 µg/dl
Total iron-binding capacity	H	51–103 µmol/l	284–572 µg/dl	30–72 µmol/l	170–400 µg/dl
Copper	H	15.7–19 µmol/l	100–120 µg/dl	13.3–16.5 µmol/l	85–105 µg/dl
Thyroxine (by RIA)	H	17–46 nmol/l*	1.3–3.6 µg/dl* (13–36 ng/ml)	12–52 nmol/l	0.9–4 µg/dl (9–40 ng/ml)
Cortisol					
By RIA	H	20–250 nmol/l	0.7–9 µg/dl	20–250 nmol/l	0.7–9 µg/dl
By fluorometric method	H	55–130 nmol/l	2–12 µg/dl	55–130 nmol/l	2–12 µg/dl
Insulin (by RIA)	H	36–180 pmol/l	5–25 µU/ml	36–180 pmol/l	5–25 µU/ml
Urinary specific gravity					
Normal range		1.015–1.045		1.035–1.060	
Maximum range possible		1.001–1.065		1.001–1.080	

Type of addition to blood sample or other requirement: C = citrate, E = EDTA, F = fluoride–oxalate (usually, although can interfere with 'strip' tests), H = heparin, lithium (although serum, i.e. NO anticoagulant, is usually equally suitable), T = Thrombo-Wellcotest tube to obtain serum, X = test can only (or best) be performed immediately after blood collection (see Panel 4.1, p. 205).

* Significant breed and/or age differences (for details refer to the main text):
● Packed cell volume – higher in Greyhounds and similar breeds.
● Total plasma protein – slightly lower in animals under 6 months.
● Albumin – slightly higher in animals under 6 months old.
● Globulin – slightly lower in animals under 6 months old.
● Glucose – may be lower in toy and miniature breeds under 6 months old.
● Inorganic phosphate – increased in dogs under 1 year old.
● Thyroxine – two to five times higher in dogs up to 3.5 months old (peak at 1 month old).
Also some enzyme activities are age related:
● Alkaline phosphatase (ALP) activity is up to six times higher in dogs and cats under 1 year old.
● Creatine kinase (CK) activity is up to two times higher in dogs under 6 months old.

† Interpretation of ESR values is best made after correction for the effects of the PCV; unfortunately correction factors are only available for canine blood that has been measured in a Wintrobe tube.

Appendix III

Conversion factors: SI units/gravimetric units

	To convert From	To convert To	Multiply by ↓	To convert From	To convert To	Multiply by
Packed cell volume (PCV)	% (or ml/dl)	l/l	0.01	l/l	% (or ml/dl)	100
Haemoglobin	g/l	g/dl	0.1	g/dl	g/l	10
	mmol/l	g/dl	1.61	g/dl	mmol/l	0.62
Urea†	mg/dl	mmol/l	0.17	mmol/l	mg/dl	6
Creatinine	mg/dl	μmol/l	88.4	μmol/l	mg/dl	0.0113
Proteins (total protein, albumin or globulin)	g/dl	g/l	10	g/l	g/dl	0.1
Bilirubin	mg/dl	μmol/l	17.1	μmol/l	mg/dl	0.059
Triglycerides	mg/dl	mmol/l	0.0114	mmol/l	mg/dl	87.5
Cholesterol	mg/dl	mmol/l	0.026	mmol/l	mg/dl	38.7
Glucose*	mg/dl	mmol/l	0.056	mmol/l	mg/dl	18
Xylose	mg/dl	mmol/l	0.067	mmol/l	mg/dl	15
Ammonia	μg/dl	μmol/l	0.57	μmol/l	μg/dl	1.7
Sodium	mEq/l	mmol/l	1	mmol/l	mEq/l	1
	mg/dl	mmol/l	0.44	mmol/l	mg/dl	2.3
Potassium	mEq/l	mmol/l	1	mmol/l	mEq/l	1
	mg/dl	mmol/l	0.26	mmol/l	mg/dl	3.9
Chloride	mEq/l	mmol/l	1	mmol/l	mEq/l	1
	mg/dl	mmol/l	0.29	mmol/l	mg/dl	3.5
Total carbon dioxide content (bicarbonate)	mEq/l	mmol/l	1	mmol/l	mEq/l	1
Calcium	mEq/l	mmol/l	0.5	mmol/l	mEq/l	2
	mg/dl	mmol/l	0.25	mmol/l	mg/dl	4
Inorganic phosphate	mEq/l	mmol/l	0.56	mmol/l	mEq/l	1.8
	mg/dl	mmol/l	0.32	mmol/l	mg/dl	3.1
Iron	μg/dl	μmol/l	0.179	μmol/l	μg/dl	5.58
Total iron-binding capacity	μg/dl	μmol/l	0.179	μmol/l	μg/dl	5.58
Copper	μg/dl	μmol/l	0.157	μmol/l	μg/dl	6.35
Thyroxine	μg/dl	nmol/l	12.87	nmol/l	μg/dl	0.078
	ng/ml	nmol/l	1.287	nmol/l	ng/ml	0.78
Cortisol	μg/dl	nmol/l	27.6	nmol/l	μg/dl	0.0362
	ng/ml	nmol/l	2.76	nmol/l	ng/ml	0.362
	μmol/l	nmol/l	1000	nmol/l	μmol/l	0.001
Insulin	μU/ml	pmol/l	7.18	pmol/l	μU/ml	0.14

↓ These columns contain the units that are currently in common usage.
* Urinary glucose: 1% = 56 mmol/l
† To convert blood urea nitrogen (BUN) to urea, multiply by 2.14.
    To convert urea to blood urea nitrogen (BUN), multiply by 0.47.
mg/dl = mg/100 ml.

Glossary of acronyms used

ACD	acid citrate dextrose
ACP	acid phosphatase
	also acetylpromazine
ACT	activated clotting time
ACTH	adrenocorticotrophic hormone
ADH	antidiuretic hormone
A:G	albumin:globulin
AIHA	autoimmune haemolytic anaemia
AIN	acute interstitial nephritis
ALP	alkaline phosphatase
ALT	alanine aminotransferase
AMS	amylase
ANA	antinuclear antibody
APTT	activated partial thromboplastin time
ARF	acute renal failure
AST	aspartate aminotransferase
ATN	acute tubular necrosis
ATP	adenosine triphosphate
BCG	bromocresol green
BFU-E	burst-forming unit–erythroid
(γ)BHC	(gamma)-benzene hexachloride (lindane)
BSP	bromsulphthalein
BT-PABA	benzoyl tyrosine para-aminobenzoic acid
BUN	blood urea nitrogen
CD	canine distemper
CFU-B	colony-forming unit–basophil
CFU-E	colony-forming unit–erythroid
CFU-Eos	colony-forming unit–eosinophil
CFU-GM	colony-forming unit–granulocyte, monocyte
CFU-M	colony-forming unit–megakaryocyte
CK	creatine kinase
CNS	central nervous system
CPK	creatine phosphokinase
CRF	chronic renal failure
	also corticotrophin-releasing factor
CRH	corticotrophin-releasing hormone
CRT	capillary refill time

o,p'-DDD	mitotane
DIC	disseminated intravascular coagulation
DMSO	dimethyl sulphoxide
ECF	extracellular fluid
ECG	electrocardiograph
EDTA	ethylenediaminetetraacetic acid
ELISA	enzyme-linked immunosorbent assay
EPI	exocrine pancreatic insufficiency
ESR	erythrocyte sedimentation rate
FDPs	fibrinogen degradation products
FeLV	feline leukaemia virus
FIA	feline infectious anaemia
FIE	feline infectious enteritis
FIP	feline infectious peritonitis
FIV	feline immunodeficiency virus
FPL	feline panleucopenia
FTLV	feline T-lymphocyte lentivirus
FUS	feline urological syndrome
GFR	glomerular filtration rate
GGT	gamma-glutamyltransferase
GOD/POD	glucose oxidase/peroxidase
GOT	glutamic oxaloacetic transaminase
GPT	glutamic pyruvic transaminase
GTP	gamma glutamyltranspeptidase
GTT	glucose tolerance test
Hb	haemoglobin
Hct	haematocrit
HDL	high-density lipoprotein
HHDI	hypothalamic–hypophyseal diabetes insipidus
HPF	high power field
HPLC	high performance liquid chromatography
HVS	hyperviscosity syndrome
ICF	intracellular fluid
ICH	infectious canine hepatitis
Ig	immunoglobulin (i.e. IgA, IgE, IgG, IgM)
IMT	immune-mediated thrombocytopenia
IRI	immunoreactive insulin
IRT	immunoreactive trypsin
ITP	idiopathic thrombocytopenic purpura
KA	King Armstrong
LCT	long chain triglyceride
LD	lactate dehydrogenase
LDH	lactate dehydrogenase

LDL	low-density lipoprotein
LE	lupus erythematosus
LPD	lymphoproliferative disorder
LPL	lipoprotein lipase
MCH	mean corpuscular haemoglobin
MCHC	mean corpuscular haemoglobin concentration
MCV	mean corpuscular volume
M:E	myeloid:erythroid
MPD	myeloproliferative disorder
MPS	mononuclear phagocyte system
MSU	mid-stream urine
NEQAS	National external quality assessment scheme
NHS	National health service
OCT	ornithine carbamyltransferase
OGTT	oral glucose tolerance test
OSPT	one-stage prothrombin time
PABA	para-aminobenzoic acid
PCV	packed cell volume
PF-3	platelet factor 3
PIE	pulmonary infiltrates with eosinophilia
PK	pyruvate kinase
PSP	phenolsulphonphthalein
PT	prothrombin time
QBC-V	quantitative buffy coat analysis – veterinary
RBC	red blood cell
RD	relative density
RDW	red cell size distribution width
RIA	radio-immunoassay
RNA	ribonucleic acid
RPI	reticulocyte production index
SAP	serum alkaline phosphatase
SALT	serum alanine aminotransferase
SAST	serum aspartate aminotransferase
SC	serum creatinine
SDH	sorbitol dehydrogenase
SGOT	serum glutamic oxaloacetic transaminase
SGPT	serum glutamic pyruvic transaminase
SI	Système Internationale
SIAP	steroid-induced alkaline phosphatase
SLDH	serum lactate dehydrogenase
SLE	systemic lupus erythematosus
SUN	serum urea nitrogen

T$_3$	tri-iodothyronine
T$_4$	thyroxine
TCO$_2$	total carbon dioxide
TCT	thrombin clotting time
TIBC	total iron-binding capacity
TLI	trypsin-like immunoreactivity
TPP	total plasma protein
TRF	thyrotrophin-releasing factor
TRH	thyrotrophin-releasing hormone
TSF	thrombocyte stimulating factor
TSH	thyroid stimulating hormone
TT	thrombin time
TTC	triphenyltetrazolium chloride
UK	United Kingdom
UKEQAS	United Kingdom external quality assessment scheme
UTI	urinary tract infection
USA	United States of America
VIII-RAg	factor VIII-related antigen
VLDL	very-low-density lipoprotein
vWF (VIII:vWF)	von Willebrand's factor
WBC	white blood cell

References

Aliakbari, K. (1975) A clinical and experimental investigation of haematopoiesis in the cat with particular reference to drug toxicity. *PhD thesis*, University of London

Allen, T. A. and Wilkie, W. L. (1988) Polyuria and polydipsia. In R. B. Ford (Ed.) *Clinical Signs and Diagnosis in Small Animal Practice*, pp. 55–73. New York: Churchill-Livingstone

Barsanti, J. A. and Finco, D. R. (1979) Protein concentration in urine of normal dogs. *Am. J. Vet. Res.* **40**, 1583–1588

Berman, E. (1974) Hemogram of the cat during pregnancy and lactation and after lactation. *Am. J. Vet. Res.* **35**, 457–460

Bobade, P. A. and Nash, A. S. (1987) A comparative study of the efficiency of acridine orange and some Romanowsky staining procedures in the demonstration of *Haemobartonella felis* in feline blood. *Vet. Parasitol.* **26**, 169–172

Breitschwerdt, E. B. (1988) Infectious thrombocytopenia in the dog. In R. B. Ford (Ed.) *Clinical Signs and Diagnosis in Small Animal Practice*, pp. 117–122. New York: Churchill-Livingstone

Bush, B. M. (1988) Polyuria and polydipsia. In A. R. Michell (Ed.) *Renal Disease in Dogs and Cats*, pp. 48–74. Oxford: Blackwell

Canfield, P. J. (1986) Screening tests available for use by the practitioner. *Proceedings no. 93. Clinical Pathology*, pp. 83–91. Post-graduate Committee in Veterinary Science, University of Sydney

Carlson, G. P. and Kaneko, J. J. (1971) Simultaneous estimation of renal function in dogs using sodium sulfanilate and sodium iodohippurate-^{131}I. *J. Am. Vet. Med. Assoc.* **158**, 1229–1234

Chastain, C. B. and Ganjam, V. K. (1986) *Clinical Endocrinology of Companion Animals*, p. 401. Philadelphia: Lea and Febiger

Chastain, C. B. and Nichols, C. E. (1984) Current concepts in the control of diabetes mellitus. *Vet. Clin. North Am.: Small Anim. Pract.* **14**, 859–872

Chew, D. J. and Meuten, D. J. (1982) Disorders of calcium and phosphorus metabolism. *Vet. Clin. North Am.: Small Anim. Pract.* **12**, 411–438

Davis, P. E. and Paris, R. (1983) Haematology of the racing greyhound. *Proceedings no. 64. Refresher course for veterinarians – Greyhounds*, pp. 63–127. University of Sydney

de Bruijne J. J. (1979) Biochemical observations during total starvation in dogs. *Int. J. Obesity* **3**, 239–247

de Bruijne, J. J. (1982) Ketone-body metabolism in fasting dogs. *PhD thesis*, Univeristy of Utrecht

Doxey, D. L. (1966) Some conditions associated with variations in circulating oestrogens – blood picture alterations. *J. Small Anim. Pract.* **7**, 375–385

Eckersall, P. D. and Douglas, T. A. (1988) New biochemistry tests. *Vet. Rec.* **122**, 240

Eiler, H. and Oliver, J. (1980) Combined dexamethasone suppression and cosyntropin (synthetic ACTH) stimulation test in the dog: a new approach to testing of adrenal gland function. *Am. J. Vet. Res.* **41**, 1243–1246

Feldberg, W. and Symonds, H. W. (1980) Hyperglycaemic effect of xylazine. *J. Vet. Pharmacol. Therap.* **3**, 197–202

Feldman, B. F. (1986) Anemias associated with blood loss and hemolysis. *Vet. Clin. North Am.: Small Anim. Pract.* **11**, 265–275

Feldman, E. C. and Nelson, R. W. (1987) *Canine and Feline Endocrinology and Reproduction*, p. 286. Philadelphia: W. B. Saunders

Finco, D. R. (1971) Simultaneous determination of phenolsulfonphthalein excretion and endogenous creatinine clearance in the normal dog. *J. Am. Vet. Med. Assoc.* **159**, 336–340

Finco, D. R. (1980) Kidney function. In J. J. Kaneko (Ed.) *Clinical Biochemistry of Domestic Animals*, 3rd edn, p. 389. New York: Academic Press

Finco, D. R. (1983) Interpretations of serum calcium concentrations in the dog. *Compend. Contin. Educ.* **5**, 778–788

Finco, D. R. and Duncan, J. R. (1976) Evaluation of blood urea nitrogen and serum creatinine as indicators of renal dysfunction. *J. Am. Vet. Med. Assoc.* **168**, 593–600

Fletch, S. M., Smart, M. E., Pennock, P. W. and Subden, R. E. (1973) Clinical and pathologic features of chondrodysplasia (dwarfism) in the Alaskan malamute. *J. Am. Vet. Med. Assoc.* **162**, 357–361

Franckel, T. and Hawkey, C. M. (1980) Haematological changes during sedation in cats. *Vet. Rec.* **107**, 512–513

Greco, D. S., Turnwald, G. H., Adams, R., Gossett, K. A., Kearney, M. and Cassey, H. (1985) Urinary gamma-glutamyl transpeptidase activity in dogs with gentamicin-induced nephrotoxicity. *Am. J. Vet. Res.* **46**, 2332–2335

Greenwood, L. and Finco, D. R. (1979) Unpublished observations. In J. J. Kaneko (Ed.) *Clinical Biochemistry of Domestic Animals,* 3rd edn, p.389. New York: Academic Press

Hall, L. W. (1985) Laboratory evaluation of liver disease. *Vet. Clin. North Am.: Small Anim. Pract.* **15**, 3–19

Harvey, J. W. (1980) Canine hemolytic anemias. *J. Am. Vet. Med. Assoc.* **176**, 970–974

Hitt, M. E. and Jones, B. D. (1986) Effects of storage temperature and time on canine plasma ammonia concentrations *Am. J. Vet. Res.* **47**, 363–364

Holt, P. E., Lucke, V. M. and Pearson, H. (1987) Idiopathic renal haemorrhage in the dog. *J. Small Anim. Pract.* **28**, 253–263

Jansen, B. S. and Lumsden, J. H. (1985) Sensitivity of routine tests for urine protein to hemoglobin. *Can. Vet. J.* **26**, 221–223

Jones, N. R., Johnstone, A. C. and Hancock, W. S. (1986) Inherited hyperchylomicronaemia in the cat. In C. S. G. Grunsell, F. W. G. Hill and M-E. Raw (Eds) *The Veterinary Annual 26*, pp. 330–340. Bristol, Scientechnica

King, L. G., Giger, U., Diserens, D. and Nagode, L. A. (1992) Anemia of chronic renal failure in dogs. *J. Vet. Int. Med.* **6**, 264–270

Lees, G. E. and Rogers, K. S. (1986) Diagnosis and localization of urinary tract infection. In R. W. Kirk (Ed.) *Current Veterinary Therapy IX, Small Animal Practice*, pp. 1118–1123. Philadelphia: W. B. Saunders

Lewis, H. B. (1932) The occurrence of cystinuria in healthy young men and women. *Ann. Intern. Med.* **6**, 183–192

Littlewood, J. D. and Bevan, S. (1989) Canine blood coagulation. *Vet. Rec.* **125**, 97

Lording, P. M. (1983) Haematology and biochemistry profiles. *Proceedings no. 64. Refresher course for veterinarians – Greyhounds,* pp. 491–506. University of Sydney

McKerrell, R. E., Blakemore, W. F., Heath, M. F., Plumb, J., Bennett, M. J., Pollitt, R. J. and Danpure, C. J. (1989) Primary hyperoxaluria (L-glyceric aciduria) in the cat: A newly recognised inherited disease. *Vet. Rec.* **125**, 31–34

Mattheeuws, D., Rottiers, R., Baeyens, D. and Vermeulen, A. (1984) Glucose tolerance and insulin response in obese dogs. *J. Am. Anim. Hosp. Assoc.* **20**, 287–293

Mia, A. S., Koger, H. D. and Tierney, M. M. (1978) Rapid turbidimetric determination of serum pancreatic lipase in the dog. *Am. J. Vet. Res.* **39**, 317–318

Michell, A. R. (1988) Renal function, renal damage and renal failure. In A. R. Michell (Ed.) *Renal Disease in Dogs and Cats,* pp. 5–29. Oxford: Blackwell

Mikiciuk, M. G. and Thornhill, J. A. (1989) Control of parathyroid hormone in chronic renal failure. *Compend. Contin. Educ.* **11**, 831–837

O'Connor, W. J. and Potts, D. J. (1988) Kidneys and drinking in dogs. In A. R. Michell (Ed.) *Renal Disease in Dogs and Cats,* pp. 30–47. Oxford: Blackwell

Parry, B. W. (1987) Laboratory evaluation of anaemias in dogs and cats. In C. S. G. Grunsell, F. W. G. Hill and M. E. Raw (Eds) *The Veterinary Annual 27*, pp. 270–292. Bristol: Scientechnica

Pemberton, P. L. (1983) Azoturia in the greyhound. *Proceedings no. 64. Refresher course for veterinarians – Greyhounds,* pp. 183–189, University of Sydney

Perman, V. (1974) Unpublished data. Cited in Perman, V. and Schall, W. D. (1983) Diseases of the red blood cells. In S. J. Ettinger (Ed.) *Textbook of Veterinary Internal Medicine: Diseases of the Dog and Cat,* 2nd edn, pp. 1938–2000. Philadelphia: W. B. Saunders

Veterinary Internal Medicine: Diseases of the Dog and Cat, 2nd edn, pp. 1733–1792. Philadelphia: W. B. Saunders

Siest, G. and Galteau, M-M. (1988) *Drug Effects on Laboratory Test Results,* p. 56. Littleton: PSG Publishing Co.

Simpson, J. W. and Doxey, D. L. (1983) Quantitative assessment of fat absorption and its diagnostic value in exocrine pancreatic insufficiency. *Res. Vet. Sci.* **35**, 249–251

Slappendel, R. J. (1986) Interpretation of tests for immune-mediated blood diseases. In R. W. Kirk (Ed.) *Current Veterinary Therapy IX, Small Animal Practice,* pp. 498–505. Philadelphia: W. B. Saunders

Snow, D. H., Harris, R. C. and Stuttard, E. (1988) Changes in haematology and plasma biochemistry during maximal exercise in greyhounds. *Vet. Rec.* **123**, 487–489

Steward, A. P. and Macdougall, D. F. (1981) Assay for fibrinogen–fibrin degradation products in urine. *Vet. Rec.* **109**, 179–180

Strombeck, D. R. (1979) *Small Animal Gastroenterology,* pp. 318, 366, Davis: Stonegate Publishing

Tvedten, H. W. (1981) Hematology of the normal dog and cat. *Vet. Clin. North Am.* **11**, 209–217

Weaver, A. D. (1981) Fifteen cases of prostatic carcinoma in the dog. *Vet. Rec.* **109**, 71–74

Werner, L. I. (1980) Coombs' positive anaemias in the dog and cat. *Compend. Contin. Educ.* **2**, 96–101

Williams, D. A. and Batt, R. M. (1983) Diagnosis of canine exocrine pancreatic insufficiency by the assay of serum trypsin-like immunoreactivity. *J. Small Anim. Pract.* **24**, 583–588

Williams, D. A., Reed, S. D. and Perry, L. (1990) Fecal proteolytic activity in clinically normal cats and in a cat with exocrine pancreatic insufficiency. *J. Am. Vet. Med. Assoc.* **197**, 210–212

Yeary, R. A. and Wise, K. J. (1975) Plasma diasapperance of sulfobromphthalein or indocyanine green in unconjugated hyperbilirubinemia. *Res. Commun. Chem. Path. Pharmacol.* **12**, 125–136

Zerbe, C. A. (1986) Canine hyperlipemias. In R. W. Kirk (Ed.) *Current Veterinary Therapy IX, Small Animal Practice,* pp. 1045–1053. Philadelphia: W. B. Saunders

Sources of information

Although information was gathered from a large number of papers and textbooks certain sources proved to be particularly valuable; these are listed below.

Major sources

Bovée, K. C. (Ed.) (1984) *Canine Nephrology*. Philadelphia: Harwal Publishing Company

Duncan, J. R. and Prasse, K. W. (1986) *Veterinary Laboratory Medicine,* 2nd edn. Ames: Iowa State University Press

Ettinger, S. J. (Ed.) (1983) *Textbook of Veterinary Internal Medicine: Diseases of the Dog and Cat,* 2nd edn. Philadelphia: W. B. Saunders

Feldman, E. C. and Nelson, R. W. (1987) *Canine and Feline Endocrinology and Reproduction.* Philadelphia: W. B. Saunders

Greene, C. E. (Ed.) (1984) *Clinical Microbiology and Infectious Diseases of the Dog and Cat.* Philadelphia: W. B. Saunders

Holzworth, J. (Ed.) (1987) *Disease of the Cat: Medicine and Surgery,* Vol. 1. Philadelphia: W. B. Saunders

Jain, N. C. (1986) *Schalm's Veterinary Haematology,* 4th edn. Philadelphia: Lea & Febiger

Jain, N. C. and Zinkl, J. G. (Eds) (1981) *Clinical Haematology, Vet. Clin. North Am. Small Anim. Pract.* **11**, (2)

Kaneko, J. J. (Ed.) (1979) *Clinical Biochemistry of Domestic Animals,* 3rd edn. New York: Academic Press

Lorenz, M. D. and Cornelius, L. M. (Eds) (1987) *Small Animal Medical Diagnosis.* Philadelphia: J. B. Lippincott

Osborne, C. A. and Stevens, J. B. (1981) *Handbook of Canine and Feline Urinalysis.* St Louis: Ralston Purina Company

Twedt, D. C. (Ed.) (1985) *Liver Diseases. Vet. Clin. North Am. Small Anim. Pract.* **15**, (1)

Index